Immunoglobulin Therapy

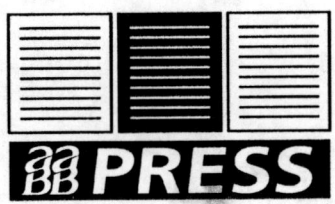

Mention of specific products or equipment by contributors to this AABB Press publication does not represent an endorsement of such products by the AABB Press nor does it necessarily indicate a preference for those products over other similar competitive products.

Efforts are made to have publications of the AABB Press consistent in regard to acceptable practices. However, for several reasons, they may not be. First, as new developments in the practice of blood banking occur, changes may be recommended to the AABB *Standards for Blood Banks and Transfusion Services*. It is not possible, however, to revise each publication at the time such a change is adopted. Thus, it is essential that the most recent edition of the *Standards* be consulted as a reference in regard to current acceptable practices. Second, the views expressed in this publication represent the opinions of authors. The publication of this book does not constitute an endorsement by the AABB Press of any view expressed herein, and the AABB Press expressly disclaims any liability arising from any inaccuracy or misstatement.

The AABB Press publishes books and CDs on many topics of interest to those in the blood banking, transfusion medicine, and cellular therapy fields.

To purchase books or to inquire about other book services, including chapter reprints and large-quantity sales, please contact our sales department:
- 866.222.2498 (within the United States)
- +1 301.215.6499 (outside the United States)
- +1 301.951.7150 (fax)
- www.aabb.org>Bookstore

AABB customer service representatives are available by telephone from 8:30 am to 5:00 pm ET, Monday through Friday, excluding holidays.

Immunoglobulin Therapy

Editors

Alan H. Lazarus, PhD
University of Toronto
Toronto, Ontario, Canada

John W. Semple, PhD
University of Toronto
Toronto, Ontario, Canada

AABB Press
Bethesda, Maryland
2010

Copyright © 2010 by AABB. All rights reserved. Reproduction or transmission of text in any form or by any means, electronic or mechanical, including photocopying, recording, or by any information storage and retrieval system is prohibited without permission in writing from the Publisher.

The Publisher has made every effort to trace the copyright holders for borrowed material. If any such material has been inadvertently overlooked, the Publisher will be pleased to make the necessary arrangements at the first opportunity.

AABB
8101 Glenbrook Road
Bethesda, Maryland 20814-2749

ISBN NO. 978-1-56395-304-0
Printed in the United States

Library of Congress Cataloging-in-Publication Data

Immunoglobulin therapy / editors, Alan H. Lazarus, John W. Semple.
p. ; cm.
Includes bibliographical references and index.
ISBN 978-1-56395-304-0
1. Immunoglobulins—Therapeutic use. 2. Intravenous therapy. I. Lazarus, Alan H. II. Semple, John W.
[DNLM: 1. Immunization, Passive. 2. Immunoglobulins, Intravenous—therapeutic use.
3. Isoantibodies—therapeutic use. QW 945 I33 2010]
RM282.I44I46 2010
615'.37—dc22

2010022529

AABB Press
Editorial Board

Miguel Lozano, MD, PhD
Richard J. Davey, MD
Susan T. Johnson, MSTM, MT(ASCP)SBB
Marisa B. Marques, MD
Sally V. Rudmann, PhD, MT(ASCP)SBB
Clarence Sarkodee-Adoo, MD, FACP
John W. Semple, PhD
Yanyun Wu, MD, PhD

Contributors

Davor Brinc, PhD
St. Michael's Hospital
Toronto, Canada

James B. Bussel, MD
New York Presbyterian Hospital
Weill Cornell Medical Center
New York, New York

Harald Arno Butterweck, PhD
Baxter Innovations GmbH
Vienna, Austria

Andrew R. Crow, BRT
Canadian Blood Services
St. Michael's Hospital
Toronto, Canada

Marinos C. Dalakas, MD
Imperial College
London, United Kingdom

Robert O. Dillman, MD, FACP
Hoag Cancer Center
Newport Beach, California
University of California Irvine
Irvine, California

Richard O. Francis, MD, PhD
Columbia University Medical Center
New York Presbyterian Hospital
New York, New York

John Freedman, MD, FRCPC
St. Michael's Hospital
Toronto, Canada

M. Bernadette Garvey, MD, FRCPC
St. Michael's Hospital
Toronto, Canada

Edward C. Gordon-Smith, MD
St. George's Hospital
London, United Kingdom

Paul Imbach, MD
University of Basel
University Children's Hospital Basel
Basel, Switzerland

Thomas R. Kreil, PhD
Baxter Innovations GmbH
Vienna, Austria

Kevin B. Laupland, MD, MSc, FRCPC
University of Calgary
Calgary, Canada

Alan H. Lazarus, PhD
Canadian Blood Services
St. Michael's Hospital
University of Toronto
Toronto, Canada

Ursula Mais-Paul, PhD
Baxter Innovations GmbH
Vienna, Austria

W. Beau Mitchell, MD
New York Blood Center
New York, New York

Robert K. Oldham, MD, FACP
Southeast Missouri Hospital
Cape Girardeau, Missouri
University of Missouri School of Medicine
Columbia, Missouri

Ruth Pettengell, MD
St. George's Hospital
London, United Kingdom

Gerhard Poelsler, PhD
Baxter Innovations GmbH
Vienna, Austria

John W. Semple, PhD
St. Michael's Hospital
University of Toronto
Canadian Blood Services
Toronto, Canada

Muriel S. Shannon, MD
St. George's Hospital
London, United Kingdom

Roberto Stasi, MD, PhD
St. George's Hospital
London, United Kingdom

Wolfgang Teschner, PhD
Baxter Innovations GmbH
Vienna, Austria

C. Ellen van der Schoot, MD, PhD
University of Amsterdam
Amsterdam, the Netherlands

Fenella Willis, MD, FRCP, FRCPath
St. George's Hospital
London, United Kingdom

Table of Contents

Preface .... **xiii**

About the Editors .... **xv**

1. **Basic Concepts and Practical Considerations of Intravenous Immunoglobulin Therapy** 1

   Paul Imbach, MD

   From Subcutaneous and Intramuscular Immune Serum Globulin to Intravenous Immunoglobulin 1
   Insight from the Substitutive Use of IVIG 3
   The Immunomodulatory Effects of IVIG 3
   Unresolved Issues and Future Directions 10
   References 11

2. **Manufacturing of IVIG** 13

   Wolfgang Teschner, PhD; Gerhard Poelsler, PhD; Harald Arno Butterweck, PhD; Ursula Mais-Paul, PhD; and Thomas R. Kreil, PhD

   History 13
   IVIG Development Strategy 17
   Manufacturing Process 20
   Pathogens and IVIG Safety 27
   Outlook 34
   References 36

3. **IVIG: Potential Mechanisms of Action** 43

   Andrew R. Crow, BRT, and Alan H. Lazarus, PhD

   IVIG and Activating Fcγ R 44
   Inhibitory Receptor FcγRIIB 46
   Idiotypic Antibodies 47
   Immunomodulation and Apoptosis 48
   Cytokine Modulation 49
   Complement 50
   FcRn 51

Dendritic Cells 52
   What Are the Molecular Targets of IVIG? 54
   Other Mechanisms 55
   Conclusions 56
   References 56

4. **IVIG for Hematologic Disorders** 67
   W. Beau Mitchell, MD, and James B. Bussel, MD

   Immune Thrombocytopenia 67
   Posttransfusion Purpura 72
   Autoimmune Neutropenia 72
   Evans Syndrome 73
   Autoimmune Hemolytic Anemia 73
   Other Hematologic Diseases 73
   Toxicity 74
   Conclusions 74
   References 75

5. **Clinical Use of IVIG in Neurology** 79
   Marinos C. Dalakas, MD

   Introduction 80
   Mechanisms of Action of IVIG in Autoimmune Neurologic Disorders:
      General Issues 80
   Status of IVIG in Autoimmune Neuromuscular Disorders: Evidence from
      Controlled Clinical Trials 82
   Novel and Promising Applications 92
   Treatment Considerations Using IVIG in Neurology 93
   References 95

6. **Clinical Use of IVIG in Infectious Diseases and Inflammatory
   Response Syndromes** 101
   Kevin B. Laupland, MD, MSc, FRCPC

   Prevention in Neonates 102
   Prevention in Critically Ill and High-Risk Surgical Patients ... 102
   Treatment 102
   Summary and Conclusion 108
   References 108

7. **Use of IVIG in Other Disorders** 113
   John Freedman, MD, FRCPC, and M. Bernadette Garvey, MD, FRCPC

   Rheumatologic Diseases 115
   Dermatologic Disorders 117
   Solid Organ Transplantation 120
   Cardiac Disorders 124

    Miscellaneous Disorders 125
    Conclusions 129
    References 129

8. Anti-D: Basic Concepts and Mechanisms of Action in Hemolytic Disease of the Fetus and Newborn 139

Davor Brinc, PhD, and Alan H. Lazarus, PhD

    Historical Overview 140
    Immune Response to the D Antigen and Immune Response Suppression 141
    Anti-D Studies in Humans 142
    Anti-D in Animal Models 142
    Monoclonal/Recombinant Anti-D 143
    Antibody-Mediated Immune Suppression 144
    Mechanisms of Anti-D 145
    Future Considerations 149
    Conclusion 150
    References 150

9. Anti-D: Basic Concepts and Mechanisms of Action in Autoimmunity 159

John W. Semple, PhD

    Immune Thrombocytopenia 160
    Overview of Anti-D 160
    Reticuloendothelial System Blockade 161
    Cytokines and Anti-D 161
    Idiotype Antibodies 165
    Anti-D and Signaling Mechanisms within the RES 166
    Monoclonal Anti-D Preparations 167
    Recombinant Polyclonal Anti-D 167
    Summary 168
    References 168

10. The Clinical Use of Anti-D 175

C. Ellen van der Schoot, MD, PhD

    Production, Infectious Risk, and Pharmacology of Anti-D 176
    Postnatal Immune Prophylaxis 177
    Antenatal Prophylaxis 178
    After Transfusion of D+ Blood Components 180
    Treatment of Primary Immune Thrombocytopenia 181
    Conclusion 183
    References 183

11. Monoclonal Antibodies in Hematology 187

Roberto Stasi, MD, PhD; Fenella Willis, MD, FRCP, FRCPath; Ruth Pettengell, MD; Muriel S. Shannon, MD; and Edward C. Gordon-Smith, MD

Rituximab 188
Alemtuzumab 196
Eculizumab 198
Gemtuzumab Ozogamicin 199
Ibritumomab Tiuxetan 204
^{131}I-Tositumomab 206
Conclusions and Future Directions 207
References 208

12. Monoclonal Antibody Therapy of Solid Malignancies 217

Robert O. Dillman, MD, FACP, and Robert K. Oldham, MD, FACP

Historical Background for Antibody Therapy 217
Mechanisms of Antibody-Mediated Antitumor Effects 218
Considerations for Monoclonal Antibody Therapy 219
Therapeutic Monoclonal Antibodies Commercially Available for Treatment of Solid Tumors 223
Trastuzumab (Herceptin) 224
Cetuximab (Erbitux) 232
Panitumumab (Vectibix) 239
Bevacizumab (Avastin) 242
Conclusions 251
References 251

Index 269

Preface

THERAPEUTIC IMMUNOGLOBulins have been in use for many years across a broad spectrum of clinical specialties. The number of diseases in which intravenous immunoglobulin (IVIG) is used increases annually, often with inadequate scientific evidence. Concurrently, the literature on this therapeutic agent increases exponentially. Given that this product is purified from the plasma of thousands of blood or plasma donors and is used at a very high dose, there is concern that supply will not be able to keep up with demand. One of the reasons for developing this book was to provide a one-source compilation of the current uses of immunoglobulins, both IVIG and anti-D, with a discussion on the hypothesized mechanisms of action and rationales for their use. We hope that this will encourage appropriate and rational use of these immunoglobulin products and contribute to immunoglobulin conservation. While we have included other therapeutic immunoglobulins (eg, monoclonal antibodies), the main focus is on the commonly used IVIG and anti-D.

Adequacy of supply and cost are major issues, but there is also concern about the possibility of the transmission of infectious disease to the recipient. Although current manufacturing processes are thought to be relatively safe, this risk is intrinsic to plasma-derived proteins, and the general population remains potentially vulnerable to the emergence of new pathogens. Administration of these therapies may also be associated with other adverse effects, some minor and some serious. The recent observations of occasional significant hemolytic reactions with these products are of particular concern. For these reasons and others, a non-human-donor-derived substitute therapy is desirable. Our understanding of the mechanisms of action of IVIG and anti-D is, however, incomplete, and the design of recombinant therapeutic substitutes is not at present straightforward. Even whether these products work by the same or similar mechanisms in different diseases is a matter of speculation. Nonetheless, as we move forward in the modern era of therapeutic immunoglobulin use, it is appropriate that the last two chapters of this book address the use of monoclonal antibodies as therapeutics for various diseases. As the reader will see, these monoclonal antibodies are not actually substitutes for IVIG but can achieve therapeutic efficacy in a number of clinical situations.

This book is written to be understandable by physicians and other allied health professionals who have a good general knowledge of basic medicine. With the burgeoning interest in therapeutic immunoglobulins, it is inevitable that even within the short time frame of this book's preparation and publication, new evidence will accumulate, both expanding and reducing current therapeutic indications, with varying levels of supportive evidence. The authors have attempted to review the current state of knowledge in the area to serve as a guide for sound clinical management.

We express our gratitude to all of the contributing authors as well as to Jay Pennington and Jennifer Boyer, who did an outstanding job in making this book a reality.

Alan H. Lazarus, PhD
John W. Semple, PhD
Editors

About the Editors

Alan H. Lazarus completed his BSc in biology and chemistry at Concordia University in Montreal in 1982. He received his PhD in microbiology and immunology from McGill University in 1987. From 1987 to 1993 he trained as a postdoctoral fellow at the Banting and Best Department of Medical Research at the Charles H. Best Institute, University of Toronto. He joined St. Michael's Hospital in 1993 and received his initial scholarship funding from the National Blood Foundation (Bethesda, MD) in 1994. In 1995 he received a 5-year scholarship from the Bayer/Canadian Red Cross Society/Medical Research Council of Canada program.

Dr. Lazarus is currently a scientist at The Canadian Blood Services, a scientist at The Keenan Research Centre in The Li Ka Shing Knowledge Institute of St Michael's Hospital, and an associate professor in the Department of Medicine of the University of Toronto. He also holds a cross-appointment in the Department of Laboratory Medicine and Pathobiology at the University of Toronto. He is actively engaged in training graduate students and postdoctoral fellows.

He has published over 80 original research papers in a number of high-impact medical journals such as *Nature Medicine, Journal of Clinical Investigation, Blood, TRANSFUSION,* and others. His main area of research has been the mechanism of action of intravenous immunoglobulin in the amelioration of the autoimmune disease immune thrombocytopenia (ITP). He is also involved in research related to the mechanism of action of anti-D in preventing hemolytic disease of the fetus and newborn. Dr. Lazarus is actively engaged in the discovery of new therapeutic agents to replace IVIG in the treatment of ITP and other autoimmune diseases.

John W. Semple studied biomedical sciences at the University of Guelph, and in 1986, he received his PhD in immunology from Queen's University at Kingston, Ontario. He then trained as a Diabetes Canada and Juvenile Diabetes fellow in the Banting and Best Department of Medical Research at the Charles H. Best Institute, University of Toronto, from 1986 to 1990. He joined St. Michael's Hospital in 1990 as a staff scientist.

Currently, he is head of transfusion medicine research and a senior staff scientist at St. Michael's, and a professor of pharmacology, medicine, and laboratory medicine and pathobiology at the University of Toronto. Dr. Semple is also an adjunct scientist with The Canadian Blood Services.

His research activities include several areas of platelet immunology, including the recognition of platelets by innate and adaptive immune mechanisms and how platelets mediate immunity via, for example, Toll-like receptors. His laboratory has also elucidated several novel theories as to how anti-D therapy raises platelet counts in patients with ITP. He routinely lectures at national and international meetings and in the last 20 years has published over 120 articles relating to platelet immunology.

1

Basic Concepts and Practical Considerations of Intravenous Immunoglobulin Therapy

Paul Imbach, MD

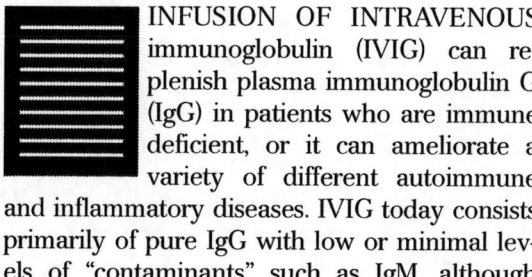INFUSION OF INTRAVENOUS immunoglobulin (IVIG) can replenish plasma immunoglobulin G (IgG) in patients who are immune deficient, or it can ameliorate a variety of different autoimmune and inflammatory diseases. IVIG today consists primarily of pure IgG with low or minimal levels of "contaminants" such as IgM, although early preparations of this plasma-derived product were much more crude in nature.

From Subcutaneous and Intramuscular Immune Serum Globulin to Intravenous Immunoglobulin

In 1946 at Harvard Medical School, Cohn and colleagues separated plasma and serum by cold ethanol precipitation into fractions of "protein and lipoprotein"[1] and subsequently developed more purified fractions containing "antibodies, isoagglutinins, prothrombin, and plasminogen."[2] The antibody fraction was known as immune serum globulin (ISG). When administered intravenously, ISG formed aggregates that caused severe adverse effects; therefore, it was subsequently administered only subcutaneously or intramuscularly.

In 1962, Barandun et al[3] at the University of Bern identified the anticomplementary activities of IgG aggregates as the main cause of the side effects of ISG administration. The anticomplementary activitiy could be reduced by pepsin digestion, which splits the IgG molecule into two antigen-binding fragments, $F(ab')_2$ and the Fc fragments[4,5] (see Fig 1-1). Other IgG production procedures such as the use of plasmin or sulfonation[6,7] also suppressed complement acti-

---

Paul Imbach, MD, Emerited Professor and Head of Division of Pediatric Hematology-Oncology, Medical Faculty of the University of Basel, University Children's Hospital Basel (UKBB), Basel, Switzerland
The authors have disclosed no conflicts of interest.

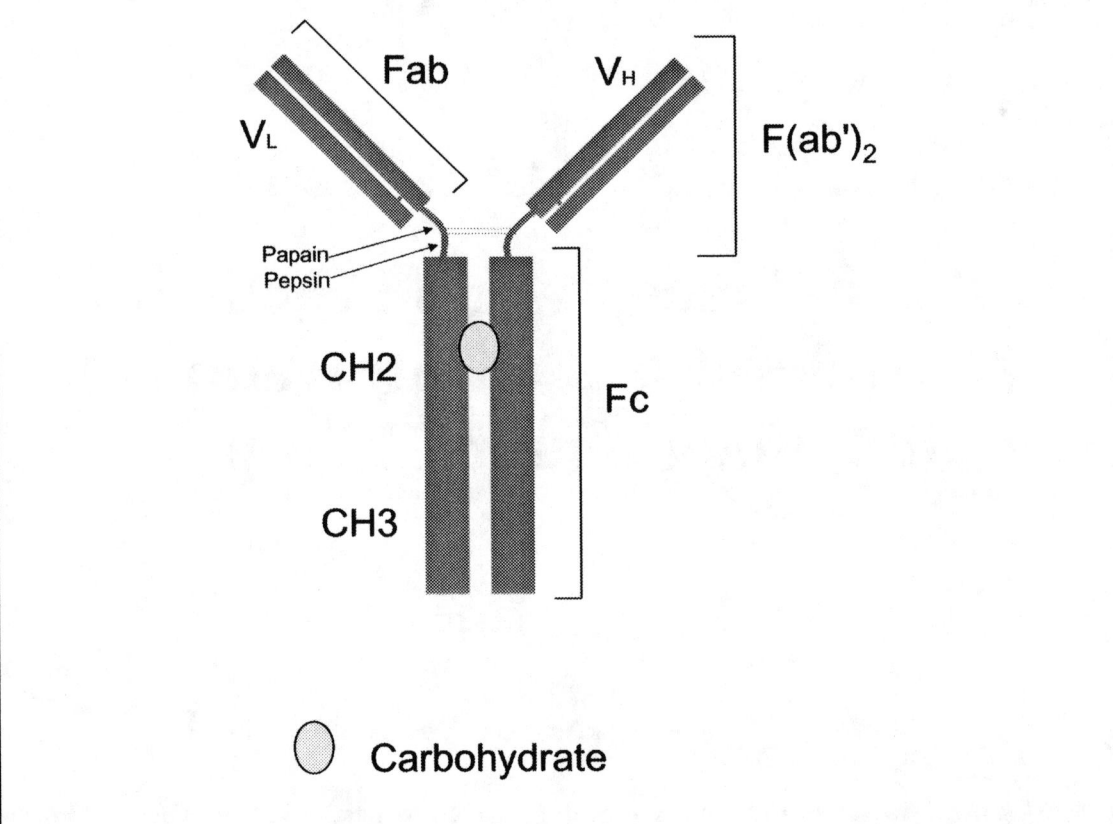

Figure 1-1. Structure and function of immunoglobulin G (IgG) antibodies. In the Fab portion of the diagram, antibody combines with antigenic determinants, representing the recognition function. In the Fc portion of the diagram, complement activation and binding to cell receptors represent the effector function. An efficient and safe intravenous immunoglobulin ensures normal cooperation between antigenic binding and humoral and cellular mechanisms of particle removal. Side reactions are minimal.

vation but simultaneously reduced some of the important biological functions of IgG. The chance observation of acidification by pH 4 at the Central Laboratory of the Swiss Red Cross, Bern, led to a reduction in anticomplementary effects in ISG without impairing the IgG functions.[8] It was later found that contamination of ISG with other potentially adverse reagents such as prekallikrein, plasminogen, and others could be reduced or eliminated by using an anion exchange chromatography purification step; this allowed the purified IgG molecules to remain intact.[9] It was around this time that ISG was renamed IVIG.

Today, IVIG is extracted from the pooled plasma of between 3000 and 60,000 blood or plasma donations, depending on the country and the manufacturer. The safety of IVIG is ensured by the careful ongoing selection and deferral of donors, by testing and validation of product lots during production, and by continual enhancements in purification and virus inactivation techniques.[10] For example, the last outbreak of hepatitis C caused by an IVIG product was caused by inappropriate virus inactivation in 1993.[11] Patient tolerability of IVIG depends on the volume and rate of infusion, the osmolality of the product, and the content of additives (eg, sugar, sodium). Details concerning current commercial IVIG preparations are given in Table 1-1 and by Hooper.[12]

Insight from the Substitutive Use of IVIG

In 1952, Bruton subcutaneously administered human immunoglobulin to a boy with immeasurable serum gammaglobulin levels and recurrent pneumococcal infections.[13] The boy's infections disappeared, and his serum gammaglobulin levels became measurable. Today, this boy's disorder is known as X-linked agammaglobulinemia and is caused by a defect in the Bruton tyrosine kinase gene, which encodes an enzyme that is central for B-lymphocyte development. Although IVIG is often used as an immunomodulatory agent today, before 1980 the only registered indications for ISG or IVIG were primary or secondary immunodeficiencies.

It may be seen retrospectively that some early observations supported an immunomodulatory effect of IVIG before 1980. These include observation of a child with immune thrombocytopenia (ITP) who was receiving corticosteroid treatment and became infected with varicella in 1964. The child received standard gammaglobulin intravenously for a treatment against varicella and displayed a dramatic increase in platelet counts.[14] In 1978, two adult patients with agammaglobulinemia developed hemolytic anemia and thrombocytopenia, and the known complications of agammaglobulinemia appeared to subside under intense substitutive treatment with IVIG.[15] In 1980 at the University Children's Hospital in Bern, IVIG administration was observed to influence the thrombocytopenia of a child with Wiskott-Aldrich syndrome but not the thrombocytopenia of two children with aplastic anemia.[16] This latter observation provided the impetus to use IVIG to treat a patient who had severe ITP, which became a key case.

The Immunomodulatory Effects of IVIG

ITP is a bleeding disorder characterized by platelet destruction because of antibody opsonization of the platelets, resulting in Fc-receptor-mediated platelet phagocytosis. A causative factor in the plasma of ITP patients was first demonstrated by Harrington et al in 1951,[17] when he injected plasma from patients with ITP into healthy volunteers and observed that they developed transient thrombocytopenia [see Fig 1-2 (A)]. Subsequently, it was documented that the causative factor of thrombocytopenia was associated with the 7S fraction of ITP plasma,[18] consistent with an IgG antibody targeted against platelet antigens. (For a historical review, see Imbach et al.[19]) It is now firmly established that the rapid destruction of platelets in ITP is caused by the presence of either immune complexes that bind to Fc receptors on the platelet or autoantibodies that bind to antigenic sites on the platelet. In addition, other elements of the immune system make the pathophysiology of ITP even more complex, involving humoral and cellular immune responses against the platelet as well as inappropriate platelet production in ITP. With these elements combined, the pathophysiologic picture supports the concept that chronic ITP is a true autoimmune disorder, although the etiology of ITP remains unknown. The maintenance of self-tolerance and the immune response may be affected in the presence of inflammatory or autoimmune processes.

The key observation supporting the immunomodulatory efficacy of IVIG was made in the case of a 12-year-old boy with severe hemorrhagic chronic ITP who, as a result of long-term treatment with vincristine and steroids, became lymphocytopenic and therefore developed secondary hypogammaglobulinemia. Because of the disturbed immune response and the need to correct this child's secondary hypogammaglobulinemia, the child received the newly available IVIG. He displayed a dramatic increase in platelet count within 24 hours, which continued with the administration of the additional four doses of 0.4 g IVIG/kg body

Table 1-1. Production and Properties of Commercial Immunoglobulins*

Trade Names	Manufacturer	Registrations	Manufacturing Procedure	Composition	Comments
Gammagard S/D	Baxter Heathcare	United States, Canada, European Union	Cold ethanol fractionation, DEAE chromatography, S/D, pH 6.8 ±0.4, freeze-dried	50 mg/mL; 8.5 mg/mL NaCl, 0.3 M glycine, 20 mg/mL PEG, 3 mg/mL albumin, 20 mg/mL glucose	<1 µg/mL IgA
Gammagard Liquid, KIOVIG	Baxter Heathcare	United States, European Union	Cold ethanol fractionation, DEAE chromatography, S/D, nanofiltration, pH 4.85 ±0.25, liquid	100 mg/mL; 0.25 M glycine	—
Intratect	Biotest	Germany, European Union	Cold ethanol fractionation, octanoic acid/calcium acetate treatment, S/D, liquid	50 mg/mL; 0.3 M glycine	—
Vigam	Bio Products Laboratory	England	—	50 mg/mL; IgG, 20 mg/mL human albumin, sucrose, glycine, pH 4.8-5.1	In US clinical trials (Gammaplex)
Carimune NF	CSL Behring AG	United States, European Union	Cold ethanol fractionation, pepsin treatment, nanofiltration, pH 6.6 ±0.2, freeze-dried	30, 60, 90, or 120 mg/mL; 100 mg/mL sucrose; 1.2 mg/mL NaCl	—
Sandoglobulin NF liquid, Carimune NF liquid	CSL Behring AG	Canada	Cold ethanol fractionation, pepsin treatment, DEAE Sephadex batch adsorption, nanofiltration, pH 5.3, liquid	120 mg/mL; 100 mM L-isoleucine, 120 mM L-proline, 80 mM nicotinamide	—

Product	Manufacturer	Country	Manufacturing process	Formulation	Comments
Privigen	CSL Behring AG	United States	Cold ethanol fractionation, octanoic acid fractionation, anion exchange chromatography, nanofiltration, pH 4.8 ±0.2, liquid	100 mg/mL; 0.25 M proline	—
Vivaglobulin	CSL Behring AG	United States	Cold ethanol, fatty alcohol, DEAE chromatography, activated carbon, heated 10 h at 60 C, pH 6.8 ±0.4, liquid	160 mg/mL; 3 g/L NaCl, 0.25 M glycine	Formulated for subcutaneous injection
Flebogamma 5%	Instituto Grifols, SA	United States, Spain	Cold ethanol, PEG precipitation, ion exchange chromatography, 10 h at 60 C, pH 5.5 ±0.5, liquid	50 mg/mL; 50 mg/mL D-sorbitol, <6 mg/mL PEG	—
Flebogamma 5% DIF	Instituto Grifols, SA	United States	Cold ethanol, PEG precipitation, ion exchange chromatography, pH 4 at 37 C, 10 h at 60 C, S/D, nanofiltration, pH 5.5 ±0.5, liquid	50 mg/mL; 50 mg/mL D-sorbitol, <3 mg/mL PEG	4 virus elimination steps
Octagam	Octapharma Pharmazeutika Produktionsges mbH	United States, European Union	Cold ethanol fractionation, S/D, 24 h at pH 4, pH 5.5 ±0.4, liquid	50 mg/mL; 100 mg/mL maltose	—
Omr-IgG-am	Omrix Biopharmaceuticals, Ltd	Israel	Cold ethanol fractionation, S/D, 24 h at pH 4, pH 5.5 ±0.4, liquid	50 mg/mL; 100 mg/mL maltose	In US clinical trials
Gamunex	Talecris Biotherapeutics, Inc	United States, European Union	Cold ethanol fractionation, caprylate precipitation, Q Sepharose-ANX Sepharose chromatography, pH 4.25 ±0.25, liquid	100 mg/mL; 0.2 M glycine	—

*Reproduced with permission from Hooper.[12]
S/D = solvent/detergent (treatment); DEAE = diethylaminoethyl; PEG = polyethylene glycol; NF = nanofiltration; DIF = dual inactivation and filtration.

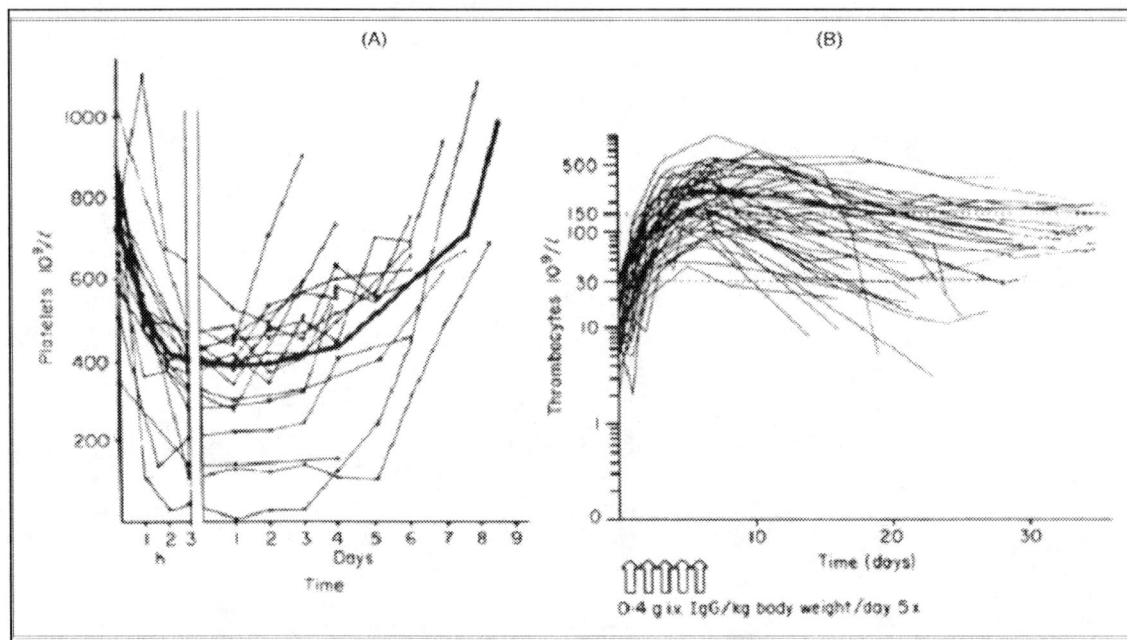

Figure 1-2. (A) Platelet counts of volunteers after infusion of ITP plasma.[17] (B) Platelet counts of 42 children with previously treated ITP during and after IVIG therapy.[23] (Reproduced with permission from Harrington et al[17] and Imholz et al.[23])
ITP = immune thrombocytopenia; IVIG = intravenous immunoglobulin.

weight (Fig 1-3, patient 1). Immediately following that observation, a pilot study in 12 consecutive children with newly diagnosed or chronic ITP who did not have hypogammaglobulinemia showed similar dramatic platelet effects in response to IVIG (Fig 1-3).[20] Consequently, the first randomized controlled multicenter study comparing corticosteroid and IVIG administration was initiated in children with ITP, and the results confirmed that IVIG was an effective therapy for raising platelet counts.[21]

Dosage of IVIG in ITP

Soon after the above mentioned studies were completed, it was realized that a lower total dose of 0.8 g IVIG/kg/dose had a similar beneficial effect in children with newly diagnosed ITP. In a cooperative randomized Canadian multicenter study, children with newly diagnosed ITP having platelet counts below 20 × 10^9/L were studied to compare treatments with IVIG, oral corticosteroids, and intravenous anti-D. In the case of IVIG, the study determined that treatment with a single dose of 0.8 g/kg body weight of IVIG showed a fast recovery to a safe platelet level in comparison with patients on 2 × 1 g/kg IVIG.[22]

Parallel Increase of Serum IgG and IgM after IVIG

In an early randomized study of IVIG vs corticosteroids,[21] five doses of 0.4 g/kg IVIG increased the serum IgG concentration by a factor of two from an average pretreatment level of 12.5 g/L to an average peak of 25.9 g/L (Fig 1-4). In patients randomized to corticosteroids, the serum IgG concentration fell significantly over 5 weeks from an average level of 12.0 g/L to 7.8 g/L. The serum IgM level increased significantly in both groups, but the increase was greater (33%) in patients random-

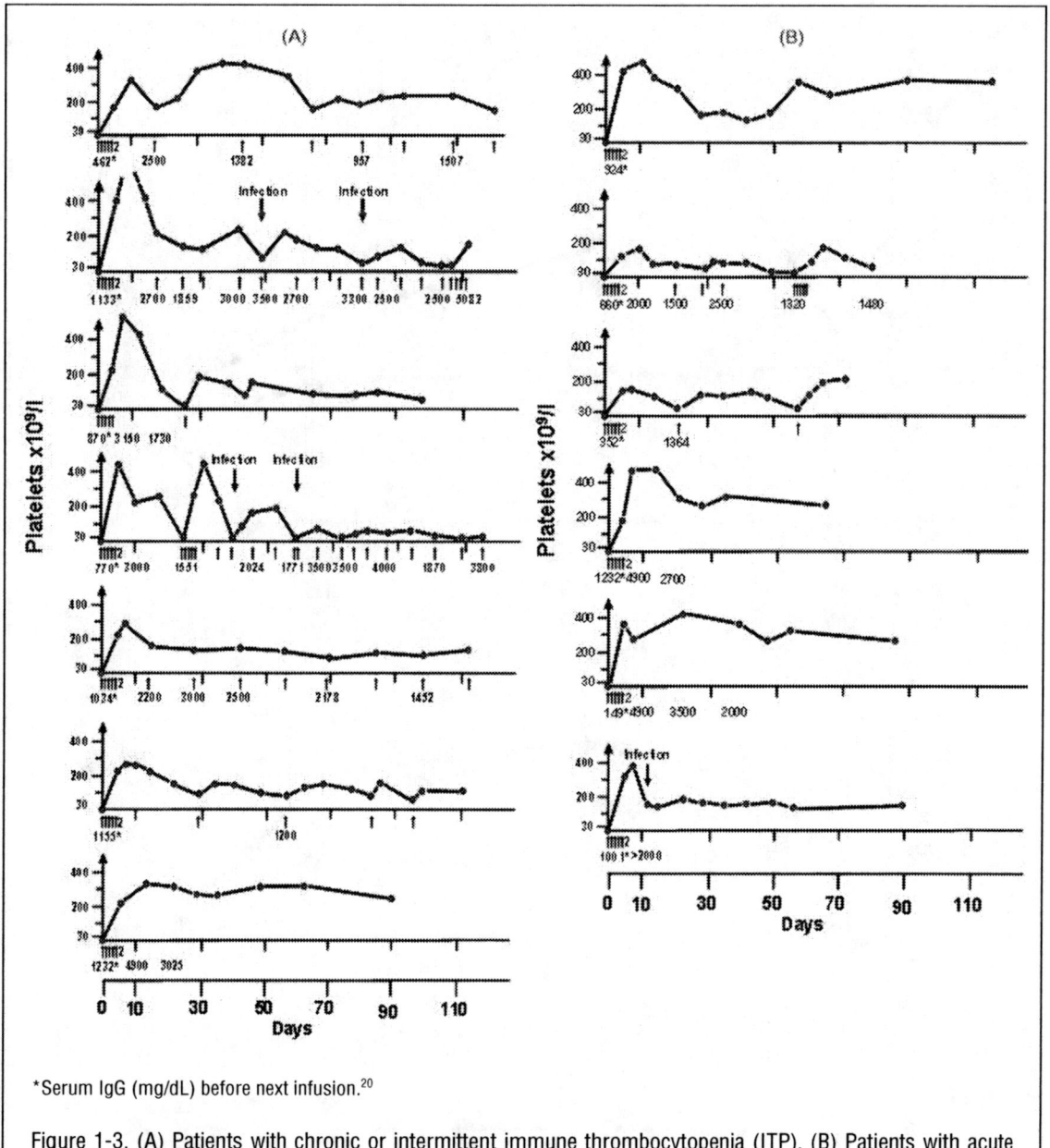

*Serum IgG (mg/dL) before next infusion.[20]

Figure 1-3. (A) Patients with chronic or intermittent immune thrombocytopenia (ITP). (B) Patients with acute ITP. Upward-pointing arrows indicate Ig-SRK, 0.4 g/kg body weight/day. (Reprinted with permission from Imbach et al.[20])
Pred = prednisone; Cyclo = cyclophosphamide; VCR = vincristine.

ized to IVIG in comparison to those randomized to corticosteroids (see Fig 1-4).

A similar phenomenon was observed in a prospective IVIG study of children with previously treated ITP [see Fig 1-5 (B)].[23] Five doses of 0.4 g/kg IVIG daily induced a significant and temporary increase in serum IgG levels, with a continuous increase in IgM levels up to day 21 despite the fact that IVIG contained only traces of IgM.

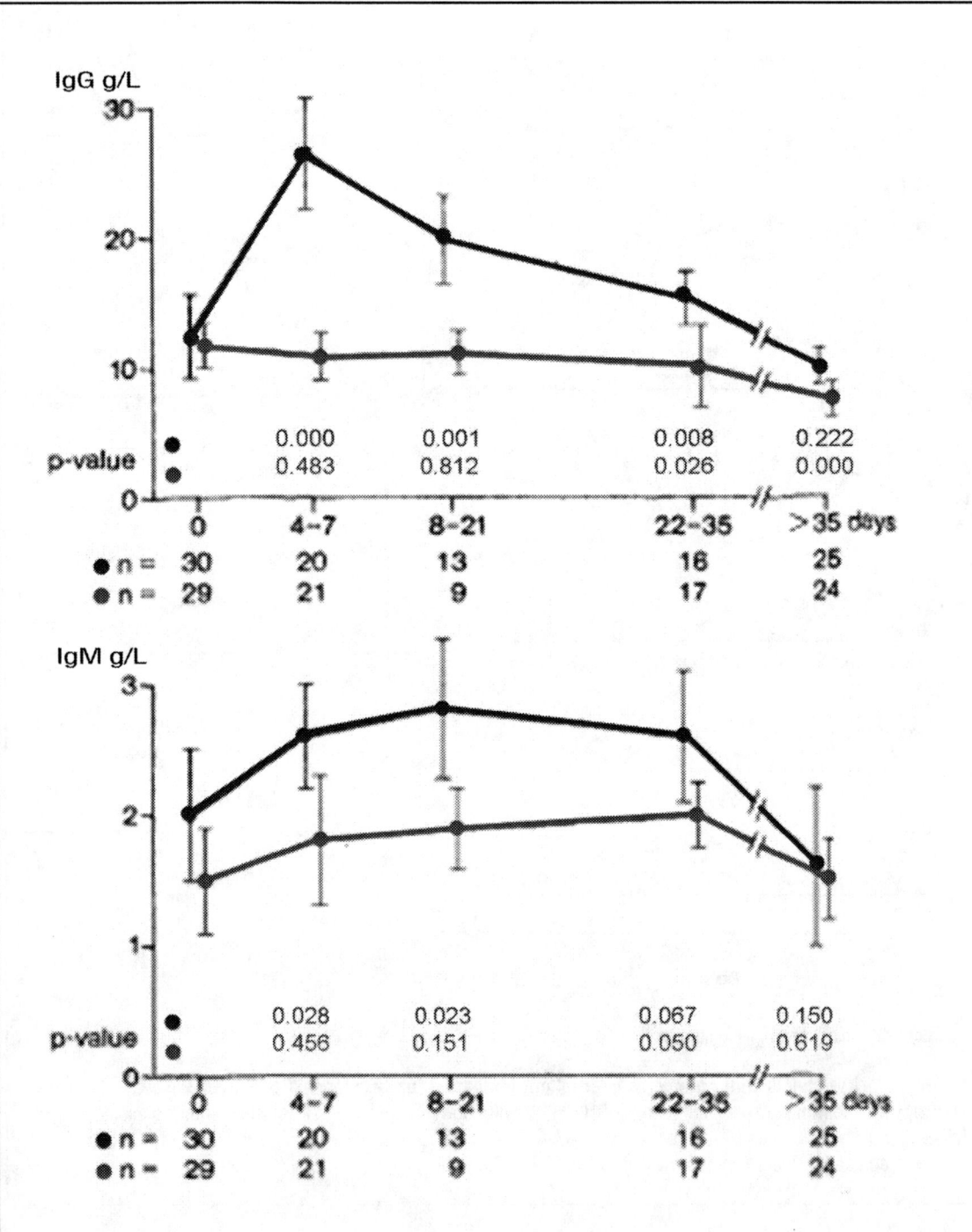

Figure 1-4. Serum IgG and IgM before, during, and after IgG (●) and corticosteroid (○) therapy. (Reprinted with permission from Imbach et al.[21])

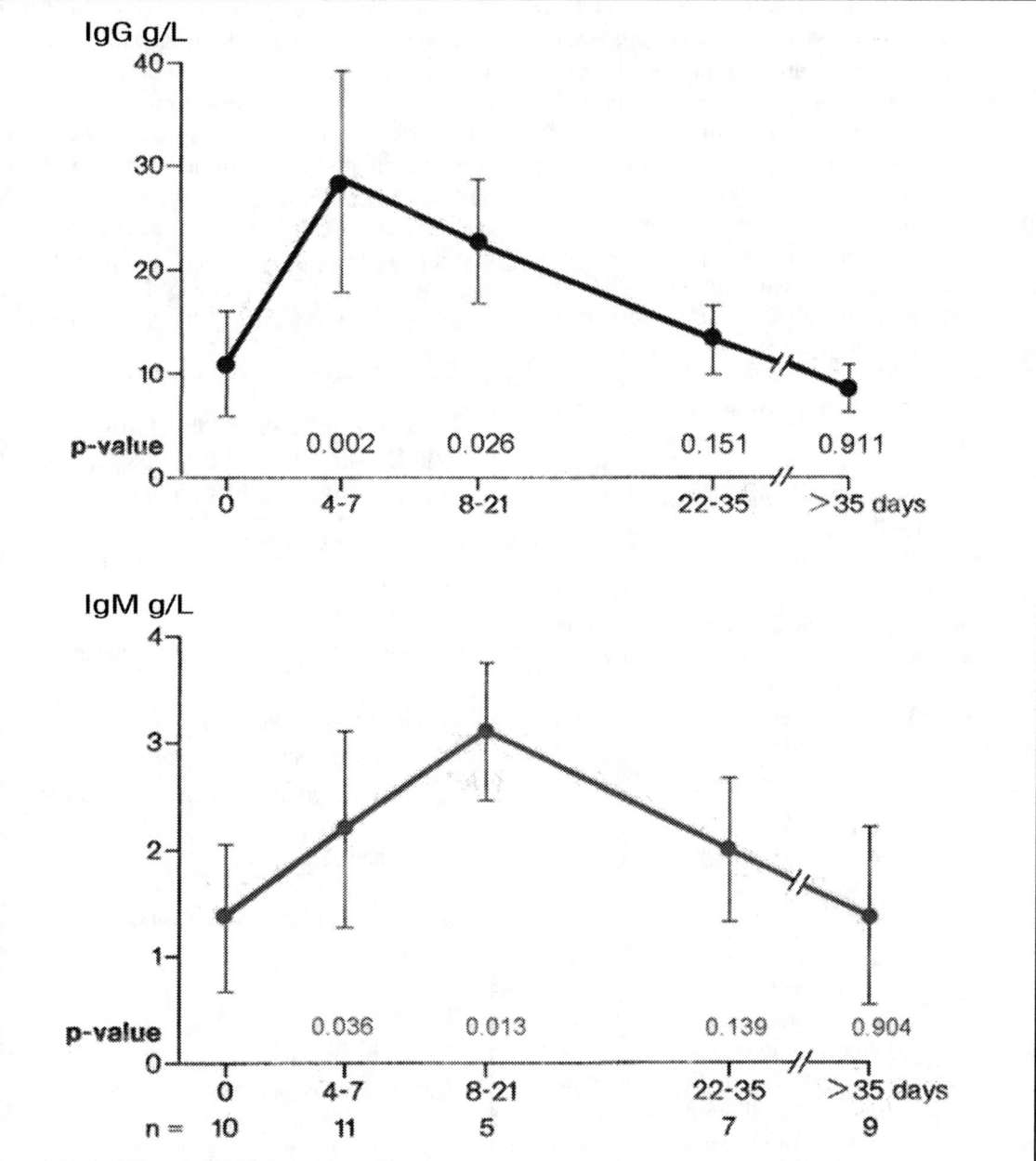

Figure 1-5. Variation of serum IgG and IgM after 5 × 0.4 g IVIG/kg body weight (mean values ±1 standard deviation); p values are in relation to the original value. (Reprinted with permission from Imholz et al.[23])

The unexpected increase of serum IgM levels during IVIG treatment of ITP remains unexplained; it might be the result of a stimulation of IgM synthesis or an alteration in IgM function and/or IgM turnover.

Background for Anti-D Immunoglobulin Treatment in ITP

One early concept of the mechanism of action of IVIG treatment was a blockade of Fc-receptors on the monocyte/macrophage system by the patient's sensitized red cells (presumably caused by red cell antibodies present in the infused IVIG).[24] This theory was first suggested by Salama et al[25] and became the basis of anti-D IgG treatment in ITP.

In summary, at least two controversial effects of antibodies have been recognized in patients with ITP. First, targeted platelet-associated IgG destroys platelets in the disorder. Second, IVIG from healthy blood donors can rapidly increase the platelet counts in ITP (see Fig 1-2).

From another perspective, somewhat similar destructive pathogeneses have been shown to be responsible for several other chronic inflammatory and autoimmune disorders (see Table 1-2). Clinical and laboratory studies have documented that IVIG may be also clinically beneficial in these disorders and that the mechanism of action of IVIG likely occurs on many different levels of the immune response.[26-30] Together, these clinical results have fueled the high demand for the product, and worldwide use of IVIG thus increased from 300 kg in 1980 to over 70,000 kg per year by 2008.

Unresolved Issues and Future Directions

As in ITP, the majority of chronic inflammatory and autoimmune disorders (Table 1-2) are characterized by extensive clinical and immunopathogenic heterogeneities, including those of the patient's clinical presentation, age, gender, and history. These differences coupled with the spectrum of innumerable antibodies present in IVIG concentrates make the treatment of chronic autoimmune diseases a complex enterprise. A concern is that rare antibodies that may contribute to the beneficial effects of IVIG are potentially diluted because of pooling. Moreover, it is possible that some antibodies present in IVIG contribute to its clinical efficacy, whereas other antibodies antagonize these functions. A resolution to this issue remains to be found.

An additional concern for IVIG is that Phase III studies for new indications (prior to approval by authorities) have not always been performed, and many unlabeled uses of IVIG are in use. IVIG dose-finding studies have not been systematically performed either, and the plasma level of IVIG necessary for optimal efficacy is not well defined. In fact, it is possible that a peak level of IVIG may be more significant than simply maintaining constant IVIG levels for some diseases. IVIG dosage has var-

Table 1-2. Examples of Disorders with Disturbed Immune Responses and Documented Effects by IVIG

Hematologic disorders:
Immune thrombocytopenia
Kawasaki syndrome
Graft-vs-host disease, allogeneic transplantation
Hemophagocytic syndrome
Acquired hemophilia
Autoimmune lymphoproliferative syndrome

Dermatomyositis

Antineutrophil cytoplasmic autoantibody vasculitis

Neurologic disorders:
Guillain-Barré syndrome
Multifocal motor neuropathy
Myasthenia gravis
Relapsing-remitting multiple sclerosis
Alzheimer disease (experimental)

Dermatologic disorders:
Pemphigus vulgaris, pemphigus foliacus
Pemphigus bullosis acquisita
Toxic epidermal necrolysis/Steven Johnson syndrome

ied among patients and various diseases treated, ranging from 0.2 to 2.0 g/kg body weight. In clinical studies, the efficacy of IVIG is highly variable, due in part to disease heterogeneity and the complexity of different immunopathogeneses as well as to the variety and extent of the different molecular specificities present in IVIG.

In clinical trials of IVIG, a difficulty has been that study objectives and endpoints have often not been based on standardized, validated assessments and scoring systems. Retrospective analysis, opinion-based guidelines, and surveys[31-34] are controversial and are not well followed in practice. Prospective studies are required, and appropriate laboratory analyses and pharmacoeconomic evaluations need to be performed.

To address these issues in ITP, the Intercontinental Cooperative ITP Study Group (ICIS) has established an international network of physicians and scientists, collaborating in prospective registries and studies (see www.itpbasel.ch), that will define less heterogeneous patient subgroups for randomized controlled trials. Studies with a well-defined subgroup of an autoimmune disorder and with clear study endpoints may find evidence-based results. Furthermore, the new Pediatric and Adult Registry on Chronic ITP (PARC-ITP; see www.parc-itp.net) has the objective of defining subgroups within ITP on the basis of natural history, genetics, quality of life, and other criteria. One of the PARC-ITP studies will focus on genetic aspects of ITP.[35,36]

Future research will need to focus on 1) registries for subgroup definitions in inflammatory and autoimmune disorders; 2) laboratory studies on the etiology, immune pathogenesis, and mechanisms of action of IVIG; 3) other biologically targeted treatments (eg, monoclonal antibodies); and 4) newer forms of immunomodulation. More appropriate patient selection and interventional trials with IVIG alone or IVIG with other medications will be helpful. It is anticipated that indications for the use of IVIG will become better defined with increased efficacy and reduced rates of product use and adverse effects.

References

1. Cohn EJ, Strong LE, Hughes WL Jr, et al. Preparation and properties of serum and plasma proteins III: A system for the separation into fractions of the protein and lipoprotein components of biological tissues and fluids. J Am Chem Soc 1946;68:459-75.
2. Oncley JL, Melin M, Richert DA, et al. The separation of the antibodies, isoagglutinins, prothrombin, plasminogen and beta-lipoprotein into subfractions of human plasma. J Am Chem Soc 1949;71:541-50.
3. Barandun S, Kistler P, Jeunet F, et al. Intravenous administration of human gamma globulin. Vox Sang 1962;7:157-74.
4. Schultze HE, Schwick G. Uber neue Möglichkeiten intravenöser gammaglobulinapplikation. Dtsch Med Wochenschr 1962;87:1643-50.
5. Burdach SE, Evers KG, Geursen RG. Treatment of acute idiopathic thrombocytopenic purpura of childhood with intravenous immunoglobulin G: Comparative efficacy of 7S and 5S preparations. J Pediatr 1986;109:770-5.
6. Stephan W. Undergraded human immunoglobulin for intravenous use. Vox Sang 1975;28:422-37.
7. Masuho Y, Tomibe K, Matsuzawa K, et al. Development of an intravenous gamma-globulin with Fc activities I: Preparation and characteristics of S-sulfonated human gamma-globulin. Vox Sang 1977;32:175-81.
8. Haessig A. 50 Jahre Blutspendedienst des Schweizerischen Roten Kreuzes. Schweiz Med Wochenschrift 1991;121:156.
9. Hooper JA, Alpern M, Mankarious S. Immunoglobulin manufacturing procedures. In: Krijnen HW, Strengers PFW, van Aken WG, eds. Immunoglobulins. Amsterdam: Central Laboratory of the Netherlands Red Cross Blood Transfusion Service, 1988:361-80.
10. Schleis TG. The process: New methods of purification and viral safety. Pharmacotherapy 2005;25(11 pt 2):73S-7S.
11. Bjoro K, Froland SS, Yun Z, et al. Hepatitis C infection in patients with primary hypogammaglobulinemia after treatment with contaminated immune globulin. N Engl J Med 1994;331:1607-11.
12. Hooper JA. Intravenous immunoglobulins: Evolution of commercial IVIG preparations. Immunol Allergy Clin North Am 2008;28:765-78.

13. Bruton OC. Agammaglobulinemia. Pediatrics 1952;9:722-7.
14. Gugler E. Die kindlichen Thrombopenien. In: Rossi E, ed. Päd Fortbildungskurse. Basel, Switzerland: Krager, 1964;11-12:143-58.
15. Barandun S, Imbach P, Morell A, Wagner HP. Traitement du purpura thrombocytopénique idiopathique par des immunoglobulines. Méd et Hyg 1982;40:1774-8.
16. Imbach P, Barandun S, Baumgartner C, et al. High-dose intravenous gammaglobulin therapy of refractory, in particular idiopathic thrombocytopenia in childhood. Helv Paediat Acta 1981;46:81-6.
17. Harrington WJ, Minnich V, Hollingsworth JW, et al. Demonstration of a thrombocytopenic factor in the blood of patients with thrombocytopenic purpura. J Lab Clin Med 1951;38:1-10.
18. Shulman NR, Marder VJ, Weinrach RS. Similarities between known antiplatelet antibodies and the factor responsible for thrombocytopenia in idiopathic purpura: Physiologic, serologic and isotopic studies. Ann NY Acad Sci 1965;124:499-542.
19. Imbach P, Kühne T, Signer E. Historical aspects and current knowledge of idiopathic thrombocytopenic purpura. Br J Haematol 2002;119:894-900.
20. Imbach P, Barandun S, d'Apuzzo V, et al. High-dose intravenous gammaglobulin for idiopathic thrombocytopenic purpura in childhood. Lancet 1981;1:1228-31.
21. Imbach P, Berchtold W, Hirt A, et al. Intravenous immunoglobulin versus oral corticosteroids in acute immune thrombocytopenic purpura in childhood. Lancet 1985;2:464-8.
22. Blanchette V, Imbach P, Andrew M, et al. Randomised trial of intravenous immunoglobulin G, intravenous anti-D, and oral prednisone in childhood acute immune thrombocytopenic purpura. Lancet 1994;344:703-7.
23. Imholz B, Imbach P, Baumgartner C, et al. Intravenous immunoglobulin (i.v. IgG) for previously treated acute or for chronic idiopathic thrombocytopenic purpura (ITP) in childhood: A prospective multicenter study. Blut 1988;56:63-8.
24. Fehr J, Hofman V, Kappler U. Transient reversal of thrombocytopenia in idiopathic thrombocytopenic purpura by high-dose intravenous gamma globulin. N Engl J Med 1982;306:1254-8.
25. Salama A, Kiefel V, Amberg R, Mueller-Eckhardt C. Treatment of autoimmune thrombocytopenic purpura with Rhesus antibodies [anti RhO(D)]. Blut 1984;49:29-35.
26. Lemieux R, Bazin R, Néron S. Therapeutic intravenous immunoglobulins (review). Mol Immunol 2005;42:839-48.
27. Stangel M, Pul R. Basic principles of intravenous immunoglobulin (IVIg) treatment. J Neurol 2006;253(Suppl 5):V18-24.
28. Negi VS, Elluru S, Sibéril S, et al. Intravenous immunoglobulin: An update on the clinical use and mechanisms of action (review). J Clin Immunol 2007;27:233-45.
29. Gold R, Stangel M, Dalakas MC. Drug insight: The use of intravenous immunoglobulin in neurology—therapeutic considerations and practical issues (review). Nat Clin Pract Neurol 2007;3:36-44.
30. Jolles S, Hughes J. Use of IGIV in the treatment of atopic dermatitis, urticaria, scleromyxedema, pyoderma gangrenosum, psoriasis, and pretibial myxedema (review). Int Immunopharmacol 2006;6:579-91.
31. George JN, Woolf SH, Raskob GE, et al. Idiopathic thrombocytopenic purpura: A practice guideline developed by explicit methods for The American Society of Hematology. Blood 1996;88:3-40.
32. Guidelines for the investigation and management of idiopathic thrombocytopenic purpura in adults, children and pregnancy. Br J Haematol 2003;120:574-96.
33. Vesely S, Buchanan GR, Cohen A, et al. Self-reported diagnostic and management strategies in childhood idiopathic thrombocytopenic purpura: Results of a survey of practicing pediatric hematology/oncology specialists. J Pediatr Hematol Oncol 2000;22:55-61.
34. Bolton-Maggs PHB, Moon I. Assessment of UK practice for management of acute childhood idiopathic thrombocytopenic purpura against published guidelines. Lancet 1997;350:620-3.
35. Foster CB, Zhu S. Erichsen HC, et al. Polymorphisms in inflammatory cytokines and Fcgamma receptors in childhood chronic immune thrombocytopenic purpura: A pilot study. Br J Haematol 2001;113:596-9.
36. Smith AJ, Keen LJ, Billingham MJ, et al. Extended haplotypes and linkage disequilibrium in the IL1R1-IL1A-IL1B-IL1RN gene cluster: Association with knee osteoarthritis. Genes Immun 2004;5:451-60.

In: Lazarus AH, Semple JW, eds.
Immunoglobulin Therapy
Bethesda, MD: AABB Press, 2010

2

Manufacturing of IVIG

Wolfgang Teschner, PhD; Gerhard Poelsler, PhD; Harald Arno Butterweck, PhD; Ursula Mais-Paul, PhD; and Thomas R. Kreil, PhD

IMMUNOGLOBULIN PRODUCTS manufactured from human plasma are used in a growing number of indications and have reached a historically unprecedented margin of safety with respect to the transmission of blood-borne pathogens. In addition to descriptions of manufacturing processes, this chapter provides a synopsis of the history of immunoglobulin manufacturing from human plasma, starting with the Cohn ethanol fractionation procedure, and development strategies to fulfill high-quality standards with a specific focus on viral safety. The outlook is promising: even after a long tradition of plasma fractionation, new clinical indications are on the horizon, and these will be behind efforts to further improve the efficiency of the manufacturing processes, yet without jeopardizing current levels of safety.

History

In the first half of the last century, Edwin J. Cohn (1892-1953) developed cold ethanol fractionation on an industrial scale for isolating blood plasma fractions rich in pharmaceutically relevant proteins.[1] The process is based on the differential solubility of albumin, immunoglobulins, and other plasma proteins, which is influenced by pH, ethanol concentration, temperature, ionic strength, and protein concentration. Albumin has the highest solubility and the lowest isoelectric point of the major plasma proteins, and it is also the most abundant. As a

---

Wolfgang Teschner, PhD, Director, Plasma Product Development/Product Support; Gerhard Poelsler, PhD, Manager II, Global Pathogen Safety; Harald Arno Butterweck, PhD, Manager, Plasma Product Development/Product Support; Ursula Mais-Paul, PhD, Manager, Plasma Product Development/Product Support, Global Pre-Clinical Research and Development; and Thomas R. Kreil, PhD, Associate Professor of Virology and Senior Director, Viral Vaccines and Global Pathogen Safety, Baxter Innovations GmbH, Vienna, Austria

The authors have disclosed no conflicts of interest.

result, albumin can be purified by ethanol fractionation in large quantities.

Cohn originally developed the process in World War II primarily to extract albumin, which is stable at room temperature, for use as a substitute for human plasma. When administered to wounded soldiers or other patients who had suffered heavy blood losses, albumin helped to expand the volume of blood and led to rapid clinical improvement.[2-4] As early as 1941, when the US naval base at Pearl Harbor was attacked, albumin fractionated from human plasma by Cohn was successfully used to stabilize blood pressure in seven casualties with severe burns. As a result, the US Navy requested large quantities of the product. Albumin manufacturing was then refined to remove heat-sensitive components and to further stabilize the preparation for heat treatment to destroy viruses.[5-9] At the time, about 23,000 cases of hepatitis in the armed forces were known to have resulted from the injection of a yellow fever vaccine stabilized with human serum.[10] A preliminary clinical study completed in 1948 by Gellis et al showed that hepatitis was not transmitted when human albumin was heat-treated in the presence of stabilizers at 60 C for 10 hours—the first effective virus-inactivation step developed for a plasma product.[11]

In parallel with the development of a stable human albumin preparation, in 1942, Cohn fraction II+III was found to contain antibodies against viruses like polio or measles. Oncley developed a process for purifying the primarily IgG-containing fraction II[12] from fraction II+III, and it was successfully used to protect children during the measles epidemic in 1943.

In 1952, Colonel Bruton,[13] who was then working at the Walter Reed Army Hospital, described a young boy suffering from recurrent sepsis, whom he diagnosed with agammaglobulinemia. After an initial subcutaneous injection of human immunoglobulin, which resulted in an increase in serum gammaglobulin from 0 to 4.6% of plasma protein, the boy was treated with monthly injections, and the frequency of sepsis decreased from 19 episodes over 4 years to no episodes over 14 months. As a result of this successful treatment, immunoglobulin administration became the standard care for patients with hypogammaglobulinemia.

In the beginning, intramuscular or subcutaneous administrations of IgG were the methods of choice[14]; much later, intramuscular preparations were favored.[15] However, much larger volumes can be delivered by the intravenous (IV) route to provide the physiologic levels of IgG needed for the effective treatment of various diseases such as primary immune deficiencies, immune (idiopathic) thrombocytopenia (ITP), and Kawasaki syndrome.[16,17] The products for intramuscular administration could, however, not fulfill the clinical requirements for IV delivery because the rapid uptake of the product into the circulation was accompanied by serious anaphylactoid reactions such as dyspnea, nausea, vomiting, lumbar pain, and hypotension, followed by high fever.[18] Thus, the fractionation of immunoglobulins had to be further refined to reach the purity and tolerability required for IV administration.

In 1962, Barandun et al proposed spontaneous complement activation by IgG aggregates as the principal cause of adverse reactions after IV IgG injection.[18] The first attempts to produce intravenous immunoglobulins (IVIGs) with reduced anticomplementary activity employed enzymatic methods such as treatment with pepsin, trypsin, chymotrypsin, and plasmin or chemical modification of the IgG, but these treatments of immunoglobulins to suppress spontaneous complement activation also had unintended consequences[19]—ie, antibodies were rapidly removed from the circulatory system by the reticuloendothelial system when chemically and physically altered during the manufacturing process.[20] In addition, some antibody preparations that were pepsin- or papain-digested or chemically modified showed reduced bacteria-opsonizing activities.[21-24]

Clearly, new purification techniques had to be developed to obtain unmodified monomeric IgGs in IVIG preparations. Apart from the use of different precipitating agents such as polyethylene glycol (PEG)[25] or octanoic acid, other methods, especially involving chromatography, were successfully established starting from plasma itself or from intermediates derived via

Cohn, Oncley, or Kistler and Nitschmann processes.[12,26,27] Polson et al initially published a report showing the feasibility of plasma fractionation by PEG precipitation.[25] Later, Steinbuch and Audran[28] and Audran et al[29] described the use of caprylic acid precipitation for the purification of IgG. Hoppe et al[30] were among the first groups to publish a chromatographic process suitable for industrial-scale production. Further processes were developed that combined some of these methods and provided functional, fully intact products with IgG of a subclass distribution similar to that of plasma.[31] Suomela as well as Falksveden presented ion exchange chromatographic processes for the isolation of IgG.[32,33] Falksveden combined cation and anion exchange chromatography after pretreatment with PEG, and Suomela introduced an affinity chromatographic step to remove proteolytic activities and further improve the quality of the final preparation. The requirements for IgG preparations designed for IV administration, in terms of low anticomplementary activity, aggregate content, and improved stability, were better fulfilled by the implementation of these methods.

In addition, alternative precipitating agents (eg, PEG) have been used, starting with Cohn intermediate fractions for the production of gammaglobulin preparations.[34,35] Gamimune-N (Bayer, Leverkusen, Germany) and Intragam (CSL Limited, Broadmeadows, Australia) are products manufactured with an anion chromatography step, preceded by precipitation and filtration processes, and are examples of the successful implementation of such methods in routine production. In 1991, Sarno presented a method to produce IgG starting from the cold ethanol fraction I+II+III treated with PEG and solvent/detergent (S/D), then further purified with cation exchange chromatography, followed by polishing with an anion exchange resin.[36] Gammagard S/D (Baxter, Deerfield, IL) is another example of an IVIG product manufactured in a similar manner. A more recent US patent by Kothe et al describes a process for yielding an immunoglobulin preparation for IV administration that uses octanoic acid precipitation, which eliminates proteolytic activities and vasoactive substances, in combination with anion or cation exchange or hydrophobic interaction chromatography.[37]

Prevention of Virus Transmission

Because of the large number of plasma blood donations required to produce a single immunoglobulin lot, a key aspect in the development of IV products has been the prevention of virus transmission. Nevertheless, an unfortunate series of hepatitis C virus (HCV) infections transmitted by IVIG occurred before donors were regularly screened for antibodies to HCV.[38,39] Also, a number of immunoglobulin lots had to be withdrawn from the market because of the presumed risk of transmitting Creutzfeldt-Jakob disease (CJD) associated with some plasma donors.[31] A strategy that relies on three pillars is used, as for all plasma products, to ensure high margins of safety with respect to transmission of viruses and prions (see Fig 2-1).

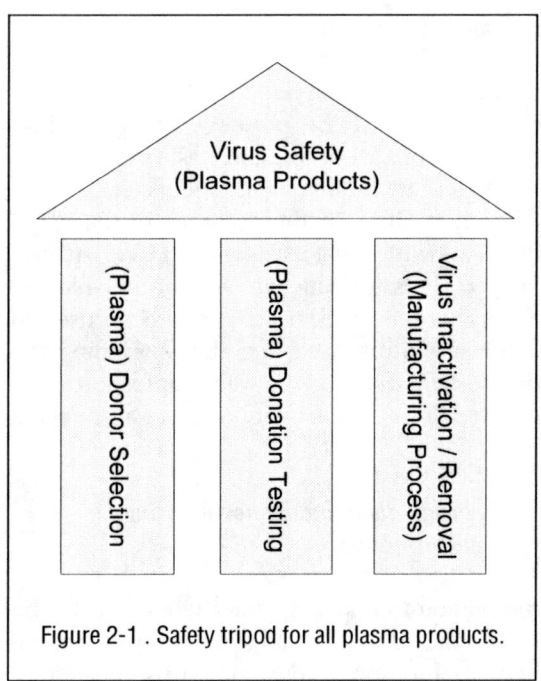

Figure 2-1. Safety tripod for all plasma products.

Donor Selection

To reduce the risk of disease transmission, donors are required to complete a detailed questionnaire that can be used to assess their risk profiles. For viruses, some questions address certain higher-risk behavior; for variant CJD (vCJD), others address residency and medical history. Plasma collected in the United Kingdom and donations from people who have lived in the United Kingdom for more than 3 months between 1980 and 1996 or who have received blood transfusions in the United Kingdom cannot be used for fractionation in the United States.

A large proportion of plasma is collected from plasmapheresis donors who receive monetary compensation. In accordance with industry standards, plasmapheresis plasma is accepted only from repeat donors, a group which has historically showed lower incidence rates of virus transmission than first-time donors.[40] According to a position statement of the European Union (EU) regulatory agency, "there is no evidence...that donor remuneration increases the risk of viral transmission via plasma-derived medicinal products."[41]

Testing of Donor Plasma

Donor plasma is screened for surrogate markers indicative of the presence of agents that cause various diseases, such as virus-induced antibodies to human immunodeficiency virus (HIV) and HCV, or the presence of the agent itself, as with hepatitis B virus (HBV) surface antigen (HBsAg). Since 1994, the polymerase chain reaction (PCR) test has also been used to detect the virus itself, thereby shortening the diagnostic window between infection and occurrence of specific antibodies in an infected host.

Virus Inactivation and Removal during the Manufacturing Process

In addition to selecting ethically motivated and lower-risk donors and screening donated plasma for indications of virus infections, numerous methods for the inactivation or removal of any residual viruses are increasingly being developed and integrated into the manufacturing processes of immunoglobulins. The Cohn-Oncley cold ethanol fractionation itself is already an effective method for virus removal and inactivation.[31] Further state-of-the art virus inactivation or removal steps integrated into the purification processes include the use of chemical agents as, for instance, during S/D treatment[42]; harsh physical conditions, such as low pH (Gamimune-N) or high temperature during pasteurization[43]; and the removal of viruses by digestion with proteases or by exploiting the difference in size between viruses and the target protein, as, for example, with nanofiltration.[44]

Beyond this state of affairs, the discovery of new viruses and increasing quality requirements for plasma products have led to the development of production processes with a growing number of virus reduction steps.[17] Whereas earlier purification schemes made use of only a single virus-inactivation or -removal step, state-of-the-art manufacturing schemes include at least two steps, both effective against lipid-enveloped viruses and at least one of them effective also against nonenveloped viruses. For instance, Hirao et al have patented a process for the purification of an immunoglobulin preparation using heat treatment (pasteurization), low pH incubation, and optional size exclusion (nanofiltration) as virus removal or inactivation steps.[45] Similarly, Baxter developed an IVIG[46] with S/D treatment, nanofiltration, and low-pH treatment [Gammagard Liquid (US brand name) or KIOVIG (brand name outside the United States)], and Grifols (Barcelona, Spain; formerly Mitsubishi) developed an IVIG (Flebogamma DIF) with pasteurization, S/D treatment, and nanofiltration as dedicated virus-inactivation/removal steps.

Product Overview

Commercial products are available as freeze-dried or liquid IgG preparations, and the past few years have seen a general transition from lyophilized to liquid products, which are more convenient for customers because they do not have to be dissolved before administration. Immunoglobulin preparations on the market contain sugars, amino acids, albumin, or other agents that function as stabilizers. Clinical implications have been reported for some of these agents—eg, for sucrose.[47] The formulation of an immunoglobulin preparation is primarily directed at maintaining the stability of the active ingredient over a prolonged storage period, which thus also determines the shelf-life of the product. Usually, the preparations are stable for longer periods when kept refrigerated.[48]

A variety of products can be purchased in the United States and Europe. Examples of lyophilized products are Gammagard SD, a neutral, low-IgA immunoglobulin preparation, and Carimmune NF (formerly Sandoglobulin; CSL Behring AG, Bern, Switzerland), a sugar-free, pH-neutral immunoglobulin preparation. Tenold, from Cutter laboratories and Green Cross Corporation, filed US patents in 1981 and 1988, respectively, that described the first attempts to formulate safe and stable liquid IgG products for IV administration.[49,50] Gamimune-N is the 10% liquid, sugar-free, low-pH preparation related to Tenold's patent, and Venoglobulin (Grifols) was developed from the Green Cross patent. Venoglobulin is a lyophilized product that has been upgraded to liquid formulations and is stabilized with D-sorbitol. It is claimed to be stable even at room temperature, unlike Gamimune-N.

A growing number of suppliers are now shifting their production toward liquid products (See Chapter 1, Table 1-1). Grifols, initially a European company, distributed Alphaglobin in a 5% liquid formulation stabilized with sorbitol. Alphaglobin was then followed by Flebogamma 5%, which was more recently upgraded to Flebogamma 5% (or 10%) DIF, stabilized with D-sorbitol at a pH around 5 to 6 (by Grifols USA, Los Angeles, CA). Other examples are the 5% liquid product Octagam (Octapharma, Vienna, Austria), supplemented with maltose, and Baxter's Gammagard Liquid/KIOVIG. Gammagard Liquid was the first 10% liquid IV product that offered triple dedicated virus inactivation/reduction. Additional licensed products in the United States are the IVIG (human) 10% preparations by CSL Behring AG and by Talecris Biotherapeutics (Research Triangle Park, NC; previously Bayer), whose products are caprylate/chromatography purified (IVIG-C or IGIV-C). Most of the IVIGs are provided by global member companies of the Plasma Protein Therapeutics Association (PPTA, a consortium of leading manufacturers of plasma products)—ie, Baxter BioScience, Biotest Pharmaceuticals, CSL Behring, Grifols, Kedrion, Octapharma, and Talecris Biotherapeutics. A complete list of licensed products and establishments is provided on the Web site of the US Food and Drug Administration (FDA).[51] In Europe, German hospital pharmacists published a summary of IVIG products based on information provided in package inserts and product monographs.[52]

CSL Behring (King of Prussia, PA) recently launched Privigen, which is claimed to be a well-tolerated and effective 10% liquid IVIG, formulated with 0.25 M L-proline that is stable at room temperature for its entire 24-month shelf-life.[48,53]

IVIG Development Strategy

In the development of an IVIG product, specific regulatory requirements must be considered for preclinical investigations and clinical studies. This section first addresses tolerability, formulation, process efficiency, and market supply at a basic level before discussing specific regulatory requirements for product quality.

Requirements for an IVIG Product

Apart from maintaining unquestionable margins of virus safety and strategic fit with manufacturing management, the following additional prerequisites must be considered.

Tolerability

A major requirement for a new IV product is that it is tolerated by patients. IVIG products are indicated as the treatment of choice in a number of immune-mediated disorders, including inflammatory and autoimmune diseases, and are generally well tolerated.[14,31] IV infusions have been found to restore physiologic immunoglobulin blood levels, cause fewer side effects, and require fewer injections than intramuscular infusions.[14] However, tolerance to a given IVIG product does not necessarily predict the same level of comfort with a similar upgraded product. Purification methods and virus inactivation procedures may alter the integrity of the IgG molecule and, hence, its biologic activity as well as the amount and composition of trace proteins, all of which affect tolerability of the product. Although a wide variety of tests are applied to characterize the final product during the development phase, the possibility of alterations that impact tolerability cannot be excluded. For example, Ameratunga et al[54] reported an increased risk of adverse events after the manufacturing process of Intragam had been upgraded. Chromatography purification steps had been added to the Cohn fractionation process to reduce the amount of aggregates and, as another benefit, the amount of residual IgA was lowered. Furthermore, the new Intragam P has been found to have a superior virus inactivation profile compared with that of its predecessor. No major adverse events have been reported in an open label study, resulting in the transition to the new product. Nevertheless, Ameratunga et al found significant side effects such as serum sickness during the first injections. The cause of the increased rate of side effects was not clear and no batch-related problems were found. Consequently, they emphasized that first-time users switching from old to new products should be monitored closely. It is also important that changes in manufacturing processes be reported extensively to prescribing physicians so that precautions can be taken.

Formulation

Customer convenience is a major concern when formulating a new product. Ready-to-use liquid formulations and room-temperature storage are favored. Although, in the last decade, IV preparations were the main focus, lately there appears to be a growing interest in subcutaneous products. Patients report a preference for the higher flexibility, linking it with greater independence because of the possibility of home-care treatment, less emotional stress, and less time involved in administration.[15] Patients who have problems with IV infusions (eg, poor venous access), side effects, or rapid IgG catabolism also prefer to receive subcutaneous administration. However, self-administration by patients must be addressed carefully because the patient must be able to achieve a high compliance level and be ready to accept responsibility. In Scandinavia, a 16.5% subcutaneous product was found to have good tolerability and to be preferred over an IV product by most patients. Until recently in the US, no such product was on the market, but a study (Stiehm et al[55]) in which three commercially available 10% IVIG products were used (Gamimune N, Gammagard, Venoglobulin S) found that the eight patients enrolled suffered from, for example, poor venous access or mild side effects after IV treatment. The peak serum level that is usual after 4 days of IV infusion was not observed. Patients with a rapid IgG catabolism profited from the slow release from the injection site.[55] With this new administration form, patients who had issues with IV infusion again had access to a safe and effective therapy. Currently, Baxter and CSL are planning on launching 20% IgG products for subcutaneous use to the market for maximal customer convenience.

Process Efficiency and Market Supply

Yield is an important factor when developing a new manufacturing process for immunoglobulins, not only for the manufacturer but also for market supply. For example, in 1998 two factors were considered responsible for a shortage of IVIG product in the United States: lack of compliance with good manufacturing practice (GMP) and withdrawal of some lots because of the assumption of a possible transmission of CJD.[31] Today, the demand for immunoglobulins is booming, with new indications for IVIG such as applications in autoimmune diseases, particularly in the field of hematology and neurology,[56] and the successful exploration of other potential fields. However, plasma products are derived from a limited source material, and regulatory requirements for their production are complex, resulting in high manufacturing costs. In an audit of hospitals to demonstrate the value of immunoglobulin therapy and gain a better understanding of where and which immunoglobulins are used in clinical practice, it was concluded that the use of immunoglobulins was well justified, and far more patients could benefit from this therapy if it were used to a greater extent.[56]

Regulatory Quality Requirements

The requirements for a polyclonal immunoglobulin product are specified in the US Pharmacopoeia (USP), the European Pharmacopoeia (EP), and guidelines provided by the European Medicines Agency (EMA). The specific monographs of the pharmacopoeias regulate the minimal standard of purity and sterility of the final immunoglobulin dose that each lot must fulfill. In addition, products with a low IgA content, defined subclass distribution, or hyperimmune immunoglobulins that contain high antibody titers against one specific entity (eg, tetanus or cytomegalovirus) have to meet the licensed target approved for them by the relevant regulatory authorities. These regulations ensure that the batches released for sale meet specifications and guarantee maximal safety for the patients.

The USP monograph "Immune Globulin" (USP 32-NF 27) states that an IgG preparation must meet the FDA regulations but describes only a product for subcutaneous or intramuscular administration. The product discussed is defined as a sterile, nonpyrogenic solution containing antibodies derived from human plasma. This human plasma can be obtained from blood, plasma, serum, or placentas from not less than 1000 donors. The protein concentration of this product should be at least 96% gammaglobulins and stabilized with 0.3 M glycine at pH 6.8 ±0.4. Furthermore, the product must be heat stable, and the pH must be verified. Potency tests concerning specific antibodies are also defined (ie, antibodies for diphtheria antitoxin, measles, and polio virus).

According to the EP monograph, steps to remove or inactivate known agents of infections are a prerequisite for production. Residues of added substrates that inactivate these agents should not provoke any adverse events in the patients.

The final product has to comply with the following tests:
- Solubility.
- pH: between 4.0 and 7.4.
- Osmolality: minimum = 240 m Osmol/kg.
- Total protein: minimum = 30 g/L and between 90% and 110% of the protein quantity stated on the label.
- Protein composition (by zone electrophoresis).
- Molecular size distribution: monomer and dimer peak >90% of the total area; polymers and aggregates <3% of the total area of chromatogram.
- Anticomplementary activity: consumption of complement ≤50%.
- Prekallikrein activator: maximum = 35 IU/mL.
- Anti-A and anti-B hemagglutinins, anti-D, and anti-HBsAg: minimum = 0.5 IU/g of immunoglobulin.
- Water.
- Sterility.
- Test of pyrogens.
- IgA (the amount has been regulated since January 2009): content must not be greater than the maximal content stated on the label.

Product specification information should include the exact amount of immunoglobulin in mg and the purity as a percentage; the route of administration; and, where applicable, the amount of albumin added as stabilizer. The distribution of the IgG subclasses must be mentioned as well as the maximum IgA content, which is very important for IgA-deficient patients.

The liquid form for IVIG should be clear or slightly opalescent and colorless to pale yellow. In contrast, the liquid preparation for subcutaneous or intramuscular administration should be clear and colorless to pale yellow or light brown and might contain a small amount of particulate matter, which could have been formed during storage.

Preclinical Investigations and Clinical Studies

Apart from those described above, another requirement is to demonstrate that the product is well tolerated regardless of the route of administration. This is accomplished by suitable animal tests and evaluation during clinical trials. Tests for the following characteristics must be conducted in specified animal models:
- Efficacy (eg, by the protective activity test in mice).
- Pharmacokinetics (eg, in rats or dogs).
- Acute toxicity (eg, in mice or rats).
- Safety (eg, by the Wessler test in rabbits evaluating the thrombogenic potential).
- Hypertensive activity in rats.

The immunoglobulin preparation must be shown through clinical trials to be safe and effective in humans for specific indications (eg, primary immune deficiency, ITP). A further requirement is proof of stability. The stability requirements are summarized in the International Conference on Harmonization guidelines provided by the EMA.[57]

Manufacturing Process

The manufacturing process should be designed, operated, and continuously documented under the regulations for GMP.[58] The minimal requirements of the manufacturing method include the following:
- At least two different antibodies should be concentrated by threefold from the source material with no effect on the integrity of the globulins.
- The process should be sufficiently robust to yield a product that is safe for injection.
- The product should be free from transmissible viral hepatitis.

Development Essentials

Development starts usually on a small scale by exploring various possibilities to improve the process and the product. From the beginning, attention should be given to establishing a robust process by which final products can meet the specification requirements. Small-scale equipment should be chosen that allows upscaling.

Next, the results from small-scale experiments must be confirmed with regard to process scalability and robustness on the larger scale. If these results are comparable to the bench scale, the next step is the production of preclinical lots to provide material for studies in animals. Stability studies on 1) stress and accelerated testing and 2) formulation are performed even on experimental batches.

Finally, the shift to large-scale manufacturing in the GMP environment can be conducted to provide material for clinical studies in humans. At this stage, ongoing stability testing is required. Process changes after clinical lot production should be avoided or at least reduced to a minimum; otherwise, further information must be presented to the regulatory authorities regarding the effect of the changes on the product.

The last step, before the product can be launched and the final data submitted to the authorities, is to demonstrate proof of reproducibility in full manufacturing scale.

Fractionation and Purification Methods

Anderson and Anderson estimated in 2002 that there are about 500 different plasma proteins.[59] Purification of these proteins using various separation techniques is based on their different physical and chemical properties, such as their ampholytic character, isoelectric point, and molecular mass. Regardless of the method, precipitation of a protein is favored near or at its isoelectric point, and large proteins tend to precipitate first with less precipitating agent.

Technical problems of plasma fractionation have been outlined in detail by Schultze and Heremans.[60] The removal of lipoproteins and proteolyic enzymes are important challenges for the fractionation process. Human plasma contains about 8% lipoproteins, which tend to accumulate on interfaces during purification. Furthermore, enzymes may be linked to lipoproteins, which can damage the protein of interest.[60] It is favorable to remove and/or reduce lipoproteins before chromatography steps. For this purpose, adsorbents with a large surface area, such as glass powder, bentonite, or fumed silica, are used. Activation of inactive precursors of proteolytic enzymes present in the fractions can also occur under precipitating conditions or in the presence of adsorbing agents. Citrate or EDTA are used as chelating agents to remove the metal ions acting as cofactors of enzymes.

Other factors influencing the fractionation process are pH, ionic composition, ionic strength, protein concentration, and temperature.

Precipitation with Inorganic Salts

Since Hofmeister published his observations concerning the effects of various salts on protein solubility,[61] the principles of the chosmotropic effect of inorganic salts on protein precipitation have been investigated and the basic mechanism well established, mainly by Timasheff and Fasman[62] and Arakawa and Timasheff.[63,64] They found that precipitating salts are hydrated by withdrawing water from the surface of proteins so that proteins are forced to share their hydration shells. As a result of the increased demand for solvent molecules, the protein-protein interactions are stronger than the solvent-solute interactions, and the protein precipitates. This process is known as salting out. The differences among the ions were explained by their different interactions with the surface of the protein molecules. The ions called chosmotropic are strongly excluded from protein surfaces, stabilize the structure of proteins, and favor protein precipitation in higher concentrations. The ions called chaotropic are able to penetrate the hydration shells of the protein surface, unfold proteins, destabilize hydrophobic aggregates, and increase the solubility of hydrophobes. Ammonium sulphate was previously used commonly for this precipitation technique but was abandoned because of its toxicity and the advantages of other precipitation agents.

Precipitation by Removal of Electrolytes

This technique, also known as "euglobulin" precipitation, had already been investigated in the 19th century and was characterized by the precipitation of proteins through enhancement of protein-protein interaction by the removal of ions.[65] IgM is one of the first to precipitate in an environment with low ionic strength because of its low solubility. As a side effect, other proteins, especially IgG, are lost when coprecipitating with these aggregates.

Precipitation by Polyethylene Glycol

The mechanism of this purification technique is the exclusion of solvent molecules by the polymer, thereby decreasing the solubility of the protein.[66] PEG precipitation combined with other separation techniques was used to prepare an IgG fraction enriched with IgA and IgM and, therefore, enhanced in antibodies to bacteria.[29] PEG is still in use in plasma fractionation, for instance for the removal of aggregates from IVIG intermediates,[67] because it is considered nontoxic and allows precipitation at room temperature.

Precipitation with Fatty Acids

In 1960, Chanutin and Curnish reported precipitation of plasma proteins by short chain (C_6-C_{12}) fatty acids at pH 4.2.[68] Differences were detected in the precipitating capacities of these acids—eg, caprylic acid precipitates gamma-globulin less than alpha and beta globulins at optimal pH conditions (between 4.8 and 5.0). With Steinbuch's method (1980), an IgG purity of 90% and high yield were obtained with one precipitation step under optimal pH, salt, protein, and reagent concentrations.[69] Octanoate and heptanoate treatments at pH 4.6 to 4.95 are used by Octapharma in purifying II+III paste.[70,71] The use of caprylate (octanoate) is employed by Talecris.[72] All these methodologies were based on publications by McKinney and Parkinson,[73] Perosa et al,[74] and Reik et al.[75]

Precipitation with Ethanol

Addition of organic solvents reduces the dielectrical constant of the solution.[26] The most critical variables in precipitation with organic solvents are temperature, organic solvent concentration, pH, ionic strength, protein concentration, and the molecular mass of the target protein. This method is often combined with precipitation using inorganic salts. Ethanol is the agent of choice.

Ethanol causes protein precipitation mainly because it significantly lowers the dielectric constant of the aqueous solution. The different precipitation steps have to be performed at temperatures below 0 C to avoid protein denaturation. Precipitation of proteins with increasing amounts of ethanol at temperatures below 0 C inhibits bacterial growth and, thus, the formation of pyrogenic substances as a further benefit.

In addition to ethanol's already mentioned low dielectric constant, it is miscible with water; lowers the freezing temperature of the solution; has high volatility, which can be used to redistill the ethanol from waste supernatants of the Cohn process (eg, fraction II supernatant and fraction V supernatant); is low in toxicity; is chemically relatively inert; and does not form explosive gas mixtures under ambient working conditions. Ethanol is also inexpensive and easily available.

Cohn and his coworkers established a system of five variables for the separation of plasma proteins based on pH, conductivity, ethanol concentration, temperature, and protein concentration.[1,12] Separation can be carried out in either of two ways: 1) conditions are selected to maximize the solubility of the protein of interest and minimize the solubility of the others, thereby precipitating them out, or 2) the desired protein is precipitated selectively.[76] The Cohn separation methods result in five main precipitates. Fraction I, which consists mainly of fibrinogen, is obtained by using either plasma or cryosupernatant after separation of cryoprecipitate and/or after carrying out adsorption of blood coagulation factors and inhibitors (as, for example, described for the Baxter product Gammagard Liquid/KIOVIG), adding 8% alcohol, and adjusting the temperature to approximately −2 C. Fraction II consists of mainly IgG purified out of fractionation II+III paste, which is generated by separating raw immunoglobulin and raw albumin. Fraction III is a waste fraction containing lipid-bearing beta globulins and IgA. Fraction IV, consisting of alpha globulins, can be obtained in two steps: fraction IV-1, which is enriched in alpha-1-antitrypsin, and fraction IV-4, which is used for further purification of transferrin or, most recently, butyrylcholinesterase.[77] Fraction V is composed mainly of albumin.

Since Cohn published his Method 6 of plasma fractionation[1] (Fig 2-2), many plasma fractionation companies such as Baxter have developed purification schemes based on this method (with minor changes for II+III precipitate). Further fractionation of the II+III precipitate was found to be critical for IgG yield. Consequently, many different fractionation schemes were developed to increase the IgG yield and/or purity throughout fractionation—eg, from Deutsch et al[76] (Fig 2-3) and Oncley et al[12] (Fig 2-4) to Kistler and Nitschmann[27] (Fig 2-5).

Chromatographic Methods

The production of fraction III in the Cohn method leads to a considerable yield loss in the range of 20%.[78] Most modern purification methods for immunoglobulins from plasma therefore start with II+III paste and apply chromatographic purification methods after resuspending the paste and clarifying the suspension by filtration or centrifugation. The performance of chromatography media in terms of capacity, selectivity, and pressure flow are critical for successful downstream processing. Lifetime, security of supply, and low batch-to-batch variations of the media are of special importance for immunoglobulins from human plasma

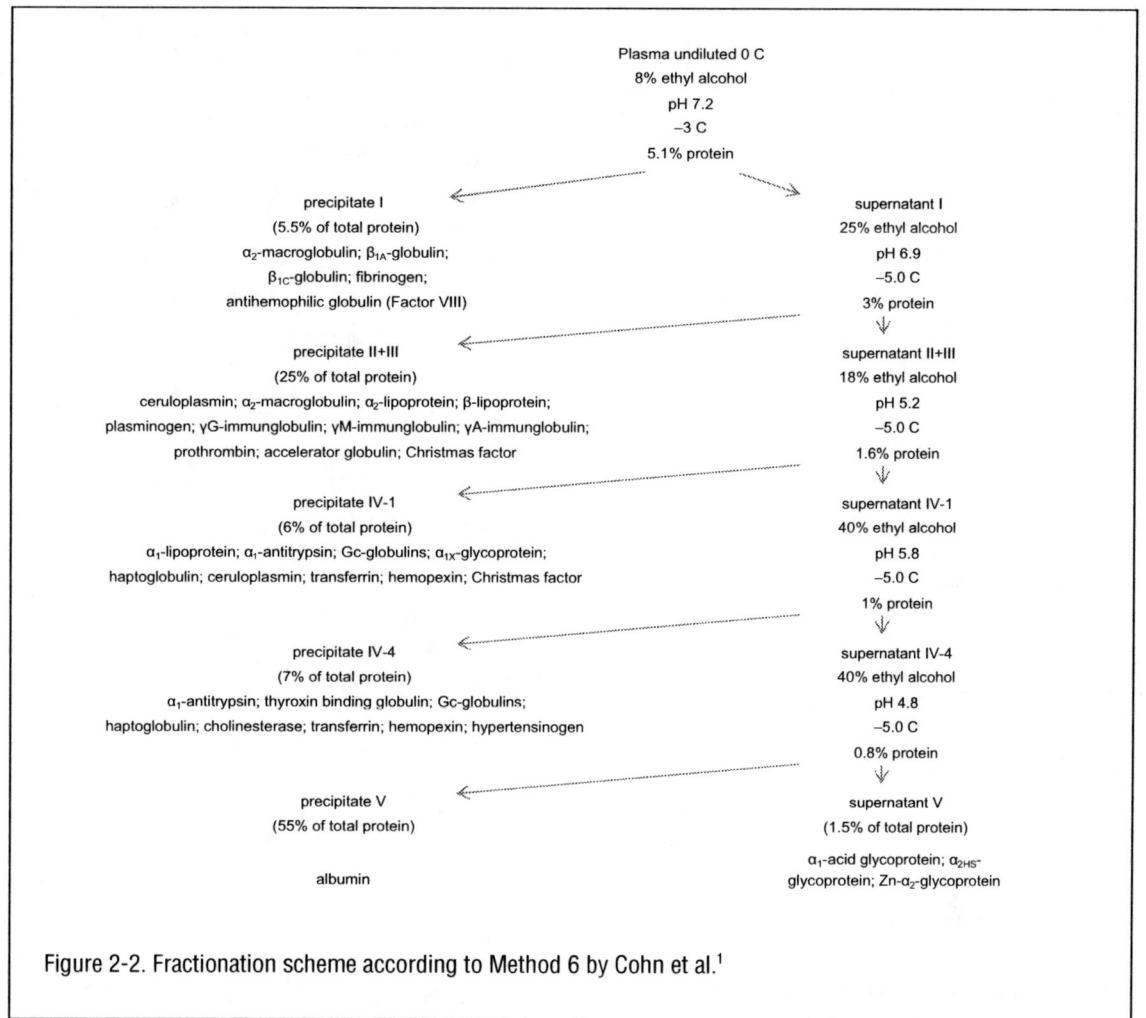

Figure 2-2. Fractionation scheme according to Method 6 by Cohn et al.[1]

because large producers manufacture several tons of this product per year. The chromatography resin consists of a base matrix and the ligand. The base matrix is characterized by particle and pore size. Coarse or medium grade particles are selected, particularly for large-scale manufacturing, because they have less back pressure in large columns. The pore size is selected in a way that the molecule of interest is able to enter the pores and effectively counteract with the ligand. The three different types of base matrices used are 1) inorganic substances such as silica, glass, carbon, or ceramic; 2) synthetic polymers such as polystyrene, acylamide, or metacrylate; and 3) biopolymers such as agarose, cellulose, and dextrane.

In the past, matrices were based mainly on biopolymers. The very first ones, such as Sephadex G (Separation Pharmacia Dextran Gel, GE Healthcare Bio-Sciences, Piscataway, NJ), were introduced 50 years ago.[79] Agarose is a hydrophilic, chemically stable resin with an open pore structure. As a soft gel, it is susceptible to pressure-induced volume changes. To overcome this disadvantage, the agarose was cross-linked to provide more mechanical stability without losing the favorable material properties.[80] This resulted in the development of Sepharose fast-flow resin (GE Healthcare), Ultrogel (Pall Lifesciences, Port Washington, NY) and, most recently, Capto high-flow resin (GE Healthcare). Lately, inorganic and syn-

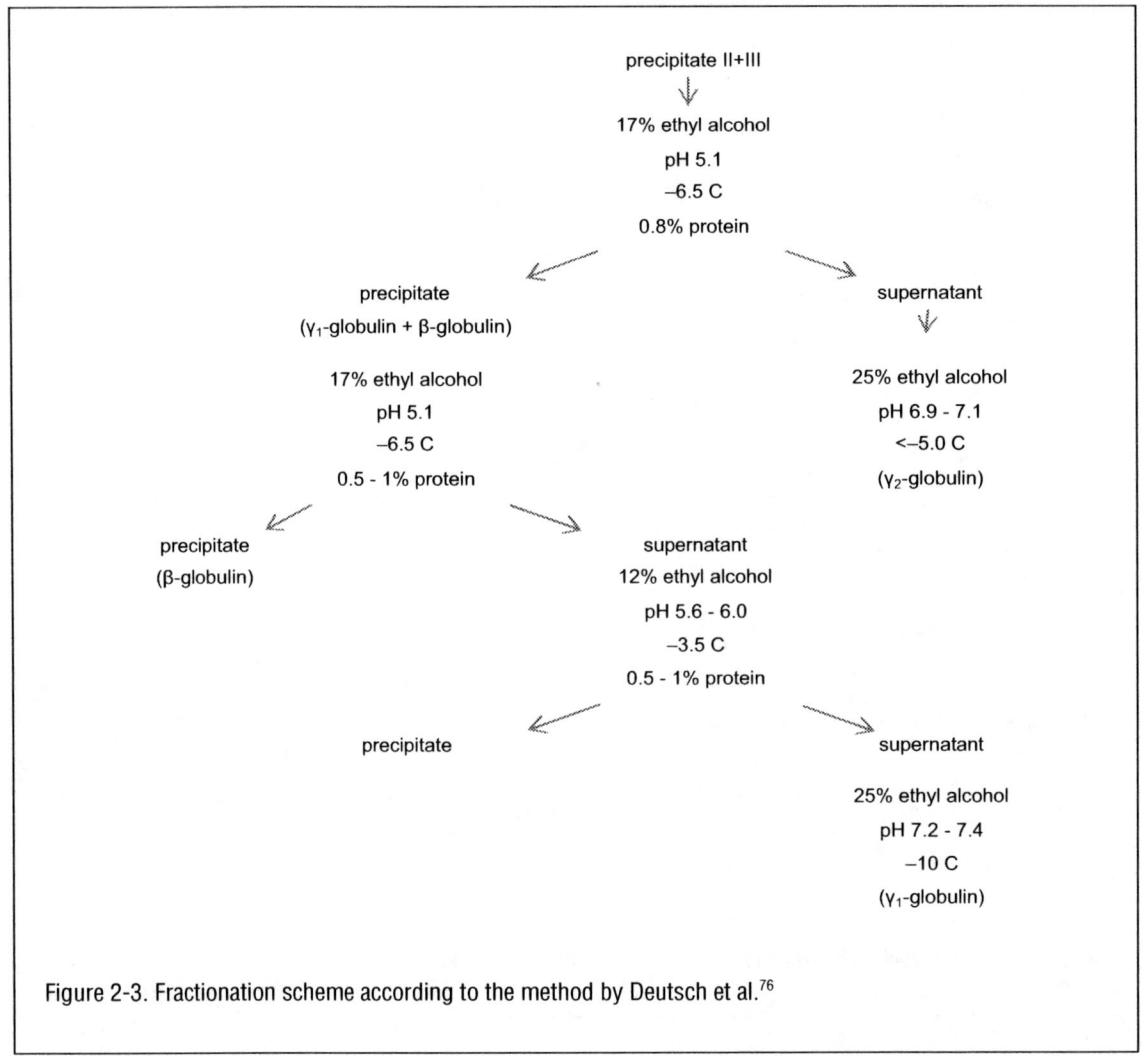

Figure 2-3. Fractionation scheme according to the method by Deutsch et al.[76]

thetic polymers have entered the market. Because they are rigid, noncompressible sorbents, they can be packed easily and provide high dynamic binding capacity at a high-flow rate. Cleaning and depyrogenation are also easily performed with sodium hydroxide because of their caustic stability. Ceramic HyperD sorbents (Pall Corp), which are made using a rigid porous ceramic bead, coated and permeated with a functionalized hydrogel, are one example of these newer resins. The bead provides good rigidity and flow performance as well as high mass transfer and dynamic properties. The complete lack of shrinking or swelling eliminates the need for repacking the columns.

Currently, ion exchange media are the most widely used resins. IgG can be bound easily on weak cation exchange resins such as CM-Sepharose fast-flow, and impurities are washed out. This resin is used, for example, to separate S/D reagents from IgG[17] as well as for reversed phase chromatography.[81] When anion exchange resins are the resin of choice, IgG is found mostly in the flow-through, whereas other proteins, especially IgA and IgM, stick to the resin.[82] By combining cation and anion exchange resins, a purification scheme starting

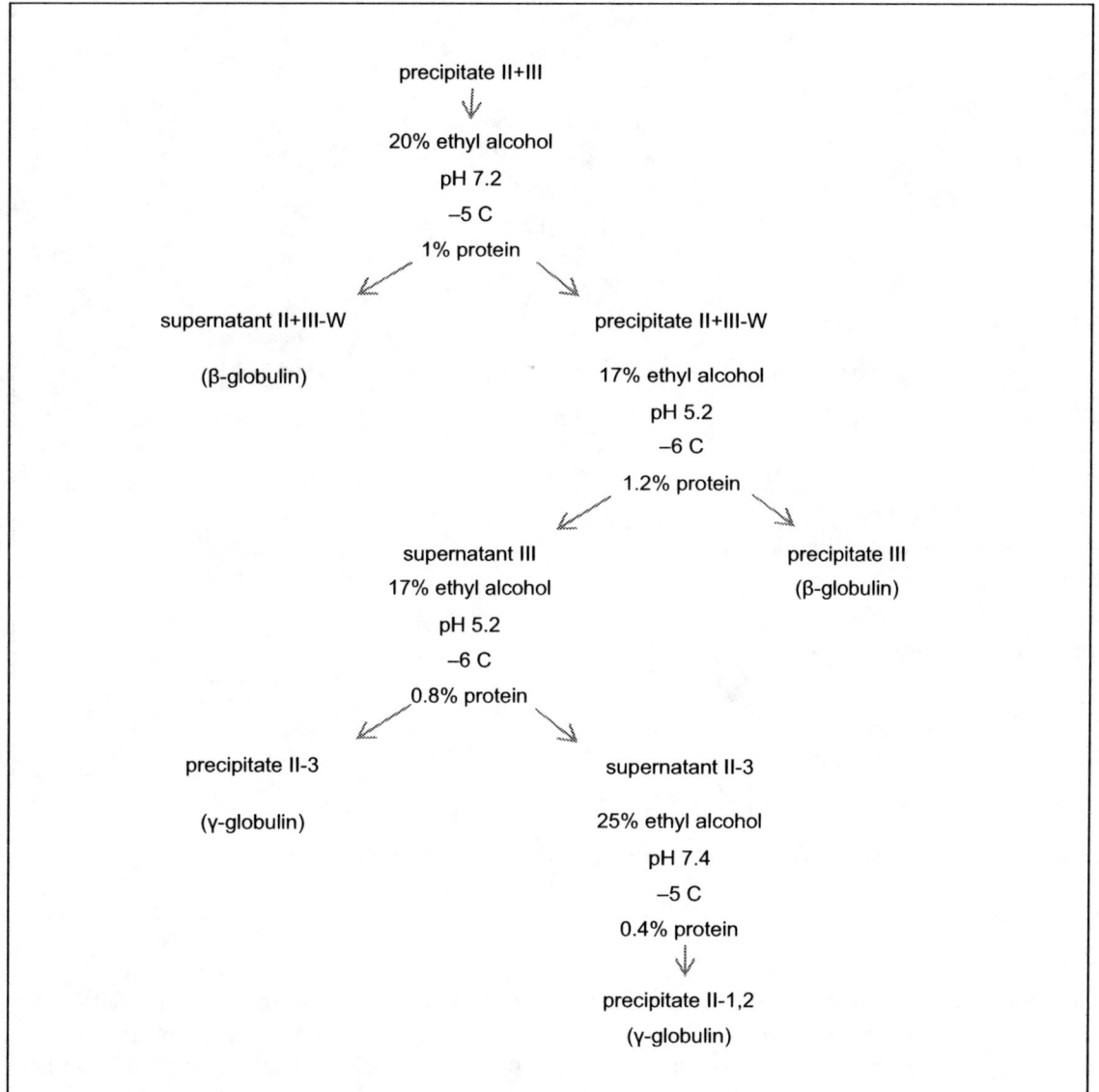

Figure 2-4. Fractionation scheme according to the method by Oncley et al (Method 9),[12] leading to the IgG-enriched fraction II.

from clarified II+III paste can be developed, leading to a product that meets all requirements for an intravenously administrable immunoglobulin product.[17] LFB Biotechnologies (Les Ulis, France) presented a new IgG manufacturing process that includes an anion exchange chromatography step binding IgG in order to remove S/D and separate IgG from other impurities like IgA and IgM by specific elution in a single step. The advantages of conventional ion exchange media over, for example, affinity resins are 1) sanitization with up to one molar sodium hydroxide, 2) reusability, and 3) moderate price.[83]

Some resins carry affinity ligands for IgG binding. For example, protein A and protein G

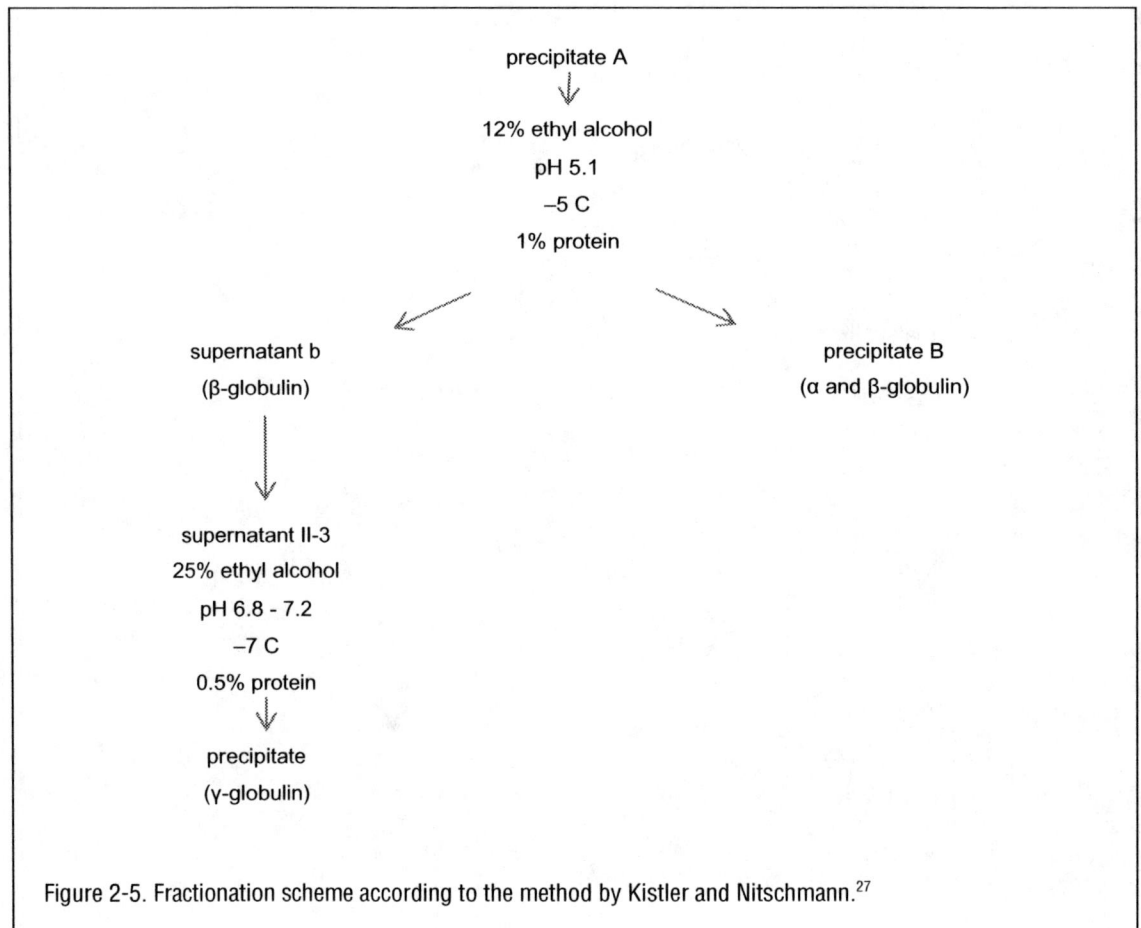

Figure 2-5. Fractionation scheme according to the method by Kistler and Nitschmann.[27]

were the first resins used as a standard capturing media in the purification of monoclonal antibodies. These two ligands have the disadvantage that the IgG has to be eluted at a low pH (below pH 3.5), resulting in protein aggregation and even modification of functionality, including modified peptide-binding properties.[84,85] To overcome this hurdle, an affinity resin using the BAC technology (Bio Affinity Company, BV, Naarden, the Netherlands) was introduced as IgSelect by GE Healthcare.[86] The ligand is a 14-kDa recombinant IgG fragment protein produced in *Saccharomyces cerevisiae* (animal-free production) that should bind all human IgG subclasses. The recombinant protein is bound to the matrix via a long hydrophilic spacer to facilitate the interaction of the IgG for capture from the loading solution and the ligand. Although this resin has a high potential to capture IgG from crude suspensions, the disadvantage of its low binding capacity, possible ligand leakage, and lack of stability against sodium hydroxide will limit its use in plasma fractionation. Affinity chromatography thus has a number of limitations but is nevertheless widely used for the production of recombinant antibodies.[83]

Multimodal and advanced affinity ligands are more recent developments. Multimodal chromatography combines more than one type of interaction with the protein from the range of ionic and hydrophobic interaction, hydrogen bonding, or thiophilic interaction. One example of a replacement for proteins A and G is the mixed-mode chromatography resin 4-MEP (4-mercapto-ethyl-pyridine) HyperCel resin (Pall Corp), which is a sorbent designed for purifying antibodies, especially from cell-culture supernatants. 4-MEP is a synthetic, stable immunoglobulin-selective ligand that binds antibodies from all species and of all isotypes. Thus, 4-MEP offers an alternative to proteins A and G for purifying recombinant antibodies and Fc fusion proteins.[78] Additionally, antibody elution from 4-MEP HyperCel is milder than typically used for proteins A and G, and there is no concern about the downstream effect of leached protein A in the final product. This chemistry is also useful for hydrophobic interaction chromatography, a hydrophobic mode without organic solvents that is much more likely to retain native structure than traditional reverse-phase chromatography. GE Healthcare's CaptoAdhere, which was designed for polishing in the purification process of antibodies (after which, the IgG is nearly 100% pure), is another example of a multimodal chromatography resin. The Danish company Upfront Chromatography A/S (Copenhagen) combines this chromatography feature with expanded bed chromatography and an IgG binding gel that can be sanitized with one molar sodium hydroxide at 60 C. The method offers the advantage that an unclarified suspension can be applied to the column.[87] Prometic (Mount-Royal, QC, Canada) has developed the "cascade" technology, which is able to separate seven major plasma proteins, one of them IgG, by the use of a series of columns with different synthetic affinity ligands.[88]

Membrane chromatography is another option for reducing small amounts of unwanted proteins from IgG preparations. These membranes are easy to use, provide good batch-to-batch reproducibility and are for single use, obviating labor-intensive and costly cleaning procedures. They are also able to remove viruses. The disadvantages of membrane-based chromatography are that it is suitable only for removing trace impurities and it is expensive.

The ultrafiltration and diafiltration technique is widely used for the concentration and the final formulation of the IgG bulk. A new method called "Gradiflow" technology, using membranes in an electrical field, has been described for small-scale purification.[89] The future will show if this technology will be scalable to the plasma fractionation scale.

Pathogens and IVIG Safety

High margins of safety with respect to *any* pathogen are a basic requirement and expected for all biological pharmaceutical drugs. Although the threat of microorganisms the size of bacteria or larger is well defended against by 1) microbiologic controls in the manufacturing process, 2) a GMP environment, which reduces the risk of pathogens entering the manufacturing process, and 3) sterile filtration steps. Two classes of smaller pathogens need special consideration: viruses and prions. Because the characteristics of viruses and prions are substantially different, this section focuses on viruses and prions separately.

Introduction to Virus-Related Safety Issues

Plasma donors may carry viruses unknowingly. For example, the US Centers for Disease Control and Prevention (CDC) estimate that approximately 25% of all people infected with HIV in the United States are not aware that they carry the virus. A donation with undetected viremia would be mixed with many others in a plasma pool and could potentially affect a vast number of products derived from that pool.

During the HIV crisis in the 1980s when some plasma-derived blood clotting factors transmitted the virus to patients with hemophilia, the medical community and the general public became aware (again) that insufficient virus inactivation or removal in the manufacturing process of plasma products can lead to their contamination. At that time, effective virus inactivation and removal methods for clotting factors were still undergoing development, which was complicated by the sensitive nature of these proteins. Nevertheless, the HIV crisis lead to increased efforts, and effective virus reduction technologies were eventually devised and implemented for all plasma products—a development process that continued well into the 1990s.

Implementation of additional manufacturing steps dedicated to virus inactivation or removal, especially the S/D treatment, led to high overall safety margins for IVIGs, where the ethanol fractionation process and other steps such as low-pH treatment had already provided for substantial virus reduction. These additions prevented further transmissions.

Virtually no transmissions of infectious viruses by plasma products have been observed in recent years. Testing is limited to selected known entities and cannot cover emerging viruses until licensed test kits are available. [For the history of West Nile virus (WNV) transmission by blood and transplants, see Alter.[90]] In addition, every approach that relies on testing has a limit of detection, and even an undetectable presence might cause infection and disease.

Regulatory Guidelines

Whereas the US FDA prefers to assess the safety of plasma products relating to viruses on a case-by-case basis, the EMA has issued specific guidelines for the European Union on virus safety requirements for plasma products and related topics. The latest EMA guideline[91] is (at the time of writing) available as a "draft for consultation," with only minor changes expected before the final version comes into effect. Overall, the US and EU interpretations of virus safety requirements for new products are relatively similar.

The World Health Organization (WHO) guidelines[92] are broadly consistent with the EMA guidelines and provide a detailed overview of existing virus inactivation and removal technologies. Because WHO does not regulate pharmaceuticals, its guidance is not binding unless cited by a national agency.

Most countries outside the United States and the European Union have requirements similar to the US and EU requirements, with some preference seen for the EU guidelines because of their explicit wording; some countries (eg, Australia) have largely adopted the respective EU guidelines, with minor modifications where deemed necessary.

Plasma Safety: The Donor and the Donation

Quantitatively, the three pillars of the "safety tripod" described earlier (Fig 2-1) do not contribute equally to virus safety. With respect to purpose, the donor selection and donation testing pillars ensure that the potential virus load in the starting material is reduced as far as possible before the start of the manufacturing process, whereas the virus inactivation or removal steps of the manufacturing process provide by far the largest contribution to overall safety margins.

Donor-Related Measures

Specific national and regional requirements apply for the acceptance of donor applicants.[93-95] Their common denominator is a physical examination and assessment of the applicant's medical history and lifestyle-related risks (including, but not limited to, sexual behavior and drug abuse) by a qualified health professional. Two topics have arisen repeatedly in donor-related discussions of safety from viruses: donor nationality and paid vs unpaid donors.

Discussions on the safety of blood and plasma products have widespread relevance, and are often emotional. Moreover, there seems to be a significant bias that products from domestic sources are "safer," and this sentiment is sometimes echoed in the medical community. For example, in December 2006, the Australian Medical Association urged its government to "…protect patients' safety by disallowing overseas tenders for Australia's blood products supply."[96] Another example is the specification in US regulations that plasma products sold in the United States must be made from US plasma only. Although the European Union accepts non-EU plasma products (eg, from the United States), EU regulations stress repeatedly that (European) community self-sufficiency in this area should be promoted. These expressions about the superior safety of domestic-source plasma products are not necessarily logical or consistent, but they do hint at certain uneasiness over the safety margins of blood and plasma products.

Currently, the only industrialized country that *discourages* the use of domestic-source plasma products for safety reasons is the United Kingdom, where, as a result of the bovine spongiform encephalopathy (BSE) crisis in the 1980s and 1990s, virtually all potential plasma donors carry a very small but not negligible risk of harboring vCJD (see section on prions later this chapter).

Perhaps more importantly, domestic-source plasma has the obvious benefit for IVIGs of providing antibodies against domestic pathogens; these antibodies might be absent in imported plasma. This benefit was demonstrated with antibodies that neutralized WNV in a comprehensive study of >30 lots of IVIGs from US plasma.[97]

Plasma for fractionation can be obtained either from whole blood donations (also called *recovered* plasma and typically collected from unpaid donors by hospitals or the Red Cross organizations) or by plasmapheresis (also called *source* plasma; the donor donates only the plasma and is reinfused with the cellular blood components), where donors are often remunerated for their time and effort. Donor remuneration has been a major issue in some jurisdictions.

Although indeed a somewhat higher disease-marker rate has been found in paid donors arriving for their first donation,[98] this difference itself is not alarming. Moreover, responsible fractionators have additional selection procedures for plasma that ensures supply with a residual risk *equivalent* to that from unpaid donors—by using only *repeat* donations from remunerated donors. (Repeat donors generally have a lower risk as demonstrated by Dodd et al.[99])

The PPTA has further improved the safety of plasma from paid donors by voluntary standards included in their International Quality Plasma Program (IQPP). IQPP requires, among other measures, that disease-marker rates of plasma centers are monitored and maintained at low levels.

In the new EMA guideline,[91] the safety differential between plasma from unpaid vs paid donors is considered from both perspectives (ie, remuneration as relevant vs irrelevant). EU member states are requested to "encourage the voluntary unpaid donation of blood and plasma" but acknowledge that "both nonremunerated and remunerated donors contribute to the supply of safe plasma-derived medicinal products."

Donation-Related Measures

Guidelines require that each individual donation is tested for antibodies against HIV-1, HIV-2 and HCV and for HBsAg.[93,100,101] After the individual units have been combined in a manufacturing pool, the pool must be tested for HBsAg, HIV antibodies, and HCV RNA (the latter by nucleic acid amplification technology, or NAT[95]). This testing was originally an industry-driven, voluntary initiative and has in the meantime been codified by the regulators.[93,102] Results for the aforementioned tests must be negative.

To ensure in advance that a manufacturing pool will not have positive NAT results (which would mean the loss of that pool), minipools are made from *samples* from individual donations and tested before the donations are formed into a manufacturing pool. Overall, therefore, testing is performed at three levels: individual donations, minipools, and manufacturing pools.

In addition, NAT testing for human parvovirus B19 (B19V) is becoming a universal requirement for plasma products.[91,103] The FDA targets a limit of 10^4 IU B19V/mL for the plasma pool, whereas the EMA requires the limit to be based on the B19V reduction capacity of the manufacturing process and a B19V risk assessment.

Further voluntary measures have been proposed by the PPTA. In its voluntary Quality Standards of Excellence, Assurance, and Leadership (QSEAL), established since 2001, participating fractionators are required to use source (ie, plasmapheresis) plasma from repeat donors only, also called "qualified donors." A donor is qualified when he or she passes all measures and donates again within 6 months. (Repeat donors have a lower risk of carrying infections such as HIV or viral hepatitis as this group consists of committed donors and excludes "test seekers.") As a further measure, called "inventory hold," plasma donations are stored for at least 60 days before manufacturing is begun. This allows for a donation to be discarded if any information that could cast doubt on the safety of that donation is received later. QSEAL also requires B19V screening at the minipool and manufacturing-pool level. Under the QSEAL program, plasma centers must adhere to "viral marker standards": viral-marker rates of donor applicants are measured, and centers significantly exceeding average rates are required to take corrective actions to ensure that they are visited by a low-risk donor population.

Plasma Safety: Virus Inactivation and Removal Processes

Viruses are generally easy to inactivate; the challenge, however, is to do this in the presence of sensitive plasma proteins without affecting their quality. The following paragraphs will focus on methods typically used for IVIGs and also provide an outlook for future options.

EU guidelines require two effective virus reduction steps for lipid-enveloped viruses, and one of these two steps has to be effective also against nonenveloped viruses. Effectiveness is defined as robust virus reduction on the order of four logs. The two steps are also required to have different mechanisms of virus reduction, so that viruses resistant to one inactivation principle will not survive the second treatment.

Chemical Methods

Solvent/Detergent Treatment. The S/D treatment, invented by Bernard Horowitz in the 1980s (then at the New York Blood Center), combines an organic solvent with low toxicity—ie, tri-n-butyl phosphate (TNBP)—with one or more detergents. (Theoretically, other solvents could be chosen, but TNBP is currently the only one used by manufacturers of plasma-derived or recombinant proteins.) The concentrations are low, typically 0.3% TNBP and 1% detergent. Nonionic detergents such as Tween-80 or Triton-X-100 are preferred as they are easier to remove in subsequent ion exchange chromatography steps (where the proteins of choice bind to the resin and the S/D components remain in the discard fraction). The choice of detergent is one of the main determinants of virus-inactivation kinetics, and S/D processes that use Tween-80 or sodium cholate only as detergents require more time for complete inactivation of viruses.

S/D treatment works by irreversible destruction of the lipid envelope of lipid-enveloped viruses and is very gentle on otherwise sensitive proteins such as clotting factors. This combination of factors has led to the near-universal implementation of S/D treatment in manufacturing processes of plasma proteins.[104] Its effectiveness and robustness is excellent, and no transmission of lipid-enveloped viruses such as HIV, HBV, or HCV has been observed for S/D-treated products. S/D treatment has no effect, however, on nonenveloped viruses.[105]

As also outlined in regulatory guidelines, particle removal before S/D treatment is essential for virus-inactivation efficacy because the particles could theoretically harbor viruses, which would then be protected from the S/D components. Filtration is typically used to ensure that such particles are absent.

Detergent-only treatments—eg, with octanoic acid—can also provide effective inactivation of lipid-enveloped viruses.[106]

Low-pH Treatment. Incubation at low pH, with and without proteinase present, was originally introduced to reduce adverse events during the IV application of immunoglobulins. A low pH also helps in achieving a stable liquid formulation of IVIG. Low-pH treatments are usually performed at pH 4 to 5; the virus inactivation capacity depends on temperature and incubation time in addition to the chosen pH. Low pH is typically effective against lipid-enveloped viruses, not always including Bovine viral diarrhea virus (BVDV), the typical HCV model used in virus-clearance studies. Effectiveness against nonenveloped viruses is more limited but may contribute two to three logs to the overall virus clearance capacity of the process.[46]

Physical Methods

Nanofiltration: Separation by Size. Nanofiltration originally referred to filters with pore sizes of 1 to 10 nm, used mostly for water purification (nanofilters discussed here for virus reduction purposes have pore sizes of roughly 15 to 50 nm). To avoid using the same term as for the water purification filters, "virus removal filtration" and similar terms have been proposed, but these have not been widely adopted. Nanofilters have somewhat larger pore sizes than ultrafilters, which are widely used to concentrate protein solutions and can separate viruses and proteins by size: proteins pass through the filter, but viruses, should they be present, are retained. Nanofiltration is basically only a filtration step. It leaves the composition of the solution unchanged and can thus, in principle, be integrated at every step of the manufacturing process where the therapeutic protein is present in solution. This makes it easier to integrate nanofiltration as an additional virus reduction step into an *already existing* process. As the pores are smaller in nanofilters than in filters used for sterile filtration, the "filterability" of intermediate fractions can be a limiting factor. Typically, nanofiltration is performed at later stages in the manufacturing process, where proteins are already present in a mostly pure form and solutions are easier to filter. A prefilter is nevertheless required in most cases. Nanofilters are expensive and currently single-use only.

As is clear from its principle, nanofiltration is problematic when small viruses need to be removed from large proteins. Often, diluting the solution and/or increasing the filter area can overcome this difficulty, as demonstrated by the successful nanofiltration of Factor VIII,[107] but this approach may not be feasible for all plasma products.

Especially relevant for IVIGs is the ability of virus-specific antibodies to bind to viruses, effectively increasing their size and thus enhancing the virus-reduction capacity of the nanofilter, as shown by Kreil et al.[108] This principle, known as "antibody-enhanced nanofiltration" has been successfully implemented in the manufacturing process of a newer IVIG, where effective removal of hepatitis A virus (HAV) and B19V could be demonstrated, although the nominal filter pore size was larger than these viruses.[46] Of course, implementing antibody-enhanced nanofiltration requires specifications for minimal titers of virus-specific antibodies.

Heating. Although heating, either in solution or as a lyophilized product, has been introduced for many processes as a virus inactivation step, so far its use for IVIGs has been rather limited. This is attributed to the tendency of immunoglobulins to form aggregates, which makes it more difficult to render the product as tolerable for IV application. Nevertheless, such aggregates can be removed by using appropriate stabilizers and/or purification steps downstream. One IVIG manufacturer includes a pasteurization step (60 C in solution, 10 hours) and claims effective inactivation of lipid-enveloped viruses, HAV, and B19V.[109]

Virus Removal by Purification (Fractionation) Steps

Fractionation steps can also contribute to the overall virus-clearance capacity of the process, but regulatory agencies have been skeptical of claims of effective virus reduction by purification steps.[91] For such steps, the critical factors—ie, those determining the virus-reduction efficacy of the step—are often difficult to define, which presents a challenge for ensuring proper control of the virus-reduction capacity on the factory floor.

The mechanism of virus reduction by alcohol fractionation is coprecipitation and removal with the discard fraction(s) rather than virus inactivation by the precipitating agent, ethanol. This is because the low temperatures involved substantially reduce the virucidal effect of alcohol (although at higher ethanol concentrations used for fractionation of albumin—eg, 40%—virucidal effects are observed even at sub-zero temperatures for more sensitive viruses such as HIV). The classic Cohn-Oncley fractionation process, specifically the precipitation and removal of fraction III from the immunoglobulin solution, typically results in overall effective virus reduction, except for BVDV, the HCV model virus.

Specific Antibodies

The product itself plays a role in safety from viruses: according to the new EMA guideline,[91] "Immunoglobulin products have a good safety record for the known nonenveloped viruses due in part to the contribution from neutralizing antibodies in the product." The contribution of antibodies is difficult to assess, however, as noted in the guideline.

Between 1993 and 1996, HCV transmissions were reported for a non-SD-treated IVIG after plasma donations were screened with second-generation (multi-antigen) anti-HCV assays. Perplexingly, no HCV transmissions were observed for lots of the same product made from unscreened plasma or plasma that tested negative by the less sensitive, first-generation anti-HCV assays[38]; at that time, the more sensitive HCV NAT testing had not yet been implemented. The production of a safer product by the less sensitive anti-HCV testing of plasma suggested the benefit of the HCV antibodies and/or was the result of a different partitioning of HCV in the manufacturing process in the presence of antibodies (meaning that HCV would be directed to a discard fraction).

In a postmarketing surveillance study, S/D-treated plasma with B19V up to $10^{3.5}$ genome copies per mL did not transmit B19V.[110] This was attributed to B19V antibodies present in S/D plasma. Modrof et al investigated the B19V neutralization capacity of plasma pools of a major plasma manufacturer and demonstrated that even the lowest anti-B19V titer measured in 2 years of screening plasma pools was able to neutralize B19V *infectivity* by at least 4 logs.[111]

It should be noted that the contribution of antibodies to safety margins could also hold in the case of a hypothetical emerging virus. As viremia during the asymptomatic phase is typically short and specific antibody levels are long-lived, there would (in a hypothetical epidemic with a new virus) soon be more people carrying antibodies than people with viremia in the asymptomatic phase of infection. Provided that fully recovered postinfection donors are allowed to donate, as in the case of WNV,[112] the plasma pool would contain more donations with specific antibodies than donations with the new emerging virus. Although it is obviously not possible to quantify the contribution of this effect for a hypothetical case in advance, a contribution of these specific antibodies could occur.

The above postulation was confirmed in the case of the WNV epidemic in the United States, where IVIG lots from US plasma were protective against an otherwise lethal WNV challenge in an in-vivo (mouse) model.[97] Subsequent investigations showed that neutralizing antibodies could be detected in IVIG lots produced early during the epidemic.[113]

Virus-Related Safety Margins and Emerging Viruses

As corroborated by clinical practice, today's IVIGs from industrialized countries can be regarded as safe with respect to pathogenic viruses. Nevertheless, the *margins of safety* often vary substantially among different products as a consequence of process design—from processes that add only an effective step for lipid-enveloped viruses on top of alcohol fractionation to more elaborate processes with three dedicated virus-reduction steps.

Virology is not a static field. Completely new viruses can appear [eg HIV in the 1980s, severe acute respiratory syndrome (SARS) and influenza A (H1N1) in this millennium], and the geographical distribution of viruses may change (eg, WNV in the United States since 1999, Chikungunya virus in southern Europe in 2008).

Virus-reduction steps are always investigated with a panel of viruses displaying different properties and different levels of resistance toward inactivation and removal. Therefore, a broadly effective step can be expected to be of equal efficacy for emerging and established viruses. Thus far, manufacturing processes in this millennium have met the challenge, and recent emerging viruses have not withstood current processes—for example, no plasma product transmitted WNV despite its widespread occurrence in the United States (meaning that a significant number of plasma pools *must have been* contaminated, but this did *not* result in any contaminated product). Subsequent virus-reduction studies confirmed the effectiveness of existing virus-reduction steps for WNV and the validity of the model virus concept.[114,115]

Although recently emerging viruses have been either removed or inactivated to date, this may not always be the case. A theoretical worst-case scenario would be a small, nonenveloped virus with high titers in the asymptomatic viremic phase of infection and substantial resistance toward physicochemical inactivation. Given past experience, such a possibility cannot be completely excluded, and an IVIG with higher safety margins would be preferable in such a situation.

TSE (Prion) Safety

Transmissible spongiform encephalopathy (TSEs) is the overarching term for a group of neurodegenerative diseases: BSE in cattle (aka, mad cow disease); scrapie in sheep and goats; and (sporadic, iatrogenic, or familial) CJD, Gerstmann-Sträussler-Scheinker syndrome, fatal familial insomnia, and kuru in humans. Although natural TSEs have been observed also for some other species such as deer and elk, they are not known for pigs, birds, dogs, rabbits, and fish. TSEs are transmitted by infectious proteins, also called prions. These prions, typically abbreviated collectively as PrP^{SC} (originally for "prion protein—scrapie" but today used for infectious prions of all TSEs), appear as a pathogenic conformation of the otherwise nonpathogenic protein, PrP^C ("^{C}" stands for "cellular"). The pathogenic form (ie, PrP^{SC}) induces further PrP^C-to-PrP^{SC} conformational changes, thus, in effect, replicating itself. After typically several years of incubation in an infected person (extremes of incubation times of >50 years have been reported for kuru[116]), clinical symptoms similar to Alzheimer disease and dementia appear, resulting finally in death. The disease is currently incurable.

In the 1980s and early 1990s at the height of the BSE epidemic in the British cattle population, millions of people in the United Kingdom, and also in countries then importing British beef, were likely exposed to BSE-contaminated meat. This exposure has so far (ie, up to 2009) led worldwide to >200 cases of vCJD (a new TSE), with the majority of cases in the United Kingdom (>80%). Four cases of probable transfusion-transmitted vCJD infections have been reported in recipients of UK-source red cell concentrates, where the donor later developed vCJD. Also, a recipient of UK-source, plasma-derived Factor VIII, where one of the donors contributing to the plasma pool later developed vCJD, was diagnosed with a vCJD infection in a postmortem examination. It should be noted, though, that this recipient of Factor VIII and one of the four recipients of red cell concentrates did not develop the clinical disease, but remained asymptomatic; nevertheless, infection was clearly demonstrated by the presence of PrP^{SC} at autopsy.

These transfusion-transmitted cases of vCJD indicate the infectivity of vCJD is different from other human TSEs (mostly spontaneous CJD), which have never been known to be transmitted by blood or plasma (products) according to comprehensive epidemiologic studies.[117] Although still rare diseases, these other human TSEs together have higher incidence rates than vCJD, according to statistics from the (UK) National Creutzfeldt-Jakob Disease Surveillance Unit. It is therefore likely that any transfusion-related transmissions of this group of diseases would have been noted, had there been any. Thus, the focus here is on vCJD, as it is the only human TSE relevant for plasma products according to available data.

Generally, PrP^{SC} titers in infected animals and humans are highest in the central nervous system, and only borderline infectivity is found in the blood; this applies especially to the asymptomatic phase of infection (only an asymptomatic person could donate plasma). A scientific committee of the European Commission has estimated that, for an asymptomatic donor, 10 infectious units per mL could be in the donor's blood as a worst case assumption, and 50% of that (ie, 5 infectious units per mL) could be expected for the plasma fraction.[118]

Together, the rarity of the disease (vCJD) and the very low level of infectivity expected for the plasma of infected but asymptomatic donors suggest that the prion risk is a priori much smaller than the risk related to viruses. Nevertheless, the vCJD risk of plasma cannot be ignored. However, screening plasma donations for PrP^{SC} is technically not an option because the concentrations in infected but asymptomatic people are very low, and no sensitive assay is available for detection of PrP^{SC} in blood or plasma. In addition, PrP^{SC} inactivation during the manufacturing process is an impossible task because of the robustness of PrP^{SC} (PrP^{SC} can be autoclaved at 121 C without being fully inactivated), and any method inactivating PrP^{SC} would also destroy the therapeutic protein. Because both screening plasma for PrP^{SC} and *inactivation* steps for PrP^{SC} are unfeasible, plasma fractionators must rely on (plasma) donor selection and PrP^{SC} *removal* during the manufacturing process to ensure products are safe.

Many fractionation steps provide for a high purification capacity, effectively removing impurities and also, according to laboratory-based experimentation, PrP^{SC}. Furthermore, as PrP^{SC} tends to precipitate easily, any fractionation step where impurities are precipitated and then removed by filtration or centrifugation from the product-containing solution can be expected to substantially remove PrP^{SC}. Because all ethanol fractionation processes for IVIGs involve such precipitation steps, they will likely also be able to remove prions, even if the manufacturer does not have process-specific prion-removal data on file.

With the detection of prions in plasma currently unfeasible, increased attention has been focused on permanently deferring donors with a potentially increased TSE risk. Donor applicants with a cumulative UK residence time of 3 months or more between 1980 and 1996 are deferred in the US[119] (EU regulations[120,121]: 12 months or more) as well as those with a medical history suggesting an increased risk (eg, recipients of human-derived growth hormone and human transplants with potential TSE risk, such as dura mater or cornea). With the proper donor deferral criteria in place, residual risks are low, according to an FDA risk assessment.[122]

As a result of the already lower risk for plasma, *less* removal capacity for PrP^{SC} is required to arrive at substantial safety margins, and regulators have not yet defined a minimal prion-clearance capacity required for a safe product. European agencies currently apply a step-wise approach leading from theoretical TSE risk assessments to process-specific TSE removal studies and further to additional measures to increase the TSE reduction capacity of the process, where deemed necessary.[120,121]

The difference in residual virus and PrP^{SC} risk is also evident from the mandatory warning statements in package inserts of plasma products. Although warning statements for viruses are mandatory, the TSE risk can be called "theoretical" according to FDA guidance,[119] and the EMA's policy does not require a mention of the TSE risk in package inserts.[123]

Outlook

IVIG demand is growing from year to year, more so because IVIG products are often used off label.[39] Fractionators always target high process efficiency, although most manufacturers have reached a fairly similar range of IgG yield, which is an indication that IgG yields might not be raised substantially over these levels in the foreseeable future. The process for a plasma-derived immunoglobulin consists of a minimum of seven steps (capture, purification, polishing, concentration, formulation, virus inactivation, and virus removal). If each step is performed with a step recovery of 95%, the overall process efficiency will results in no more than 70% recovery in the final bulk, not counting losses for sterile filtration, filling, and packaging.

A general trend is noticeable toward the revival of subcutaneous IgG treatment, which is more convenient for patients, especially in regions like Scandinavia where travelling to a hospital can be cumbersome. The number of systemic adverse events is also much lower for this mode of administration.[124] High concentrations of immunoglobulin preparations are thus a focus of current development activities, as subcutaneous administration is limited by volume and infusion rate. The much lower bioavailability of the drug, compared with intravenously administered immunoglobulin, is a possible drawback.[125] However, the very recent development with the use of human hyaluronidase (recombinant) overcomes this drawback by improving delivery to the circulation.[126] Hyaluronidase facilitates the dispersion of subcutaneously administered IVIG (Gammagard Liquid) and enables administration of a full monthly dose at a single site with improved bioavailability compared to standard subcutaneous administration in patients with immunodeficiency diseases. Future insights might also reveal an ideal form of administration, at least for some diseases.

Upgrading existing market products to state-of-the-art virus-reduction quality is another constant driving factor. Although clinical experience suggests that all current IVIGs are safe, preparations with higher margins of safety would likely be beneficial in some hypothetical scenarios with emerging viruses. As infectious diseases are often limited to certain geographies or regions, this raises the question of how immunodeficient patients can be effectively protected with IVIG preparations when the titers of the antibody preparation and the origin of the blood donations are unknown. A good example is the prevalence of WNV in the United States, with studies showing considerable fluctuations in the titer in blood plasma as well as in IVIG preparations.

Apart from these issues, the anti-inflammatory potential of IVIG is well described in the literature[127,128] and not only encourages the use of IVIG in new patient groups but also intensifies attempts by scientists to understand these preparations in more detail. The best example of the growing use of IVIG is its application in neurologic disorders. As evidence-based practice, IVIG is given to patients with multifocal motor neuropathy because physicians consider IVIG as the first-line treatment for these patients.[129,130] Ongoing clinical trials over recent years support the use of IVIG in Alzheimer disease. With promising early results, Baxter has entered a Phase III clinical trial to show that the memory loss of treated patients is significantly retarded compared with placebo-treated patient groups.

Finally, the growing understanding of the functions of immunoglobulins in the immune system is reflected in numerous approaches to investigate the possibility of replacing plasma-derived IVIG therapy by recombinant products. Analyses of the structural features of the enormously diverse IgG derived from plasma has revealed the mechanisms by which antibodies bind to receptors and antigens, leading to treatments for tumors[131,132] and for rheumatoid diseases,[133] using monoclonal antibodies or fragments of them focusing on the opsonizing or Fc-mediated signaling part, as well as for ITP, using recombinant polyclonal anti-D hyperimmune preparations.[134] The different sugar moieties on the Fc part of IgG molecules, for instance, have been found to affect their effector functionalities. Agalactosylated IgG was shown to play a role in rheumatoid arthritis.[135] Sialylation of the Fc part was reported to influence the anti-inflammatory activity.[127] Such investigations also reveal the importance of understanding the ability of a process to enrich a specific, known IgG subfraction and the importance of developing analytical procedures[136,137] to eventually prove that the molecules of interest are present in the final IVIG product.

Although some may think that the days of plasma-derived immunoglobulins will soon be over, others believe that this is only the beginning and there is much more to learn from this precious preparation. The knowledge gained will, in certain cases, reveal the possibility for recombinant therapies[138]; in other cases, it can initiate the development of a more diversified preparation of modified or domestic-plasma-derived IVIG preparations and the respective new separation processes. Ultimately, the combination of recombinant and plasma-derived antibody therapy might also be an option for certain indications.[139]

References

1. Cohn EJ, Strong LE, Hughes WL, et al. Preparation and properties of serum and plasma proteins. IV. A system for the separation into fractions of the protein and lipoprotein components of biological tissues and fluids. J Am Chem Soc 1946;68:459-75.
2. Janeway CA, Gibson ST, Woodruff LM, et al. Chemical, clinical, and immunological studies on the products of human plasma fractionation. VII. Concentrated human serum albumin. J Clin Invest 1944;23:465-90.
3. Heyl JT, Gibson JG, Janeway CA, et al. Studies on the plasma proteins. V. The effect of concentrated solutions of human and bovine serum albumin on blood volume after acute blood loss in man. J Clin Invest 1943;22:763-73.
4. Scatchard G, Gibson ST, Woodruff LM, et al. Chemical, clinical, and immunological studies on the products of human plasma fractionation. IV. A study of the thermal stability of human serum albumin. J Clin Invest 1944; 23:445-53.
5. Scatchard G, Strong LE, Hughes WL, et al. Chemical, clinical, and immunological studies on the products of human plasma fractionation. XXVI. The properties of solutions of human serum albumin of low salt content. J Clin Invest 1945;24:671-9.
6. Scatchard G, Batchelder AC, Brown A. Chemical, clinical, and immunological studies on the products of human plasma fractionation. VI. The osmotic pressure of plasma and of serum albumin. J Clin Invest 1944;23:458-64.
7. Ballou GA, Boyer PD, Luck JM, Lum FG. Chemical, clinical and immunological studies on the products of human plasma fractionation. V. The influence of non-polar anions on the thermal stability of serum albumin. J Clin Invest 1944;23:454-7.
8. Ballou GA, Boyer PD, Luck JM, Lum FG. The heat coagulation of human serum albumin. J Biol Chem 1944;153:589-605.
9. Boyer PD, Lum FG, Ballou GA, et al. The combination of fatty acids and related compounds with serum albumin. I. Stabilization against heat denaturation. J Biol Chem 1946;162:181-98.
10. Sawyer WA, Meyer KF, Eaton MD, et al. Jaundice in army personnel in the western region of the United States and its relation to vaccination against yellow fever. Am J Epidemiol 1944;39: 337-430.
11. Gellis SS, Neefe JR, Stokes J, et al. Chemical, clinical, and immunological studies on the products of human plasma fractionation. XXXVI. Inactivation of the virus of homologous serum hepatitis in solutions of normal human serum albumin by means of heat. J Clin Invest 1948;27:239-44.
12. Oncley JL, Melin M. The separation of the antibodies, isoagglutinins, prothrombin, plasminogen, and beta1-lipoprotein into subfractions of human plasma. J Am Chem Soc 1949;71:541-50.
13. Bruton OC. Agammaglobulinemia. Pediatrics 1952;9:722-8.
14. Weiler CR. Immunoglobulin therapy: History, indications, and routes of administration. Int J Dermatol 2004;43:163-6.
15. Chinen J, Shearer WT. Subcutaneous immunoglobulins: Alternative for the hypogammaglobulinemic patient? J Allergy Clin Immunol 2004;114:934-5.
16. Ballow M. Immunoglobulin therapy: Methods of delivery. J Allergy Clin Immunol 2008;122: 1038-9.
17. Teschner W, Butterweck HA, Auer W, et al. A new liquid, intravenous immunoglobulin product (IGIV 10%) highly purified by a state-of-the-art process. Vox Sang 2007;92:42-55.
18. Barandun S, Kistler P, Jeunet F, Isliker H. Intravenous administration of human gamma-globulin. Vox Sang 1962;7:157-74.
19. Romer J, Morgenthaler JJ, Scherz R, Skvaril F. Characterization of various immunoglobulin preparations for intravenous application. I. Protein composition and antibody content. Vox Sang 1982;42:62-73.
20. Hooper JA. Intravenous immunoglobulins: Evolution of commercial IVIG preparations.

Immunol Allergy Clin North Am 2008;28: 765-78.
21. Munro CS, Stanley PJ, Cole PJ. Assessment of biological activity of immunoglobulin preparations by using opsonized micro-organisms to stimulate neutrophil chemiluminescence. Clin Exp Immunol 1985;61:183-8.
22. Pollack M. Antibody activity against Pseudomonas aeruginosa in immune globulins prepared for intravenous use in humans. J Infect Dis 1983;147:1090-8.
23. Kim KS, Wass CA, Kang JH, Anthony BF. Functional activities of various preparations of human intravenous immunoglobulin against type III group B Streptococcus. J Infect Dis 1986;153:1092-7.
24. van Furth R, Braat AG, Leijh PC, Gardi A. Opsonic and physicochemical characteristics of intravenous immunoglobulin preparations. Vox Sang 1987;53:70-5.
25. Polson A, Potgieter GM, Largier JF, et al. The fractionation of protein mixtures by linear polymers of high molecular weight. Biochim Biophys Acta 1964;16;82:463-75.
26. Kistler P, Friedli H. Ethanol precipitation. In: Curling JM, ed. Methods of plasma protein fractionation. London: Academic Press, 1980:3-16.
27. Kistler P, Nitschmann H. Large scale production of human plasma fractions. Eight years experience with the alcohol fractionation procedure of Nitschmann, Kistler and Lergier. Vox Sang 1962;7:414-24.
28. Steinbuch M, Audran R. [Isolation of IgG immunoglobulin from human plasma using caprylic acid.] Rev Fr Etud Clin Biol 1969;14: 1054-8.
29. Audran R, Pejaudier L, Steinbuch M. Obtention d'une préparation d'immunoglobulines G,A,M (IgGAM) à l'usage thérapeutique. Rev Fr Transfus Immunohematol 1975;18:119-35.
30. Hoppe HH, Krebs HJ, Mester T, Hennig W. Production of anti-Rh gamma globulin for preventive immunization. Munch Med Wochenschr 1967;109:1749-52.
31. Ballow M. Intravenous immunoglobulins: Clinical experience and viral safety. J Am Pharm Assoc 2002;42:449-58.
32. Suomela H. An ion exchange method for immunoglobulin production. In: Curling JM, ed. Methods of plasma protein fractionation. London: Academic Press, 1980:107-13.
33. Falksveden LG, Lundblad G. Ion exchange and polyethylene glycol precipitation of immunoglobulin G. In: Curling JM, ed. Methods of plasma protein fractionation. London: Academic Press, 1980:93-105.
34. Uemura Y, Uriyu K, Takechi K, et al. Method of producing immunoglobulin preparations for intravenous injection. European Patent Specification 0 246 579 B1; 1993.
35. Uemura Y, Goto T, Kano Y, Funakoshi S. Process for preparing immunoglobulin suitable for intravenous injection. United States Patent 4,371,520; 1983.
36. Sarno ME, Graf C, Neslund G, et al. Process for purifying immune serum globulins. United States Patent 5,177,194; 1993.
37. Kothe N, Rudnick D, Piechaczek D, et al. Manufacturing intravenous tolerable immunoglobulin-G preparation. United States Patent 5,164,487; 1992.
38. Bresee JS, Mast EE, Coleman PJ, et al. Hepatitis C virus infection associated with administration of intravenous immune globulin. A cohort study. JAMA 1996;276:1563-7.
39. Farrugia A, Poulis P. Intravenous immunoglobulin: Regulatory perspectives on use and supply. Transfus Med 2001;11:63-74.
40. Glynn SA, Kleinman SH, Schreiber GB, et al. Trends in incidence and prevalence of major transfusion-transmissible viral infections in US blood donors, 1991 to 1996. JAMA 2000; 284:229-35.
41. Committee for Proprietary Medicinal Products (European Agency for the Evaluation of Medicinal Products). CPMP position statement: Non-remunerated and remunerated donors: Safety and supply of plasma-derived medicinal products. EMEA/CPMP/BPWG/BWP/1818/02. (May 2002) London: EMEA, 2002.
42. Horowitz B, Wiebe ME, Lippin A, Stryker MH. Inactivation of viruses in labile blood derivatives. I. Disruption of lipid-enveloped viruses by tri(n-butyl)phosphate detergent combinations. Transfusion 1985;25:516-22.
43. Uemura Y, Uriyu K, Hirao Y, et al. Inactivation and elimination of viruses during the fractionation of an intravenous immunoglobulin preparation: Liquid heat treatment and polyethylene glycol fractionation. Vox Sang 1989;56:155-61.
44. Burnouf-Radosevich M, Appourchaux P, Huart JJ, et al. A new specific virus elimination method applied to high-purity Factor IX and Factor XI concentrates. Vox Sang 1994;67: 132-8.

45. Hirao Y, Hashimoto M, Kitamura T, Uemura Y. Immunoglobulin preparation and preparation process thereof. United States Patent 6,124,437; 2000.
46. Poelsler G, Berting A, Kindermann J, et al. A new liquid intravenous immunoglobulin with three dedicated virus reduction steps: Virus and prion reduction capacity. Vox Sang 2008; 94:184-92.
47. Sherer Y, Levy Y, Shoenfeld Y. IVIG in autoimmunity and cancer—efficacy versus safety. Expert Opin Drug Saf 2002;1:1537.
48. Cramer M, Frei R, Sebald A, et al. Stability over 36 months of a new liquid 10% polyclonal immunoglobulin product (IgPro10, Privigen(c)) stabilized with L-proline. Vox Sang 2009;96: 219-25.
49. Tenold RA. Intravenously injectable immune serum globulin. United States Patent 4,396,608; 1983.
50. Hirao Y, Takechi K, Uriyu K, Uemura Y. Gammaglobulin injectable solutions containing sorbitol. United States Patent 4,876,088; 1989.
51. Food and Drug Administration. Immune globulin intravenous (IGIV) indications. Rockville, MD: FDA, 2009. [Available at http://www.fda.gov/BiologicsBloodVaccines/Blood BloodProducts/ApprovedProducts/Licensed ProductsBLAs/FractionatedPlasmaProducts/ucm133691.htm (accessed March 7, 2010).]
52. Scholze K, Fenske D. Gegenüberstellung von intravenösen Immunglobulinen. Krankenhauspharmazie 2009;30:298-304.
53. Stein MR, Nelson RP, Church JA, et al. Safety and efficacy of Privigen, a novel 10% liquid immunoglobulin preparation for intravenous use, in patients with primary immunodeficiencies. J Clin Immunol 2009;29:137-44.
54. Ameratunga R, Sinclair J, Kolbe J. Increased risk of adverse events when changing intravenous immunoglobulin preparations. Clin Exp Immunol 2004;136:111-3.
55. Stiehm ER, Casillas AM, Finkelstein JZ, et al. Slow subcutaneous human intravenous immunoglobulin in the treatment of antibody immunodeficiency: Use of an old method with a new product. J Allergy Clin Immunol 1998;101(6 Pt 1):848-9.
56. Lin MW, Kirkpatrick PE, Riminton DS. How intravenous immunoglobulin is used in clinical practice: Audits of two Sydney teaching hospitals. Intern Med J 2007;37:308-14.
57. International Conference on Harmonization of Technical Requirements for Registration of Pharmaceuticals for Human Use. Quality guidelines. Geneva, Switzerland: ICH, 2005. [Available at http://www.ich.org/cache/compo/276-254-1.html (accessed January 8, 2010).]
58. European Medicines Agency. Inspections—good manufacturing practice. London: EMA, 2010. [Available at www.emea.europa.eu/inspections/gmphome.html (accessed March 4, 2010).]
59. Anderson NL, Anderson NG. The human plasma proteome: History, character, and diagnostic prospects. Mol Cell Proteomics 2002;1: 845-67.
60. Schultze HE, Heremans JF. Molecular biology of human proteins with special reference to plasma proteins. Vol 1: Nature and metabolism of extracellular proteins. Amsterdam: Elsevier, 1966.
61. Hofmeister F. Arbeiten aus dem pharmakologischen Institut der deutschen Universität zu Prag. Zur Lehre von der Wirkung der Salze. Zweite Mittheilung. Arch exp Path Pharm 1887;24:247-60.
62. Timasheff SN, Inoue H. Preferential binding of solvent components to proteins in mixed water-organic solvent systems. Biochemistry 1968;7:2501-13.
63. Arakawa T, Timasheff SN. Mechanism of protein salting in and salting out by divalent cation salts: Balance between hydration and salt binding. Biochemistry 1984;23:5912-23.
64. Arakawa T, Timasheff SN. Preferential interactions of proteins with salts in concentrated solutions. Biochemistry 1982;21:6545-52.
65. Panum P. Neue Beobachtungen über die eiweifsartigen Körper. Virchows Archiv 1852; 4:419-67.
66. Ingham KC, Wickerhauser M. Fractional precipitation of proteins with polyethylene glycol. In: Curling JM, ed. Methods of plasma protein fractionation. London: Academic Press, 1980: 57-74.
67. Parkkinen J, Rahola A, von Bonsdorff L, et al. A modified caprylic acid method for manufacturing immunoglobulin G from human plasma with high yield and efficient virus clearance. Vox Sang 2006;90:97-104.
68. Chanutin A, Curnish RR. The precipitation of plasma proteins by short-chain fatty acids. Arch Biochem Biophys 1960;89:218-20.
69. Steinbruch M. Protein fractionation by ammonium sulphate, rivanol, and caprylic acid preparation. In: Curling JM, ed. Methods of plasma

protein fractionation. London: Academic Press, 1980:33-56.
70. Romisch J, Buchacher A, Iberer G. A method of providing a purified, virus safe antibody preparation. International Patent Application WO 2005/082937 A2; 2005.
71. Romisch J, Buchacher A, Iberer G. A method of providing a purified, virus safe antibody preparation—corrected version. International Patent Application WO 2005/082937 A3; 2005.
72. Lebing W, Alred P, Lee DC, Paul HI. Chromatographic method for high yield purification and viral inactivation of antibodies. United States Patent 6,307,028 B1; 2001.
73. McKinney MM, Parkinson A. A simple, non-chromatographic procedure to purify immunoglobulins from serum and ascites fluid. J Immunol Methods 1987;96:271-8.
74. Perosa F, Carbone R, Ferrone S, Dammacco F. Purification of human immunoglobulins by sequential precipitation with caprylic acid and ammonium sulphate. J Immunol Methods 1990;128:9-16.
75. Reik LM, Maines SL, Ryan DE, et al. A simple, non-chromatographic purification procedure for monoclonal antibodies. Isolation of monoclonal antibodies against cytochrome P450 isozymes. J Immunol Methods 1987;100:123-30.
76. Deutsch HF, Gosting LJ, Alberty RA, Williams JW. Biophysical studies of blood plasma proteins III. Recovery of gammaglobulin from human blood protein mixtures. J Biol Chem 1946;164:109-18.
77. Kolarich D, Weber A, Pabst M, et al. Glycoproteomic characterization of butyrylcholinesterase from human plasma. Proteomics 2008; 8:254-63.
78. Buchacher A, Iberer G. Purification of intravenous immunoglobulin G from human plasma—aspects of yield and virus safety. Biotechnol J 2006;1:148-63.
79. Janson JC. On the history of the development of Sephadex. Chromatographia 1987;23:361-5.
80. Andersson M, Ramberg M, Johansson BL. The influence of the degree of cross-linking, type of ligand and support on the chemical stability of chromatography media intended for protein purification. Process Biochem 1998;33:47-55.
81. Guerrier L, Flayeux I, Boschetti E, Radosevich MB. Specific sorbent to remove solvent-detergent mixtures from virus-inactivated biological fluids. J Chromatogr B Biomed Appl 1995; 664:119-25
82. Lebing W, Remington KM, Schreiner C, Paul HI. Properties of a new intravenous immunoglobulin (IGIV-C, 10%) produced by virus inactivation with caprylate and column chromatography. Vox Sang 2003;84:193-201.
83. Roque AC, Silva CS, Taipa MA. Affinity-based methodologies and ligands for antibody purification: Advances and perspectives. J Chromatogr A 2007;1160(1-2):44-55.
84. Bussone G, Dib H, Dimitrov JD, et al. Identification of target antigens of self-reactive IgG in intravenous immunoglobulin preparations. Proteomics 2009;9:2253-62.
85. Sakamoto K, Ito Y, Hatanaka T, et al. Discovery and characterization of a peptide motif that specifically recognizes a non-native conformation of human IgG induced by acidic pH conditions. J Biol Chem 2009;284:9986-93.
86. ten Haaft M, Hermans P, Dawson B. Separations in proteomics: Use of camelid antibody fragments in the depletion and enrichment of human plasma proteins for proteomics applications. In: Smejkal G, Lazarev A, eds. Separation methods in proteomics. Boca Raton, FL: CRC Taylor and Francis, 2006:29-40.
87. Hubbuch JJ, Heeboll-Nielsen A, Hobley TJ, Thomas OR. A new fluid distribution system for scale-flexible expanded bed adsorption. Biotechnol Bioeng 2002;78:35-43.
88. Bryant C, Baines D, Carbonell R, et al. A new, high yielding, affinity cascade for sequential isolation of plasma proteins of therapeutic value. Presented at the 4th Plasma Product Biotechnology Meeting, Porto Elounda, Crete, Greece, May 9-12, 2005.
89. Evtushenko M, Wang K, Stokes HW, Nair H. Blood protein purification and simultaneous removal of nonenveloped viruses using tangential-flow preparative electrophoresis. Electrophoresis 2005;26:28-34.
90. Alter HJ. Emerging, re-emerging and submerging infectious threats to the blood supply. Vox Sang 2004;87(Suppl 2):56-61.
91. European Medicines Agency, Committee for Proprietary Medicinal Products for Human Use. Note for guidance on plasma derived medicinal products (draft). CPMP/BWP/269/95/rev4. (February 19, 2009) London: EMEA, 2009.
92. World Health Organization. Annex 4: Guidelines on viral inactivation and removal procedures intended to assure the viral safety of

human blood plasma products. In: WHO Expert Committee on Biological Standardization. 52nd report. Technical report series, No. 924. Geneva: WHO, 2004.
93. European pharmacopoeia 6.2. Monograph No. 0853: Human plasma for fractionation. Strasbourg, France: European Directorate for the Quality of Medicines and HealthCare, 2008.
94. Commission Directive 2004/33/EC. Official Journal of the European Union 2004:L91/25.
95. Directive 2002/98/EC of the European Parliament and of the Council. Official Journal of the European Union 2003:L33/30.
96. Australian Medical Association. Health ministers must ensure blood supply safety. Kingston, Australia: AMA, 2006 [Available at http://www.ama.com.au/node/2555 (accessed March 6, 2010).]
97. Planitzer CB, Modrof J, Kreil TR. West Nile virus neutralization by US plasma-derived immunoglobulin products. J Infect Dis 2007; 196:435-40.
98. US General Accounting Office. Blood plasma safety: Plasma product risks are low if good manufacturing practices are followed. GAO/HEHS-98-205. (September 1998) Washington, DC: GAO, 1998.
99. Dodd RY, Notari EP, Stramer SL. Current prevalence and incidence of infectious disease markers and estimated window-period risk in the American Red Cross blood donor population. Transfusion 2002;42:975-9.
100. (US) Code of federal regulations. Title 21, CFR Part 610.40. Test requirements. Washington, DC: US Government Printing Office, 2010 (revised annually).
101. World Health Organization, Requirements for the collection, processing and quality control of blood, blood components and plasma derivatives. WHO Technical Report Series, No. 840, Annex 2. Geneva, Switzerland: WHO, 1994.
102. Food and Drug Administration. Guidance for industry: Use of nucleic acid tests on pooled and individual samples from donors of whole blood and blood components (including source plasma and source leukocytes) to adequately and appropriately reduce the risk of transmission of HIV-1 and HCV. (October 2004) Rockville, MD: CBER Office of Communication, Outreach, and Development, 2004.
103. Food and Drug Administration. Guidance for industry: Nucleic acid testing (NAT) to reduce possible risk of parvovirus B19 transmission by plasma-derived products. (July 28, 2009) Rockville, MD: CBER Office of Communication, Outreach, and Development, 2009.
104. Dichtelmuller HO, Biesert L, Fabbrizzi F, et al. Robustness of solvent/detergent treatment of plasma derivatives: A data collection from Plasma Protein Therapeutics Association member companies. Transfusion 2009;49:1931-43.
105. Horowitz B, Prince AM, Horowitz MS, Watklevicz C. Viral safety of solvent-detergent treated blood products. Dev Biol Stand 1993; 81:147-61.
106. Trejo SR, Hotta JA, Lebing W, et al. Evaluation of virus and prion reduction in a new intravenous immunoglobulin manufacturing process. Vox Sang 2003;84:176-87.
107. Furuya K, Murai K, Yokoyama T, et al. Implementation of a 20-nm pore-size filter in the plasma-derived Factor VIII manufacturing process. Vox Sang 2006;91:119-25.
108. Kreil TR, Wieser A, Berting A, et al. Removal of small nonenveloped viruses by antibody-enhanced nanofiltration during the manufacture of plasma derivatives. Transfusion 2006; 46:1143-51.
109. Package insert. Flebogamma DIF 5%. Los Angeles, CA: Grifols Biologicals, 2006. [Available at: http://www.fda.gov/downloads/BiologicsBloodVaccines/BloodBloodProducts/ApprovedProducts/LicensedProductsBLAs/FractionatedPlasmaProducts/UCM172599.pdf (accessed March 6, 2010).]
110. Brown KE, Young NS, Alving BM, Barbosa LH. Parvovirus B19: Implications for transfusion medicine. Summary of a workshop. Transfusion 2001;41:130-5.
111. Modrof J, Berting A, Tille B, et al. Neutralization of human parvovirus B19 by plasma and intravenous immunoglobulins. Transfusion 2007;48:178-86.
112. Food and Drug Administration. Guidance for industry: Assessing donor suitability and blood and blood product safety in cases of known or suspected West Nile virus infection. (June 23, 2005) Rockville, MD: CBER Office of Communication, Outreach, and Development, 2005.
113. Planitzer CB, Modrof J, Yu M, Kreil TR. Seroprevalence of West Nile virus infection reflected in intravenous immune globulins made from plasma of US blood and plasma donors. Emerg Infect Dis 2009;15:1668-70.
114. Kreil TR, Berting A, Kistner O, Kindermann J. West Nile virus and the safety of plasma derivatives: Verification of high safety margins, and

115. Kreil TR. West Nile virus: Recent experience with the model virus approach. Dev Biol (Basel) 2004;118:101-5.
116. Collinge J, Whitfield J, McKintosh E, et al. Kuru in the 21st century—an acquired human prion disease with very long incubation periods. Lancet 2006;367:2068-74.
117. Dorsey K, Zou S, Schonberger LB, et al. Lack of evidence of transfusion transmission of Creutzfeldt-Jakob disease in a US surveillance study. Transfusion 2009;49:977-84.
118. Scientific Committee on Emerging and Newly Identified Health Risks (European Commission). Opinion on the safety of human-derived products with regard to variant Creutzfeldt-Jakob disease. SCENIHR/005/06. Brussels/Luxembourg: European Commission Health and Consumer Protection Directorate-General, 2006.
119. Food and Drug Administration. Guidance for industry: Revised preventive measures to reduce the possible risk of transmission of Creutzfeldt-Jakob disease (CJD) and variant Creutzfeldt-Jakob disease (vCJD) by blood and blood products. (January 9, 2002) Rockville, MD: CBER Office of Communication, Outreach, and Development, 2002.
120. European Medicines Agency. CHMP position statement on Creutzfeldt-Jakob disease and plasma-derived and urine-derived medicinal products. EMEA/CMPM/BWP/2879/02/rev 1. (June 2004) London: EMEA, 2004.
121. European Medicines Agency. CHMP concept paper on the need to update the CHMP statement position on CJD and plasma-derived and urine-derived medicinal products. EMEA/CPMP/BWP/2879/02 Rev 1. (June 2009) London: EMEA, 2009.
122. Food and Drug Administration. Draft quantitative risk assessment of vCJD risk potentially associated with the use of human plasma-derived Factor VIII manufactured under United States (US) license from plasma collected in the US. (November 27, 2006) Rockville, MD: CBER Office of Communication, Outreach, and Development, 2006.
123. Committee for Proprietary Medicinal Products (European Agency for the Evaluation of Medicinal Products). Note for guidance on the warning on transmissible agents in summary of product characteristics (SPCs) and package leaflets for plasma-derived medicinal products. the validity of predictions based on model virus data. Transfusion 2003;43:1023-8.

CPMP/BPWG/BWP/561/03, 2003. (October 2003) London: EMEA, 2003.
124. Gustafson R, Hammarstrom L. Subkutane Immunglobulin-Substitutionstherapie. Ellipse 2002;18:37-40.
125. Ochs HD, Gupta S, Kiessling P, et al. Safety and efficacy of self-administered subcutaneous immunoglobulin in patients with primary immunodeficiency diseases. J Clin Immunol 2006;26:265-73.
126. Schiff R, Leibl H, Engl W. Recombinant human hyaluronidase facilitates dispersion of subcutaneously administered Gammagard Liquid enabled administration of full monthly dose in a single site with improved bioavailability in patients with immunodeficiency diseases. Presented at the 6th Plasma Product Biotechnology Meeting (PPB09), Punta Prima, Menorca, Spain, May 11-15, 2009.
127. Nimmerjahn F, Ravetch JV. The antiinflammatory activity of IgG: The intravenous IgG paradox. J Exp Med 2007;204:11-15.
128. Kazatchkine MD, Kaveri SV. Immunomodulation of autoimmune and inflammatory diseases with intravenous immune globulin. N Engl J Med 2001;345:747-55.
129. Gold R, Stangel M, Dalakas MC. Drug insight: The use of intravenous immunoglobulin in neurology—therapeutic considerations and practical issues. Nat Clin Pract Neurol 2007;3:36-44.
130. Elovaara I, Apostolski S, van Doorn P, et al. EFNS guidelines for the use of intravenous immunoglobulin in treatment of neurological diseases: EFNS task force on the use of intravenous immunoglobulin in treatment of neurological diseases. Eur J Neurol 2008;15:893-908.
131. Clynes R, Takechi Y, Moroi Y, et al. Fc receptors are required in passive and active immunity to melanoma. Proc Natl Acad Sci U S A 1998;95:652-6.
132. Waldmann TA. Effective cancer therapy through immunomodulation. Ann Rev Med 2006;57:65-81.
133. Gartlehner G, Hansen RA, Thieda P, et al. Drug class review on targeted immune modulators (report). Chapel Hill, NC: RTI-UNC Evidence-Based Practice Center (University of North Carolina at Chapel Hill), 2007.
134. Frandsen TP. Development of a recombinant polyclonal antibody product rozrolimupab to replace plasma derived anti-D products. Presented at the 6th Plasma Product Biotechnol-

ogy Meeting (PPB09), Punta Prima, Menorca, Spain, May 11-15, 2009.
135. Matsumoto A, Shikata K, Takeuchi F, et al. Autoantibody activity of IgG rheumatoid factor increases with decreasing levels of galactosylation and sialylation. J Biochem 2000;128:621-8.
136. Dalziel M, McFarlane I, Axford JS. Lectin analysis of human immunoglobulin G N-glycan sialylation. Glycoconj J 1999;16:801-7.
137. Stadlmann J, Weber A, Pabst M, et al. A close look at human immunoglobulin G sialylation and subclass distribution after lectin fractionation. Proteomics 2009;9:4143-53.
138. Anthony RM, Nimmerjahn F, Ashline DJ, et al. Recapitulation of IVIG anti-inflammatory activity with a recombinant IgG Fc. Science 2008;320:373-6.
139. Nydegger UE, Mohacsi PJ, Escher R, Morell A. Clinical use of intravenous immunoglobulins. Vox Sang 2000;78(Suppl 2):191-5.

3

IVIG: Potential Mechanisms of Action

Andrew R. Crow, BRT, and Alan H. Lazarus, PhD

INITIALLY USED AS A PLASMA protein replacement therapy for immune-deficient patients in the early 1950s, intravenous immunoglobulin (IVIG) has also been used for almost 30 years to treat an ever-increasing number of autoimmune and systemic inflammatory diseases. It has been approved by the Food and Drug Administration for use in only six conditions: 1) the treatment of primary immunodeficiencies, 2) the prevention of bacterial infections in patients with hypogammaglobulinemia caused by B-cell chronic lymphocytic leukemia, 3) the prevention of coronary artery aneurysms in Kawasaki disease, 4) the prevention of infections, pneumonitis, and acute graft-versus-host disease after marrow transplantation, 5) the reduction of serious bacterial infections in children with human immunodeficiency virus (HIV), and 6) the increase of platelet counts in patients with immune thrombocytopenia (ITP). However, IVIG is also used off-label to treat a multitude of other diseases, including chronic inflammatory demyelinating polyneuropathy (CIDP), toxic epidermal necrolysis, Guillain-Barré syndrome (GBS), myasthenia gravis, dermatomyositis, and many others.

ITP is an autoimmune disorder characterized by the production of platelet-reactive autoantibodies that induce platelet clearance, resulting in thrombocytopenia, which can lead to bleeding complications. The first report of the treatment of autoimmune disease with IVIG was by Imbach et al,[1] who demonstrated that high-dose administration of IVIG resulted in a rapid reversal of thrombocytopenia associated with ITP in children. Since then, IVIG has

---

Andrew R. Crow, BRT, Senior Research Assistant, Canadian Blood Services, St Michael's Hospital, and Alan H. Lazarus, PhD, Scientist, Canadian Blood Services, St Michael's Hospital, and Associate Professor of Medicine and Associate Professor, Laboratory Medicine and Pathobiology, University of Toronto, Toronto, Ontario, Canada

This work was supported by the Canadian Institutes of Health Research and the Canadian Blood Services-Canadian Institutes of Health Research Request for Proposal program.

The authors have disclosed no conflicts of interest.

been used for the treatment of a wide range of autoimmune and systemic inflammatory diseases. Despite decades of therapeutic use, its mechanism of action has remained enigmatic. Much of the work analyzing IVIG in humans as well as animal models of disease had led to a plethora of theories as to how IVIG functions, including mononuclear phagocytic system blockade/inhibition, autoantibody neutralization by idiotype antibodies, accelerated pathogenic autoantibody clearance by saturation of the neonatal Fc receptor, cytokine and immune cell modulation, complement neutralization, and immune complex formation leading to dendritic cell (DC) priming (for a more comprehensive list, see Table 3-1). Although the field of neurology is greatly assisting in understanding IVIG function, much of the information gathered on IVIG's mechanism of action has been gleaned from experience with ITP and experimental models of thrombocytopenia; thus this chapter will discuss the multiple theories of the mechanism of action of IVIG in regard to many diseases, but with an emphasis on ITP.

IVIG and Activating FcγR

It has long been theorized that the clearance of antibody-sensitized platelets in ITP occurs via Fcγ receptor (FcγR)-bearing phagocytic cells in the spleen and sometimes the liver (cells of the mononuclear phagocytic system, or MPS). Four classes of standard activating FcγRs are expressed on phagocytic cells in the MPS: a high affinity receptor, FcγRI, which binds monomeric IgG, and the lower-affinity receptors FcγRIIA, FcγRIII, and FcγRIV, which bind complexed IgG, such as IgG-sensitized platelets or multivalent immune complexes.[2,3] Humans express FcγRI, FcγRIIA, and FcγRIII, whereas mice express FcγRI, FcγRIII, and FcγRIV. No study has yet found FcγRIV to be expressed in humans, although a report has confirmed that mouse FcγRIV is most closely related to human FcγRIII because of high-sequence homology.[4]

Preclinical and clinical studies have suggested that the activating FcγRIIA and FcγRIIIA are primarily involved in the FcγR-mediated clearance of platelets in ITP,[5-7] although some data has suggested that platelet clearance in ITP may occur via other mechanisms.[8-10] Nonetheless, it is not surprising that one of the earliest theories of the mechanism of action of IVIG in the treatment of ITP was competitive inhibition of activating FcγR on phagocytic macrophages within the MPS by IVIG-sensitized erythrocytes.[11,12] The most direct early evidence that MPS blockade by IVIG could rescue antibody-sensitized cells from phagocytosis came from experiments per-

---

Table 3-1. Potential Mechanisms of Action of IVIG

Activating FcγR inhibition/modulation
Inhibitory receptor FcγRIIB
Idiotype antibodies
Immunomodulation
Apoptosis
Cytokine modulation
Complement inhibition
FcRn-mediated, accelerated, pathogenic autoantibody clearance
Dendritic cell modulation and/or priming
Remyelination
Enhanced steroid sensitivity
Inhibition of cell migration
Normal antibody spectrum repopulation

formed by Fehr et al,[13] who showed that in patients with ITP who had not undergone splenectomy, IVIG treatment prolonged the in-vivo clearance of antibody-sensitized, radiolabeled red cells. Others have confirmed these results.[14-17] The authors' Canadian Blood Services laboratory at St Michael's Hospital has also demonstrated that IVIG[18] and therapeutic soluble immune complexes[19] can block the clearance of antibody-sensitized, labeled red cells in a murine model of ITP.

One study found that blocking of FcγRI with a monoclonal antibody had no effect in patients with ITP,[6] but Clarkson and colleagues demonstrated that an FcγRII/III-specific antibody successfully increased platelet counts in ITP patients.[5] IVIG effectively reverses ITP in mice genetically deficient in FcγRI.[20] Murine studies have further shown that administration of a monoclonal antibody (2.4G2) that blocks FcγRII and FcγRIII prevented the clearance of IgG-sensitized red cells.[21] In the authors' laboratory, it was demonstrated that 2.4G2 ameliorates murine ITP, although not as efficiently as IVIG.[22]

Other support for a role for FcγRII and FcγRIII in platelet clearance was provided in a study showing that IVIG dimers and multimers (which should bind FcγRII/III/IV) were more effective than IVIG monomer preparations in inhibiting the thrombocytopenia associated with murine ITP.[23] This same group has also suggested that monomeric IVIG may bind to FcγRII/III and antagonize these receptors.[24] However, it is not clear that true monomers were antagonistic when considering the data of Lamoureux et al, who observed that monomeric IVIG, in reactions with in-vivo antigens, may form an immune complex[25] that then ameliorates the ITP. This finding is similar to that of the authors' laboratory, which demonstrated that the therapeutic effects of IVIG could be replaced with soluble immune complexes.[19] It has also been shown that, in mice expressing a human FcγRIII, a blocking antibody to this receptor successfully inhibited murine ITP.[20] In addition, a monoclonal antibody to human FcγRIII ameliorated thrombocytopenia in a pilot study in a patient with HIV-related ITP.[26] Bussel and colleagues reported that a humanized anti-FcγRIII antibody (GMA161) successfully, though transiently, increased platelet counts in ITP patients who failed IVIG therapy.[27]

Although competitive blockade of the MPS appears to have been one of the most accepted mechanisms to explain the therapeutic effects of IVIG in ITP, observations in humans and murine models have suggested that either this mechanism may be incorrect or it may not be the only pathway by which IVIG exerts its protective effect. In particular, some patients have responded to F(ab')$_2$ fragments of IVIG, which have no FcγR-binding activity.[28,29] It has also been shown that IVIG is ineffective at treating ITP in mice that are genetically deficient in the inhibitory receptor FcγRIIB[20,30]; if IVIG indeed functions by MPS blockade, it should ameliorate thrombocytopenia in the absence of this inhibitory receptor, yet in these two murine studies, it did not. Casting further doubt on MPS blockade in murine models of ITP, the authors' laboratory determined that IVIG blocked the ability of the MPS to clear labeled, antibody-sensitized red cells in FcγRIIB-deficient mice.[31] Because thrombocytopenic mice that lack FcγRIIB do not appear to respond to IVIG treatment[20,30] but nevertheless undergo MPS blockade by IVIG,[31] either IVIG does not function via MPS blockade, or red cell clearance, as evaluated by the MPS blockade assay, may occur by a fundamentally different mechanism than platelet clearance in mice.

It has been reported that intact IVIG, but not F(ab')$_2$ fragments, can suppress FcγR-mediated phagocytosis of opsonized erythrocytes by microglia,[32] and the same study found that endocytosis of soluble myelin basic protein by microglia can be inhibited by the F(ab')$_2$ portion of IVIG. The investigators speculated that this latter effect may contribute to the immunomodulatory effects of IVIG in treating diseases of the central nervous system.[32] It has been suggested that in patients with CIDP, GBS, and inflammatory myopathies, IVIG-mediated blockade of FcγR on macrophages might inhibit the macrophage-mediated phagocytosis of antigen-bearing target cells and thus potentially prevent macrophage-mediated demyelination.[33]

IVIG treatment has been shown to downregulate the expression of FcγRI and FcγRIII on human monocytes in patients with Kawasaki disease[34] and FcγRIV on kidney-infiltrating macrophages in a murine nephritis model.[35] In addition, it has been suggested that alleviation of the incidence and severity of diabetes in mice with nonobese diabetes (NOD) by IVIG is mediated via activating FcγRs.[36] It has been demonstrated that monocyte FcγRI expression is enhanced in secondary generalized epilepsy patients undergoing IVIG therapy.[37] Also, anti-inflammatory concentrations of soluble monomeric IgG decrease FcγRIIA expression on human DCs.[38]

Inhibitory Receptor FcγRIIB

In humans, two types of FcγRII exist: 1) the activating FcγRIIA and 2) the inhibitory FcγRIIB, which contains an intracellular immunoreceptor tyrosine-based inhibitory motif; however, in mice, only the inhibitory variant is present. In animal models, evidence is accumulating in favor of an important role of FcγRIIB in the anti-inflammatory properties of IVIG: Samuelsson et al[20] have shown that IVIG requires the presence of FcγRIIB for preventing the induction of thrombocytopenia in a murine model of ITP, and that FcγRIIB expression is increased on murine splenic macrophages after in-vivo exposure to IVIG. Because the inhibitory FcγRIIB is not likely to be involved in mediating platelet phagocytosis, perhaps an altogether different mechanism may be involved in IVIG action.

The authors' laboratory has confirmed the requirement of FcγRIIB in IVIG action in murine ITP, and it has extended these observations by demonstrating that the IVIG requirement for FcγRIIB also holds true for mice with established ITP.[30] However, work by Bazin and colleagues[39] may be in line with the concept that the requirement for FcγRIIB in the amelioration of murine ITP may be dependent on the size of the IVIG complex.[19] In the Bazin study, a complex consisting of IVIG cross-linked via a monoclonal IgG antibody (total apparent molecular weight of 850 kD) was able to ameliorate murine thrombocytopenia independent of FcγRIIB expression. This may suggest that there is a diminishing role for FcγRIIB when large IgG complexes are used to treat thrombocytopenia. The authors' laboratory has previously demonstrated that large particulate immune complexes (mouse red cells + anti-red-cell IgG) ameliorate murine ITP independently of FcγRIIB expression,[40] and that a small, soluble immune complex consisting of ovalbumin (OVA) plus a monoclonal anti-OVA (~200 kD) is dependent on the expression of FcγRIIB to ameliorate murine ITP.[19] Thus, the function of FcγRIIB may indeed exist only for low-molecular-weight immune complexes.

How IVIG functions via FcγRIIB is still unclear. Lin and Kinet[41] proposed a model in which FcγRIIB mediates inhibition of ITP by the generation of inhibitory signaling via the SH2-containing inositol 5-phosphatase, SHIP1. It is known that co-cross-linking of FcγRIIB with the B-cell receptor complex or with FcεRI in mast cells results in cell inhibition, and this effect is mediated by recruitment of the inositol phosphatase SHIP1 to the cytoplasmic tail of the FcγR.[42] Whether or not this pathway is involved in IVIG function has not been established, although the authors' laboratory found that the individual expression of SHIP1 and of two other potential FcγRIIB signaling mediators, SHP-1 and Btk, are not required for IVIG to ameliorate ITP;[30] the authors speculated that IVIG might use a unique signaling pathway through FcγRIIB.

Although FcγRIIB expression appears to be required for IVIG to ameliorate murine ITP, whether IVIG actually interacts with this receptor had not been established. To attempt to answer this question, the authors' laboratory devised a novel protocol for evaluating the amelioration of murine ITP by IVIG: in brief, it was demonstrated that IVIG-primed, washed leukocytes could, upon passive transfer to naive mice, completely recapitulate the protective effects of IVIG in ITP, and that IVIG targets DCs during its amelioration of murine ITP.[43]

Using this cellular therapy, the laboratory was able to demonstrate that IVIG-primed DCs from FcγRIIB-deficient mice were able to ameliorate ITP upon transfer into recipient wild-type mice.[43] This suggests that IVIG does not bind directly to the FcγRIIB itself to mediate the IVIG effect (discussed in more detail later).

Whether modulation of FcγRIIB expression contributes to the beneficial effects of IVIG therapy in humans is questionable given that IVIG treatment does not alter FcγRIIB messenger RNA expression in circulating human monocytes in patients with Kawasaki disease[34] nor does it alter FcγRIIB expression on human DCs in vitro.[38] However, it has recently been reported that CIDP patients who respond to IVIG therapy demonstrate increased FcγRIIB expression on both B cells and monocytes.[44]

Idiotypic Antibodies

Another proposed mechanism for IVIG function involves the regulatory properties of a subset of antibodies called idiotypic antibodies, which react with the antigen-combining (or idiotypic) region of other antibodies, binding and, in effect, neutralizing them.[45,46]

IVIG contains antibodies that react with the idiotypic region of many pathogenic antibodies, including anti-Factor VIII,[47] anti-thyroglobulin,[48] antineutrophil cytoplasmic antibodies (ANCA),[49,50] endothelial cell antibodies,[51] acetylcholine receptor antibodies,[52] and many others.[53,54] It has been shown that the level of idiotypic antibodies increases in patients when IVIG is administered, and that both intact IVIG and F(ab')$_2$ fragments of IVIG can neutralize the functional activity of various autoantibodies and/or inhibit the binding of the autoantibodies to their respective autoantigens in vitro.[55] The presence of these anti-idiotypes in IVIG may contribute to the therapeutic effects of IVIG. It has been demonstrated that IVIG can block autoantibody activity in vivo in a number of autoimmune states, including anti-Factor-VIII disease and ANCA-associated diseases, in which disease activity decreased with decreasing levels of pathogenic antibodies.[49-51,56]

IVIG has been shown to improve symptoms in patients with GBS, and it has been demonstrated that IVIG and monovalent and divalent Fab fragments prepared from IVIG can successfully block neuromuscular-blocking antibodies found in these patients.[57] In patients with IgM paraproteinemic polyneuropathies, IVIG can reduce the IgM antimyelin-associated glycoprotein and sulfoglucuronyl paragloboside antibody titers in some patients, but whether this occurs through antibody neutralization or an inhibition of antibody production is not known.[58] In many clinical studies, the administration of IVIG is associated with a decrease in circulating levels of IgE,[59-61] and it has been suggested that in the treatment of allergic disease, administration of IVIG may provide anti-idiotypes that bind to IgE molecules and remove them from the circulation.[62] In addition, it has been demonstrated that both intact IVIG and F(ab')$_2$ fragments can suppress the production of IgE by human tonsillar B cells, and it was suggested that this might be caused by the presence of anti-idiotypes.[63] In acquired hemophilia, IVIG can neutralize autoantibodies against Factor VIII,[64] and in anti-phospholipid syndrome, IVIG neutralizes autoantibodies against phospholipids, such as anti-cardiolipin.[65] Idiotypic antibodies in IVIG can neutralize cytotoxic antibodies and prevent them from binding to the fetoplacental unit in cases of recurrent spontaneous abortion.[66] Oral administration of IVIG could induce tolerance in an experimental model of anti-phospholipid syndrome; it was hypothesized that this effect was caused by the action of anti-idiotypes directed against anti-β2GPI autoantibodies.[67] In addition, pemphigus vulgaris patients who are responsive to IVIG treatment demonstrate a reduction in pathogenic antibody levels.[68] In idiopathic solar urticaria, IVIG may provide idiotypic antibodies capable of suppressing histamine-releasing autoantibodies.[69]

The potential role that idiotypic antibodies may play in the treatment of ITP has been difficult to ascertain with in-vivo studies, and data have been conflicting in regard to the potential role of IVIG anti-idiotypes in the amelioration of thrombocytopenia. In particular, Berchtold et al[70] demonstrated that IVIG contains antibodies that can bind to and neutralize the effects of autoantibodies directed against integrin $α_{IIb}β3$ (glycoprotein IIb/IIIa, a major target of autoantibodies in ITP). In contrast to these findings, Barbano et al[71] found IVIG to be ineffective at autoantibody neutralization in ITP patients. Moreover, Fc fragments of IVIG, which contain no anti-idiotypic activity, have been shown to increase platelet counts in pediatric ITP patients.[72] Work from the authors' laboratory has shown that the anti-idiotypes present in IVIG were not required in the amelioration of thrombocytopenia in a murine model of ITP.[18] Specifically, IVIG depleted of idiotypic antibodies reactive with endogenous murine IgG as well as with the antibody used to induce thrombocytopenia was just as effective as unmanipulated IVIG in reversing murine ITP. In addition, the authors' laboratory found IVIG to be ineffective at neutralizing the platelet antibody used to induce murine ITP, both in vitro and in vivo,[18] and another report showed that IVIG was unable to inhibit the binding of a panel of monoclonal antibodies directed against either GPIIb/IIIa or GPIbα to mouse platelets in vitro.[10] It has also been demonstrated that IVIG was ineffective at blocking the binding of a monoclonal platelet antibody to human platelets in vitro.[73]

Immunomodulation and Apoptosis

IVIG has the ability to affect the cellular immune response itself. IVIG antibodies have been shown to react with a variety of lymphocyte antigens, including the T-cell receptor,[74] CD4,[75] CD5,[76] CD40,[77] cytokines and their receptors,[78] and HLA Class I.[79] IVIG can enhance suppressor T-cell function and can decrease autoantibody production.[80-82] Successful treatment of recurrent spontaneous abortion with IVIG has been associated with a downregulation of natural killer (NK) cell activity.[66] In inhibiting the spread of tumors in mice, some of the anti-metastatic effects of IVIG include an elevation of interleukin (IL)-12 secretion and a subsequent enhancement of NK cell activity.[83]

IVIG also has the ability to reduce CD4+ T-helper cells in vivo,[84] can induce immune tolerance in both B and T cells,[85] and is able to suppress the proliferation of T cells in both antigen-dependent and antigen-independent responses.[86] In an experimental model of myasthenia gravis, IVIG was shown to inhibit disease severity by the suppression of the responses of B cells and T-helper Type 1 (Th1) cells.[87] In the presence of IVIG, DCs from common variable immunodeficiency patients show upregulation of CD1a (a marker of differentiated DCs) and the costimulatory molecules CD40, CD80, and CD86.[88]

Binding of IgG to FcγR in vitro induces the production of soluble Fc receptors, which can neutralize autoantibodies and downregulate local Ig production.[89] Also, it has been demonstrated that IVIG can suppress IgG and IgM production in B cells in an FcγR-dependent manner.[90] Pemphigus vulgaris patients successfully treated with IVIG demonstrate decreased levels of both IgG1 and IgG4 anti-desmoglein-1 antibodies and IgG1 and IgG4 anti-desmoglein-3 antibodies, the specific antibodies that mediate the disease.[91] IVIG was shown to be effective in reducing HLA antibody levels and significantly improving transplant rates in highly-HLA-sensitized patients in a controlled clinical trial; data suggested that IVIG Fc-fragment-mediated deletion of B cells may result in long-term deletion of specific antibody-producing clones.[92]

In patients with ITP, in vitro immunoglobulin (IgG, IgM, and IgA) synthesis was decreased after IVIG therapy, along with a decrease in the CD4/CD8 T-cell ratio.[84] In addition, IVIG contains antibodies to BAFF (B-cell activation factor belonging to the tumor necrosis factor family), which can interrupt the differentiation of B cells and prevent the generation of autoantibodies.[93] IVIG can also inhibit the production of IL-6, which is required for antibody secretion by plasma cells.[94]

Matrix metalloproteinases (MMPs) are upregulated in demyelinating neuropathies such as GBS and CIDP, and they enhance inflammatory responses.[95] It has been demonstrated that MMP-2 and MMP-9 are downregulated at the protein and mRNA level in demyelinating neuropathy patients treated with IVIG,[96] and a decrease in MMP-9 has been shown in Kawasaki disease patients treated with IVIG.[97] It has been speculated that IVIG inhibits the activity of MMP and thus downregulates the inflammatory mediators associated with demyelination.[96]

Although the effects of IVIG may contribute to long-term immunomodulatory effects, at least in ITP, IVIG achieves increases in platelet counts very rapidly; thus the immunomodulatory effects may not contribute to the acute effects of IVIG. Indeed, the authors' laboratory has shown that in the rapid amelioration of murine ITP, IVIG functions in the absence of both B and T cells.[18] Some immunomodulatory effects of IVIG have been speculated to be caused by "contaminating" products present in the IVIG preparation, such as transforming growth factor (TGF)-β,[98] soluble CD200,[99] soluble CD4, CD8, and HLA molecules;[100] however the authors' data using monoclonal antibody replacement therapies (ie, where it was unlikely that these contaminating products were present) do not support this contention.[22]

One of the in-vitro effects observed with IVIG is the growth arrest of cells.[101] Although one study has suggested that this could be caused by glycolipid antibodies,[102] IVIG has also been shown to affect the apoptosis of lymphocytes and monocytes via a Fas (CD95)-dependent effect.[101,103] Indeed, IVIG inhibits toxic epidermal necrolysis (TEN) by blocking the binding of Fas to its ligand, FasL.[104] This effect was believed to be the result of naturally occurring antibodies to Fas contained in IVIG that block Fas-FasL binding.[104] However, it has been demonstrated that although lesion biopsies from TEN patients express Fas and FasL, biopsies from patients treated with IVIG showed no expression of Fas/FasL in 85.7% of patients, suggesting that IVIG may work in this disorder by downregulating the expression of Fas and FasL.[105] IVIG may protect against autoimmune blistering diseases by preventing the autoantibody-induced apoptosis and oncosis (cell swelling before necrosis) of keratinocytes.[106] IVIG can also prevent graft vs host disease in rats by the induction of apoptosis of activated alloreactive donor T cells.[107] Circulating neutrophils increase in number during the acute phase of Kawasaki disease, and it has been demonstrated that IVIG can significantly decrease the number of circulating neutrophils in these patients by accelerating their apoptosis.[108] In a murine model of ITP, the authors' laboratory has shown that IVIG can inhibit platelet-antibody-induced platelet apoptosis via inhibition of caspase-3 activation and phosphatidylserine exposure.[109]

Siglecs are a novel lectin family of inhibitory receptors, and IVIG contains antibodies to both Siglec-8 and Siglec-9.[110] These antibodies can induce cell death in both eosinophils[111] and neutrohils,[112] respectively. It has been speculated that successful use of IVIG therapy in hypereosinophilic syndrome may be caused by the presence of Siglec-8 antibodies found in IVIG.[110] Similarly, in Churg-Strauss syndrome, a disorder associated with hypereosinophilia, IVIG treatment has been shown to reduce eosinophil numbers in the blood.[113]

Cytokine Modulation

Modified cytokine production might play a role in the pathogenesis of autoimmune diseases.[114] Studies have demonstrated modulation of numerous pro- and anti-inflammatory cytokines in vivo and in vitro after exposure to IVIG.[115-117] A study by Aukrust et al has demonstrated an increase in IL-6, -8, tumor necrosis factor alpha (TNFα), and IL-1 receptor antagonist (IL-1Ra) within 1 hour of IVIG administration to patients with primary hypogammaglobulinemia.[117] In work by others, IVIG has also been shown to induce the production of IL-1Ra,[118] which in turn can inhibit inflammation and macrophage phagocytic function[119] as well as regulate the activated state of DCs.[120] Primary hypogammaglobulinemia patients treated with IVIG demonstrate significantly increased serum concentration levels of IL-6, -12, and -8 and TNFα.[121]

In a study of GBS patients, Deng et al found a decrease in soluble TNF receptor 1 (TNFR1) and IL-12 p70 levels after IVIG therapy.[122] Decreased levels of TNFα and IL-1β were also associated with the clinical improvement from IVIG treatment.[123] In a double-blind, placebo-controlled study, treatment of multiple sclerosis (MS) patients with IVIG resulted in an increase in the levels of three isoforms of the anti-inflammatory cytokine TGF: TGFβ-1, -2, and -3.[124] Increased levels of interferon gamma (IFNγ) and IL-6 were observed in secondary generalized epilepsy patients undergoing IVIG therapy.[37] Repeated muscle biopsies from patients with dermatomyositis who demonstrated an improvement after IVIG treatment exhibited a downregulation of the in-situ expression of TGFβ and TGFβ mRNA and a reduction of cytokine-induced major histocompatibility complex (MHC) Class I and intercellular adhesion molecule (ICAM)-I expression.[125] A study of pemphigus vulgaris patients who successfully responded to IVIG treatment showed a decrease in serum IL-1β, IL-6, IL-8, IFNγ, and TNFα after treatment.[126] The chemokine receptors CCR-1, -2, -3, -4, and -5 are all upregulated in patients with CIDP and other demyelinating neuropathies,[127] and there is evidence that IVIG treatment modulates these chemokine receptors and their ligands as well as macrophage inflammatory protein at the protein and mRNA levels.[128] A recent paper reported that patients with Kawasaki disease who responded to IVIG treatment exhibited decreased levels of soluble TNFR1, IL-6, vascular endothelial growth factor (VEGF), damage-associated molecular pattern molecules, the myeloid-related protein MRP14, and the calcium-modulated protein S100A12, compared to pretreatment levels.[129] In chronic heart failure patients, IVIG treatment was associated with an increase in circulatory IL-1Ra and increases in IL-10 and soluble p55-TNFR and p75-TNFR.[130] Also, in the treatment of myocarditis, IVIG therapy decreases plasma TNFα, thioredoxin, and IL-6 levels, as well as other proinflammatory cytokines carrying a possible toxic role in the pathogenesis of this condition.[131,132] IVIG reduces both TNFα and IL-1 release, contributing to its anti-inflammatory effects in vasculitis.[133] In rat models of experimental autoimmune encephalomyelitis and adjuvant arthritis, IVIG inhibits the production of the proinflammatory cytokine TNFα.[134]

IVIG was shown to selectively trigger the production of IL-1Ra in cultures of purified monocytes, without concomitant effects on the production of the proinflammatory cytokines IL-1α, IL-1β, IL-6, and TNFα.[135,136] IVIG can also modulate Th1 and Th2 cytokine production.[137] Bruhns et al demonstrated that mice defective in colony-stimulating factor (CSF)-1 (osteopetrotic mice) did not respond to the therapeutic effect of IVIG in a passive arthritis model.[138]

Cooper and colleagues reported an increase in IL-10 in ITP patients 2 hours after IVIG treatment and an increase in monocyte chemoattractant protein (MCP)-1 7 days after treatment.[115] Using a mouse model of ITP, the authors' laboratory has confirmed an increase in mouse serum levels of IL-1Ra after exposure to IVIG, yet a recombinant IL-1Ra did not ameliorate thrombocytopenia.[139] The authors' laboratory has also demonstrated that IVIG was able to function therapeutically in mice lacking specific cytokines or their receptors that can potentially affect DC/macrophage function [IL-1 receptor, IL-4, IL-10, IL-12β, TNFα, IFNγR1 (subunit), and macrophage inflammatory protein-1 alpha (MIP-1α)] or in mice deficient for the common cytokine receptor γ chain, which is required for signal transduction through the receptors for IL-2, -4, -7, -9, -15, and -21.[139] Another report has extended these observations of the apparent lack of requirement of several cytokines in the amelioration of acute murine ITP by IVIG: Aubin et al showed that mice exposed to IVIG demonstrated no modulation of mRNA expression of 84 cytokine, chemokine, or receptor mRNAs.[140]

Complement

The interaction of IVIG with complement can prevent the generation of the C5b-9 membrane attack complex and subsequent complement-mediated tissue damage; this is accomplished by clearing active complement components and redirecting complement attack from cellular targets.[141,142] IVIG has demonstrated the ability to bind anaphylatoxins C3a and C5a,[143] to inhibit complement-mediated attack on host tissues and complement-dependent clearance of cells,[144] and to inhibit complement-dependent MPS effects.[145] It has been suggested that the beneficial effect of IVIG in dermatomyositis, CIDP, GBS, and myasthenia gravis could be exerted through prevention of membrane attack complex formation and interference of complement fragment deposition on sensitized target cells.[146] There is also evidence that the use of IVIG may be of benefit in sepsis, which is thought to involve the complement system in its pathology.[147]

IVIG can prevent complement activation induced by an antibody to a specific ganglioside (a relevant autoantigen in GBS) in peripheral nerve cultures.[57] In an ischemic brain damage model, IVIG was shown to target neural complement expression, which led to decreased neuronal cell death.[148] It has also been shown that in mice, IVIG treatment inhibits progression of atherosclerotic lesions by a complement-dependent mechanism.[149] IVIG has been used successfully in patients with a severe form of IgA nephropathy, and improvement of renal function was in correlation with a decrease of glomerular C3 deposition.[150] IVIG can exert its protective effect in patients with dermatomyositis by inhibiting complement uptake and the formation and deposition of the membrane attack complex on endomysial capillaries.[151]

The role of complement in the pathogenesis of ITP is not yet clear,[152] and the potential role that IVIG-mediated complement inhibition may play in the amelioration of ITP has not been fully explored. In both adult and pediatric patients with autoimmune hemolytic anemia and autoimmune neutropenia/thrombocytopenia, a significant reduction of the number of C3 molecules on red cells and platelets, respectively, was reported following IVIG therapy (compared to pretreatment values).[153] It was demonstrated that IVIG could inhibit the number of C3 molecules on platelets in the presence of complement-activating platelet antibodies.[154]

A clinical observation showed that IVIG infusion decreased the levels of platelet-associated C3 and C4 in children with ITP.[155]

In murine models of ITP, it has been demonstrated, however, that IVIG can ameliorate thrombocytopenia in the genetic absence of complement component C3 as well as in mice lacking complement receptor CR2/CR1,[20] and the authors' laboratory has found that IVIG and soluble immune complexes were fully functional in mice depleted of complement by cobra venom factor.[19] In addition, the authors' laboratory found that a monoclonal antibody against the complement receptor CR2/CR1 did not ameliorate murine thrombocytopenia.[22]

FcRn

The long half-life of serum IgG has been attributed to the function of the neonatal Fc receptor (FcRn). This MHC-Class-I-like Fcγ receptor binds IgG, protecting it from intracellular degradation by trafficking it out of the cell, thereby prolonging its half-life.[156] Several reports have demonstrated that IVIG treatment can reduce human plasma levels of pathogenic antibodies.[157-159] Expanding on these observations, Hansen et al, using a rat model of ITP, observed that IVIG-induced clearance of pathogenic platelet antibodies was at least in part mediated by FcRn.[73]

Similar to MHC Class I, FcRn requires β_2 microglobulin (β_2M) in order to be functionally expressed.[160,161] Israel et al showed that mice lacking β_2M demonstrated an increased clearance of IgG and suggested a "protective" role for FcRn.[160] Hansen and colleagues speculated that IVIG competitively binds to and saturates FcRn, thus leaving a greater fraction of platelet antibody available for catabolism.[73] They also found that IVIG failed to enhance the clearance of platelet antibody in mice lacking β_2M,[162] suggesting that FcRn plays a role in the clearance of pathogenic antibodies. It has been speculated that accelerated pathogenic autoantibody clearance caused by IVIG saturation of FcRn may explain IVIG's beneficial effects in autoantibody-mediated neuropathies.[96] Another study found that FcRn-deficient mice exhibited a reduced response to IVIG treatment of autoimmune arthritis,[163] and Li and colleagues found an absolute requirement for FcRn in the IVIG treatment of murine models of skin-blistering diseases.[164] Based on these observations, the authors' laboratory speculated that IVIG should not ameliorate thrombocytopenia well in mice lacking β_2M, as FcRn is nonfunctional in β_2M-deficient mice.[160] Surprisingly, IVIG successfully ameliorated ITP in β_2M-deficient mice with the same platelet-recovery kinetics as wild-type mice.[31]

IVIG may well enhance the clearance of pathogenic antibodies in animal models of ITP and humans, and FcRn-mediated antibody clearance may play a role in the amelioration of thrombocytopenia in humans with ITP. However, at least for acute effects, the authors found no requirement for β_2M (and, hence, functional FcRn expression[160]) in the rapid recovery of platelet counts in murine ITP by IVIG.

Dendritic Cells

Interaction with IVIG

DCs are a heterogeneous set of antigen-presenting cells involved in the induction of immunogenic or tolerogenic immune responses.[165] Because of their ability to stimulate naive T cells, DCs have a key role in the initiation of primary immune responses and thus have been viewed as promising targets for immunotherapy.[166] IVIG can inhibit T-cell proliferation and T-cell cytokine production.[86,135] Bayry et al further investigated these qualities by showing that the immunosuppressive effects of IVIG on T-cell activation may be mediated by DCs and suggested that IVIG inhibits the maturation of DCs and modulates their activation and survival, resulting in abrogation of T-cell activation and proliferation.[167] In addition, IVIG can inhibit DC production of IL-12, while increasing production of the anti-inflammatory cytokine IL-10.[167] IL-10 can play an important role in dampening phagocytic macrophage activation[168]; in fact, increases in the levels of IL-10 in ITP patients undergoing IVIG therapy have been observed.[115,137]

Both Fc and F(ab')$_2$ fragments of IVIG are able to mediate the suppression of DCs, revealing that both FcγR- and non-FcγR-mediated signaling events may be involved in IVIG-mediated modulation of DC function.[167] In vitro, IVIG suppresses the expression of FcγRIIA on human DCs, thereby preventing their activation by immune complexes.[38] In addition, IVIG can differentially modulate the antigen-presenting molecules on DCs: the expression of MHC Class II on DCs is downregulated upon incubation with IVIG in vitro,[167] but the expression of CD1d and activation of CD1d-restricted natural killer T cells (NK-T cells) is enhanced.[169] In experimental models, IVIG has suppressed DC function via FcγR interactions in an autoimmune giant-cell myocarditis model.[170] In vitro, IVIG downregulates the expression of CD49d (a crucially important molecule in the pathogenesis of MS) on DCs from both MS patients and healthy controls.[171]

Previously, the authors' laboratory speculated that IVIG might ameliorate autoimmunity via direct interactions with DCs. The authors initially found that IVIG-primed leukocytes could, upon transfer to naive mice, completely recapitulate the protective effects of IVIG in ITP.[43] Using this cellular therapy protocol to study IVIG function, the authors' laboratory determined that CD11c+ DCs were a specific target cell of IVIG in the amelioration of murine ITP.[43] In particular, it was demonstrated that IVIG-primed CD11c+ DCs, but not CD11c− cells, could adoptively transfer the ameliorative effects of IVIG to thrombocytopenic mice, and that IVIG drives signaling through activating FcγRs on DCs as its primary mode of action in the amelioration of murine ITP. Kaneko et al found that only IVIG that is properly glycosylated has anti-inflammatory activity, and nonglycosylated IVIG did not have anti-inflammatory activity.[172] Further, nonglycosylated IgG does not bind to activating FcγRs.[173] These findings support the authors' hypothesis that IVIG ameliorates autoimmunity via interactions with activating FcγRs. Interestingly, Kaneko and colleagues also demonstrated that the level of sialylation affects both the ability of pathogenic antibodies to bind their target antigen and the anti-inflammatory activity of IVIG.[172]

Several other studies have subsequently confirmed that the IVIG effect in vivo could be similarly recapitulated by adoptive transfer of IVIG-treated cells. For example, it has been observed that adoptive transfer of splenocytes from IVIG-treated mice into recipient mice can protect from fetal resorption in a murine model of spontaneous abortion, thought to be caused by an aberrant immune response at the placenta.[174] The authors' results have also been reproduced by Anthony and colleagues, who demonstrated that passive transfer of splenocytes from IVIG-treated mice could protect from experimental inflammatory arthritis.[175] Furthermore, in NOD mice (a model of type 1 diabetes), IVIG was unable to alleviate the incidence and severity of diabetes in the absence of FcγR, suggesting that IVIG effects may be mediated via activating FcγRs.[36] However, in the latter study it is also possible that IVIG may alleviate only the diabetes-related pathology caused by activating FcγRs, rather than exert its effect via FcγRs themselves.

Dendritic Cells and Cytokines

Exactly how IVIG-primed DCs (IVIG-DCs) may reverse ITP in the murine model is currently not understood. IVIG-DCs may secrete soluble mediators, such as cytokines, capable of downregulating the macrophage response. Two groups have observed an increase in the anti-inflammatory cytokine IL-10 in ITP patients undergoing IVIG therapy.[115,137] As previously mentioned, the authors' laboratory found that in a murine model of ITP, the acute protective effect of IVIG in vivo was independent of specific cytokines or their receptors that can potentially affect DC/macrophage function. In addition, although the authors confirmed an increase in mouse serum levels of the anti-inflammatory modulator IL-1Ra (which can regulate the activated state of DCs[120]) after exposure to IVIG, a recombinant IL-1Ra did not ameliorate thrombocytopenia.[139] These results by themselves, however, do not exclude the possibility that "long-term" protection afforded by IVIG-DCs is dependent on these or other anti-inflammatory cytokines. For example, IVIG can, by binding FcγRIII, inhibit IFNγ-enhanced phagocytosis in murine and human macrophages by suppressing expression of the IFNGR2 gene, which encodes a subunit of the IFNγR.[176] This indicates that engagement of the activating FcγRIII can, paradoxically, trigger the inhibition of cellular function. Thus the induction of an IFNγ-refractory state may help to explain more sustained immunomodulatory effects of IVIG.

Interactions with Natural Killer Cells

An alternative explanation to the above is that IVIG-DCs may exert a protective effect via an intermediate cell subset, such as NK cells. Several studies have observed DC-NK cell interactions and established the role of this interaction in the immune response.[177] For example, DCs matured in the presence of IVIG can activate NK cells, enhance NK cell degranulation, and elicit NK-cell-mediated, FcγRIII-dependent lysis of the same IVIG-matured DCs.[178] On the basis of the observation that macrophage responses may be downregulated following phagocytosis of apoptotic cells,[179] it may be speculated that following adoptive transfer, IVIG-DCs trigger NK-cell-mediated apoptosis of target cells, leading to suppression of the macrophage response. It has recently been demonstrated that expression of CD1d and activation of CD1d-restricted NK-T cells is enhanced in human monocyte-derived DCs after IVIG treatment, leading to the speculation that these DCs may activate immunoregulatory NK-T cells.[169] In addition, there is evidence that DCs such as NK-DCs[180] or IFN-producing killer DCs[181,182] can induce apoptosis or lysis of target cells such as T cells or tumor cells,[183] suggesting that IVIG-DCs may remove macrophages involved in platelet clearance.

Do IVIG-Primed Dendritic Cells Promote T Regulatory Cells?

T regulatory cells (Tregs) are potent suppressors of autoimmunity[184] and can prevent T-cell as well as B-cell immune responses.[185] IVIG provided protection from autoimmune encephalomyelitis in a murine model by expanding and enhancing the function of naturally occurring CD4+CD25+FoxP3+ Tregs.[186] The number of Tregs in acute-stage GBS patients is significantly decreased, and IVIG therapy can increase the number of Tregs in the peripheral blood toward the level of healthy controls[187]; this was observed to be correlated with the ability of IVIG to stabilize the patients' condition. It has been demonstrated that IVIG markedly enhances the differentiation, expansion, and effector functions of CD25+CD4+Fox-P3+ Tregs.[188] It has also been shown that there is a low frequency of CD4+CD25+ Tregs in systemic lupus erythematosus patients,[189] and decreased levels of peripheral Tregs have been reported in patients with ITP.[190] Recent data from Yu and colleagues suggested that functional defects in Tregs may contribute to breakdown of self-tolerance in patients with chronic ITP.[191] Thus it is fully plausible that Tregs may play a role in the dampening of chronic ITP, and IVIG-DCs could stimulate the production of Tregs downstream of the acute effects seen in mouse models of ITP. Indeed, De Groot and colleagues have reported the presence of "Tregitopes," Treg-activating regions in the Fc portion of IgG.[192] This finding may assist in understanding the long-term tolerogenic effects of IVIG in autoimmunity.

What Are the Molecular Targets of IVIG?

The actual molecular target of IVIG has remained elusive. However, in the passive murine ITP model, the authors' laboratory has demonstrated that the protective effects of IVIG can be replaced by soluble immune complexes (sIC).[19] Specifically, mice treated with soluble OVA plus anti-OVA or treated with monoclonal antibodies directed to murine albumin or transferrin were successfully protected from thrombocytopenia. Similar results were reported by Bazin et al, who demonstrated amelioration of murine ITP by immune complexes formed from IVIG and a monoclonal human IgG antibody.[39] The authors therefore suspected that IVIG or sIC might interact with either activating or inhibitory FcγR. However, as IVIG-primed DCs from FcγRIIB−/− mice ameliorated ITP in normal mice,[43] it is very unlikely that FcγRIIB is a molecular target of IVIG.

Whether IVIG-primed DCs directly act to increase FcγRIIB on macrophages, or an intermediary cell is involved, is unclear. Samuelsson et al demonstrated that IVIG upregulated FcγRIIB expression on splenic macrophages.[20] The authors' laboratory has shown that FcγRIIB need not be expressed on the DCs that bind IVIG but need only be expressed in the recipient mouse.[43] In the amelioration of murine ITP, the authors suggest that IVIG directly primes DCs via interaction with activating FcγRs, which subsequently act directly, or indirectly, with phagocytic macrophages. This interaction then leads to anti-inflammatory effects, including the upregulation of macrophage FcγRIIB, resulting in the inhibition of platelet clearance.

A recent study has reported that in the amelioration of murine inflammatory arthritis, IVIG requires the expression of the macrophage c-type lectin SIGN-R1 (specific ICAM-3-grabbing, nonintegrin-related 1) for its therapeutic effects.[193] It may be speculated that IVIG uses different pathways in different models of disease or multiple pathways in the same disease; eg, in the amelioration of murine ITP, the authors show that IVIG is dependent on DCs expressing activating Fcγ receptors, and that IVIG-primed macrophages had no effect at reversing thrombocytopenia.[43] Alternately, SIGN-R1 ligation may be occurring downstream of DC priming by IVIG by an as-yet-unknown ligand.

Other Mechanisms

IVIG use has been approved for IgG replacement in primary (ie, genetic) and secondary immune deficiencies. Secondary immune deficiencies occur in such disorders as chronic B-cell leukemia, pediatric HIV, and those relevant in marrow or stem cell transplantations. The mechanism in these states is likely a mere repopulation of the normal antibody spectrum as prophylaxis against severe infections or as an adjunctive measure for sepsis. IVIGs represent a significant advantage for patients with these conditions as they have been demonstrated to be safe and effective in decreasing the risk of infections.[194-196] For example, several studies have documented a decrease in the incidence of pneumonia in primary immune deficiencies after IVIG therapy,[197-199] and it has also been demonstrated that the incidence of mycoplasma infections is significantly reduced after the introduction of IVIG.[200] IVIG can also be used to erradicate *Clostridium difficile* bacteria as a last resort in immunosupressed patients.[201]

In addition to potentially immunomodulating antibodies in IVIG, there are other antibodies present that exert different effects. IVIG contains naturally occuring antibodies to a variety of antigens, including β-amyloid protein, which has been implicated as a fundamental cause of Alzheimer disease. A study found that patients with different neurologic diseases undergoing IVIG therapy had increased levels of β-amyloid antibodies in serum and cerebrospinal fluid and subsequent decreased levels of β-amyloid protein.[202] A follow-up study using Alzheimer patients demonstrated that IVIG therapy successfully increased mini-mental state scores (results of which are used in the diagnosis of Alzheimer disease) and increased β-amyloid antibodies in cerebrospinal fluid.[203]

Separately, IVIG has been shown to promote central nervous system remyelination in a rat model of MS.[204] This same study found that human monoclonal antibodies that bound oligodendrocytes were as efficacious as IVIG at treating the disease, and it was suggested that a direct effect of the antibodies on these cells was responsible for myelination[204]; however, a direct modulation of oligodendrocytes by IVIG has not been observed.[205] Similar results have been observed with IVIG in experimental autoimmune neuritis, the animal model of GBS.[206] Little is known about the exact mechanism behind this phenomenon. It has been theorized that immunoglobulins may, through improved opsonization of myelin and axons, lead to a limited secondary cellular infiltration and thus to protection from further injury.[207] Removal of myelin-associated inhibitors that are known to be present in central nervous system and peripheral nervous system lesions may, in addition, play a role in this process. Immunoglobulins lead to increased uptake of myelin debris by macrophages in vitro,[208] and it has been speculated that the phagocytosis of myelin debris by macrophages in demyelinating diseases may lead to removal of these myelin-associated inhibitory factors.[207]

In MS, brain volume (BV) loss occurs early in the disease process and accelerates over time. So far, IVIG is the only disease-modifying agent that shows a positive effect (ie, decelerating BV loss), and it has been suggested that increased protein content from chronic IVIG treatment results in increased osmotic pressure and water content in the brain, which might be responsible for a decreased loss of BV.[209]

IVIG has also been used as an oral glucocorticoid (GC)-sparing agent in patients with steroid-dependent asthma. It has been demonstrated that the combination of IVIG and dexamethasone act to synergistically suppress lymphocyte activation, and that IVIG has the ability to significantly improve GC receptor binding affinity.[210] It has been speculated that IVIG, by virtue of its immunosuppressive or anti-inflammatory effects, results in improved binding affinity of GC receptors, which is responsible for its steroid-sparing effects.[210]

Molecular mechanisms that are required for the migration of leukocytes into tissue are an important part of inflammatory reactions and may be inhibited by IVIG. It has been demonstrated that in animal experimental autoimmune encephalomyelitis (EAE, a model of MS), IVIG was able to inhibit the recruitment of leukocytes into the brain parenchyma. It was proposed that this was mediated by interference with α4-integrin-dependent adhesion,[211] a principle shown to be effective in the treatment of MS.[212] Also in EAE, it has been demonstrated that IVIG-treated mice showed a significant decrease in leukocyte recruitment (rolling and adhesion) before and after disease onset, which was concomitant with improved clinical score; this was the result of an interference of α4 integrin-VCAM-1 (vascular cell adhesion molecule) binding.[211] IVIG has direct inhibitory effects on leukocyte recruitment, both in vitro and in vivo, through inhibition of selectin and integrin functions.[213] IVIG can also have a potent effect on suppression of vaso-occlusion by inhibition of leukocyte adhesion, as shown in a mouse model of sickle cell disease.[214] It has been hypothesized that IVIG may also provide therapeutic effects in stroke by reducing cell adhesion molecule production and subsequent infiltration of inflammatory cells, thus reducing inflammation in the infarcted region.[215]

It has been shown that IVIG can inhibit endothelial cell proliferation in a dose- and time-dependent manner and downregulate the expression of adhesion molecule mRNA (ICAM-1 and VCAM-1). It was speculated that this may explain, in part, the therapeutic effect of IVIG in vascular and inflammatory disorders.[216] In addition, IVIG has been shown to reduce adhesion of T cells to the extracellular matrix,[217] and IVIG contains antibodies to the Arg-Gly-Asp (RGD) motif, the attachment site for a number of adhesive extracellular matrix proteins and β1, β3, and β5 integrins.[218]

Conclusions

In summary, although IVIG is used worldwide to treat myriad autoimmune and inflammatory diseases, its mechanism of action in humans remains unresolved. IVIG can block or inhibit MPS function, regulate activating and inhibitory FcγR expression, modulate the immune system, inhibit complement, and prime DCs. Undoubtedly, the multiple mechanisms of action of IVIG are mutually nonexclusive, and the outcome of IVIG treatment manifests as a combination of many different effects. The cellular and molecular details underlying IVIG-mediated immunosuppression will undoubtedly reveal new insights and provide additional strategies for the design of more effective therapeutics.

References

1. Imbach P, Barandun S, d'Apuzzo V, et al. High-dose intravenous gammaglobulin for idiopathic thrombocytopenic purpura in childhood. Lancet 1981;1:1228-31.
2. Crow AR, Lazarus AH. Role of Fcγ Receptors in the pathogenesis and treatment of idiopathic thrombocytopenic purpura. J Pediatr Hematol Oncol 2003;25:S14-S18.
3. Nimmerjahn F, Ravetch JV. Fcgamma receptors: Old friends and new family members. Immunity 2006;24:19-28.
4. Hirano M, Davis RS, Fine WD, et al. IgEb immune complexes activate macrophages through FcgammaRIV binding. Nat Immunol 2007;8:762-71.
5. Clarkson SB, Bussel JB, Kimberly RP, et al. Treatment of refractory immune thrombocytopenic purpura with an anti-Fc gamma-receptor antibody. N Engl J Med 1986;314:1236-9.
6. Ericson SG, Coleman KD, Wardwell K, et al. Monoclonal antibody 197 (anti-Fc gamma RI) infusion in a patient with immune thrombocytopenia purpura (ITP) results in down-modulation of Fc gamma RI on circulating monocytes. Br J Haematol 1996;92:718-24.
7. Flesch BK, Achtert G, Neppert J. Inhibition of monocyte and polymorphonuclear granulocyte immune phagocytosis by monoclonal antibodies specific for Fc gamma RI, II and III. Ann Hematol 1997;74:15-22.
8. Nieswandt B, Bergmeier W, Rackebrandt K, et al. Identification of critical antigen-specific mechanisms in the development of immune thrombocytopenic purpura in mice. Blood 2000;96:2520-7.
9. Olsson B, Andersson PO, Jernas M, et al. T-cell-mediated cytotoxicity toward platelets in chronic idiopathic thrombocytopenic purpura. Nat Med 2003;9:1123-4.
10. Webster ML, Sayeh E, Crow M, et al. Relative efficacy of intravenous immunoglobulin G in ameliorating thrombocytopenia induced by

antiplatelet GPIIbIIIa versus GPIbalpha antibodies. Blood 2006;108:943-6.
11. Salama A, Mueller-Eckhardt C, Kiefel V. Effect of intravenous immunoglobulin in immune thrombocytopenia. Lancet 1983;2:193-5.
12. Salama A, Kiefel V, Amberg R, Mueller-Eckhardt C. Treatment of autoimmune thrombocytopenic purpura with rhesus antibodies [anti-RhO(D)]. Blut 1984;49:29-35.
13. Fehr J, Hofmann V, Kappeler U. Transient reversal of thrombocytopenia in idiopathic thrombocytopenic purpura by high-dose intravenous gamma globulin. N Engl J Med 1982;306:1254-8.
14. Bussel JB, Kimberly RP, Inman RD, et al. Intravenous gammaglobulin treatment of chronic idiopathic thrombocytopenic purpura. Blood 1983;62:480-6.
15. Uchida T, Yui T, Umezu H, Kariyone S. Prolongation of platelet survival in idiopathic thrombocytopenic purpura by high-dose intravenous gamma globulin. Thromb Haemost 1984;51:65-6.
16. Macintyre EA, Linch DC, Macey MG, Newland AC. Successful response to intravenous immunoglobulin in autoimmune haemolytic anaemia. Br J Haematol 1985;60:387-8.
17. Newland AC, Macey MG. Immune thrombocytopenia and Fc receptor-mediated phagocyte function. Ann Hematol 1994;69:61-7.
18. Crow AR, Song S, Semple JW, et al. IVIG inhibits reticuloendothelial system function and ameliorates murine passive-immune thrombocytopenia independent of anti-idiotype reactivity. Br J Haematol 2001;115:679-86.
19. Siragam V, Brinc D, Crow AR, et al. Can antibodies with specificity for soluble antigens mimic the therapeutic effects of intravenous IgG in the treatment of autoimmune disease? J Clin Invest 2005;115:155-60.
20. Samuelsson A, Towers TL, Ravetch JV. Anti-inflammatory activity of IVIG mediated through the inhibitory Fc receptor. Science 2001;291:484-6.
21. Kurlander RJ, Hall J. Comparison of intravenous gamma globulin and a monoclonal anti-Fc receptor antibody as inhibitors of immune clearance in vivo in mice. J Clin Invest 1986;77:2010-18.
22. Song S, Crow AR, Freedman J, Lazarus AH. Monoclonal IgG can ameliorate immune thrombocytopenia in a murine model of ITP: An alternative to IVIG. Blood 2003;101:3708-13.
23. Teeling JL, Jansen-Hendriks T, Kuijpers TW, et al. Therapeutic efficacy of intravenous immunoglobulin preparations depends on the immunoglobulin G dimers: Studies in experimental immune thrombocytopenia. Blood 2001;98:1095-9.
24. van Mirre E, Teeling JL, van der Meer JW, et al. Monomeric IgG in intravenous Ig preparations is a functional antagonist of FcgammaRII and FcgammaRIIIb. J Immunol 2004;173:332-9.
25. Lamoureux J, Aubin E, Lemieux R. Autoantibodies purified from therapeutic preparations of intravenous immunoglobulins (IVIG) induce the formation of autoimmune complexes in normal human serum: A role in the in vivo mechanisms of action of IVIG? Int Immunol 2004;16:929-36.
26. Soubrane C, Tourani JM, Andrieu JM, et al. Biologic response to anti-CD16 monoclonal antibody therapy in a human immunodeficiency virus-related immune thrombocytopenic purpura patient. Blood 1993;81:15-19.
27. Bussel J, Patel V, Dunbar C, et al. GMA161 treatment of refractory ITP: Efficacy of Fc{gamma}-RIII blockade (abstract). Blood 2006;108:1074.
28. Burdach SE, Evers KG, Geursen RG. Treatment of acute idiopathic thrombocytopenic purpura of childhood with intravenous immunoglobulin G: Comparative efficacy of 7S and 5S preparations. J Pediatr 1986;109:770-5.
29. Tovo PA, Miniero R, Fiandino G, et al. Fc-depleted vs intact intravenous immunoglobulin in chronic ITP. J Pediatr 1984;105:676-7.
30. Crow AR, Song S, Freedman J, et al. IVIG-mediated amelioration of murine ITP via Fc{gamma}RIIB is independent of SHIP1, SHP-1, and Btk activity. Blood 2003;102:558-60.
31. Crow AR, Song S, Siragam V, Lazarus AH. Mechanisms of action of intravenous immunoglobulin in the treatment of immune thrombocytopenia. Pediatr Blood Cancer 2006;47:710-13.
32. Stangel M, Joly E, Scolding NJ, Compston DA. Normal polyclonal immunoglobulins ('IVIG') inhibit microglial phagocytosis in vitro. J Neuroimmunol 2000;106:137-44.
33. Dalakas MC. Mechanism of action of intravenous immunoglobulin and therapeutic considerations in the treatment of autoimmune neurologic diseases. Neurology 1998;51:S2-8.

34. Abe J, Jibiki T, Noma S, et al. Gene expression profiling of the effect of high-dose intravenous Ig in patients with Kawasaki disease. J Immunol 2005;174:5837-45.
35. Kaneko Y, Nimmerjahn F, Madaio MP, Ravetch JV. Pathology and protection in nephrotoxic nephritis is determined by selective engagement of specific Fc receptors. J Exp Med 2006; 203:789-97.
36. Inoue Y, Kaifu T, Sugahara-Tobinai A, et al. Activating Fc gamma receptors participate in the development of autoimmune diabetes in NOD mice. J Immunol 2007;179:764-74.
37. Ling ZD, Yeoh E, Webb BT, et al. Intravenous immunoglobulin induces interferon-gamma and interleukin-6 in vivo. J Clin Immunol 1993;13:302-9.
38. Boruchov AM, Heller G, Veri MC, et al. Activating and inhibitory IgG Fc receptors on human DCs mediate opposing functions. J Clin Invest 2005;115:2914-23.
39. Bazin R, Lemieux R, Tremblay T. Reversal of immune thrombocytopenia in mice by cross-linking human immunoglobulin G with a high-affinity monoclonal antibody. Br J Haematol 2006;135:97-100.
40. Song S, Crow AR, Siragam V, et al. Monoclonal antibodies that mimic the action of anti-D in the amelioration of murine ITP act by a mechanism distinct from that of IVIG. Blood 2005; 105:1546-8.
41. Lin SY, Kinet JP. Immunology. Giving inhibitory receptors a boost. Science 2001;291: 445-6.
42. Ott VL, Fong DC, Cambier JC. Fc gamma RIIB as a potential molecular target for intravenous gamma globulin therapy. J Allergy Clin Immunol 2001;108:S95-8.
43. Siragam V, Crow AR, Brinc D, et al. Intravenous immunoglobulin ameliorates ITP via activating Fcgamma receptors on dendritic cells. Nat Med 2006;12:688-92.
44. Tackenberg B, Jelcic I, Baerenwaldt A, et al. Impaired inhibitory Fc{gamma} receptor IIB expression on B cells in chronic inflammatory demyelinating polyneuropathy. Proc Natl Acad Sci U S A 2009;106:4788-92.
45. Bayary J, Dasgupta S, Misra N, et al. Intravenous immunoglobulin in autoimmune disorders: An insight into the immunoregulatory mechanisms. Int Immunopharmacol 2006;6: 528-34.
46. Crow AR, Lazarus AH. The mechanisms of action of intravenous immunoglobulin and polyclonal anti-d immunoglobulin in the amelioration of immune thrombocytopenic purpura: What do we really know? Transfus Med Rev 2008;22:103-16.
47. Blanchette VS, Kirby MA, Turner C. Role of intravenous immunoglobulin G in autoimmune hematologic disorders. Semin Hematol 1992; 29:72-82.
48. Dietrich G, Kazatchkine MD. Normal immunoglobulin G (IgG) for therapeutic use (intravenous Ig) contain antiidiotypic specificities against an immunodominant, disease-associated, cross-reactive idiotype of human anti-thyroglobulin autoantibodies. J Clin Invest 1990; 85:620-5.
49. Jayne DR, Davies MJ, Fox CJ, et al. Treatment of systemic vasculitis with pooled intravenous immunoglobulin. Lancet 1991;337:1137-9.
50. Tuso P, Moudgil A, Hay J, et al. Treatment of antineutrophil cytoplasmic autoantibody-positive systemic vasculitis and glomerulonephritis with pooled intravenous gammaglobulin. Am J Kidney Dis 1992;20:504-8.
51. Hurez V, Kaveri SV, Kazatchkine MD. Normal polyspecific immunoglobulin G (IVIG) in the treatment of autoimmune diseases. J Autoimmun 1993;6:675-81.
52. Liblau R, Gajdos P, Bustarret FA, et al. Intravenous gamma-globulin in myasthenia gravis: Interaction with anti-acetylcholine receptor autoantibodies. J Clin Immunol 1991;11:128-31.
53. Roifman CM, Schaffer FM, Wachsmuth SE, et al. Reversal of chronic polymyositis following intravenous immune serum globulin therapy. JAMA 1987;258:513-15.
54. Silverman ED, Laxer RM, Greenwald M, et al. Intravenous gamma globulin therapy in systemic juvenile rheumatoid arthritis. Arthritis Rheum 1990;33:1015-22.
55. Kazatchkine MD, Dietrich G, Hurez V, et al. V region-mediated selection of autoreactive repertoires by intravenous immunoglobulin (i.v.Ig). Immunol Rev 1994;139:79-107.
56. Jordan SC. Intravenous gamma-globulin therapy in systemic lupus erythematosus and immune complex disease. Clin Immunol Immunopathol 1989;53:S164-9.
57. Buchwald B, Ahangari R, Weishaupt A, Toyka KV. Intravenous immunoglobulins neutralize blocking antibodies in Guillain-Barré syndrome. Ann Neurol 2002;51:673-80.
58. Dalakas MC, Quarles RH, Farrer RG, et al. A controlled study of intravenous immunoglobu-

lin in demyelinating neuropathy with IgM gammopathy. Ann Neurol 1996;40:792-5.
59. Jakobsson T, Croner S, Kjellman NI, et al. Slight steroid-sparing effect of intravenous immunoglobulin in children and adolescents with moderately severe bronchial asthma. Allergy 1994;49:413-20.
60. Kimata H. High dose gammaglobulin treatment for atopic dermatitis. Arch Dis Child 1994;70:335-6.
61. Mazer BD, Gelfand EW. An open-label study of high-dose intravenous immunoglobulin in severe childhood asthma. J Allergy Clin Immunol 1991;87:976-83.
62. Rabinovitch N, Gelfand EW, Leung DY. The role of immunoglobulin therapy in allergic diseases. Allergy 1999;54:662-8.
63. Zhuang Q, Mazer B. Inhibition of IgE production in vitro by intact and fragmented intravenous immunoglobulin. J Allergy Clin Immunol 2001;108:229-34.
64. Rossi F, Sultan Y, Kazatchkine MD. Anti-idiotypes against autoantibodies and alloantibodies to VIII:C (anti-haemophilic factor) are present in therapeutic polyspecific normal immunoglobulins. Clin Exp Immunol 1988;74:311-16.
65. Krause I, Blank M, Kopolovic J, et al. Abrogation of experimental systemic lupus erythematosus and primary antiphospholipid syndrome with intravenous gamma globulin. J Rheumatol 1995;22:1068-74.
66. Kwak JY, Kwak FM, Ainbinder SW, et al. Elevated peripheral blood natural killer cells are effectively downregulated by immunoglobulin G infusion in women with recurrent spontaneous abortions. Am J Reprod Immunol 1996;35:363-9.
67. Krause I, Blank M, Sherer Y, et al. Induction of oral tolerance in experimental antiphospholipid syndrome by feeding with polyclonal immunoglobulins. Eur J Immunol 2002;32:3414-24.
68. Bystryn JC, Jiao D, Natow S. Treatment of pemphigus with intravenous immunoglobulin. J Am Acad Dermatol 2002;47:358-63.
69. Hughes R, Cusack C, Murphy GM, Kirby B. Solar urticaria successfully treated with intravenous immunoglobulin. Clin Exp Dermatol 2009.
70. Berchtold P, Dale GL, Tani P, McMillan R. Inhibition of autoantibody binding to platelet glycoprotein IIb/IIIa by anti-idiotypic antibodies in intravenous gammaglobulin. Blood 1989;74:2414-17.
71. Barbano G, Saleh MN, Mori PG, et al. Effect of intravenous gammaglobulin on circulating and platelet-bound antibody in immune thrombocytopenia. Blood 1989;73:662-5.
72. Debre M, Bonnet MC, Fridman WH, et al. Infusion of Fc gamma fragments for treatment of children with acute immune thrombocytopenic purpura. Lancet 1993;342:945-9.
73. Hansen RJ, Balthasar JP. Effects of intravenous immunoglobulin on platelet count and antiplatelet antibody disposition in a rat model of immune thrombocytopenia. Blood 2002;100:2087-93.
74. Marchalonis JJ, Kaymaz H, Dedeoglu F, et al. Human autoantibodies reactive with synthetic autoantigens from T-cell receptor beta chain. Proc Natl Acad Sci U S A 1992;89:3325-9.
75. Hurez V, Kaveri SV, Mouhoub A, et al. Anti-CD4 activity of normal human immunoglobulin G for therapeutic use. (Intravenous immunoglobulin, IVIg.) Ther Immunol 1994;1:269-77.
76. Vassilev T, Gelin C, Kaveri SV, et al. Antibodies to the CD5 molecule in normal human immunoglobulins for therapeutic use (intravenous immunoglobulins, IVIg). Clin Exp Immunol 1993;92:369-72.
77. Bayry J, Lacroix-Desmazes S, Donkova-Petrini V, et al. Natural antibodies sustain differentiation and maturation of human dendritic cells. Proc Natl Acad Sci U S A 2004;101:14210-15.
78. Bendtzen K, Hansen MB, Ross C, Svenson M. High-avidity autoantibodies to cytokines. Immunol Today 1998;19:209-11.
79. Kaveri S, Vassilev T, Hurez V, et al. Antibodies to a conserved region of HLA Class I molecules, capable of modulating CD8 T cell-mediated function, are present in pooled normal immunoglobulin for therapeutic use. J Clin Invest 1996;97:865-9.
80. Delfraissy JF, Tchernia G, Laurian Y, et al. Suppressor cell function after intravenous gammaglobulin treatment in adult chronic idiopathic thrombocytopenic purpura. Br J Haematol 1985;60:315-22.
81. Dammacco F, Iodice G, Campobasso N. Treatment of adult patients with idiopathic thrombocytopenic purpura with intravenous immunoglobulin: Effects on circulating T cell subsets and PWM-induced antibody synthesis in vitro. Br J Haematol 1986;62:125-35.
82. Macey MG, Newland AC. CD4 and CD8 subpopulation changes during high dose intrave-

nous immunoglobulin treatment. Br J Haematol 1990;76:513-20.
83. Shoenfeld Y, Fishman P. Gamma-globulin inhibits tumor spread in mice. Int Immunol 1999;11:1247-52.
84. Tsubakio T, Kurata Y, Katagiri S, et al. Alteration of T cell subsets and immunoglobulin synthesis in vitro during high dose gammaglobulin therapy in patients with idiopathic thrombocytopenic purpura. Clin Exp Immunol 1983;53:697-702.
85. Chiller JM, Habicht GS, Weigle WO. Cellular sites of immunologic unresponsiveness. Proc Natl Acad Sci U S A 1970;65:551-6.
86. van Schaik IN, Lundkvist I, Vermeulen M, Brand A. Polyvalent immunoglobulin for intravenous use interferes with cell proliferation in vitro. J Clin Immunol 1992;12:325-34.
87. Zhu KY, Feferman T, Maiti PK, et al. Intravenous immunoglobulin suppresses experimental myasthenia gravis: Immunological mechanisms. J Neuroimmunol 2006;176:187-97.
88. Bayry J, Lacroix-Desmazes S, Kazatchkine MD, et al. Common variable immunodeficiency is associated with defective functions of dendritic cells. Blood 2004;104:2441-3.
89. Lowy I, Brezin C, Neauport-Sautes C, et al. Isotype regulation of antibody production: T-cell hybrids can be selectively induced to produce IgG1 and IgG2 subclass-specific suppressive immunoglobulin-binding factors. Proc Natl Acad Sci U S A 1983;80:2323-7.
90. Kondo N, Kasahara K, Kameyama T, et al. Intravenous immunoglobulins suppress immunoglobulin productions by suppressing Ca(2+)-dependent signal transduction through Fc gamma receptors in B lymphocytes. Scand J Immunol 1994;40:37-42.
91. Green MG, Bystryn JC. Effect of intravenous immunoglobulin therapy on serum levels of IgG1 and IgG4 antidesmoglein 1 and antidesmoglein 3 antibodies in pemphigus vulgaris. Arch Dermatol 2008;144:1621-4.
92. Jordan SC, Tyan D, Stablein D, et al. Evaluation of intravenous immunoglobulin as an agent to lower allosensitization and improve transplantation in highly sensitized adult patients with end-stage renal disease: Report of the NIH IG02 trial. J Am Soc Nephrol 2004;15:3256-62.
93. Le Pottier L, Bendaoud B, Dueymes M, et al. BAFF, a new target for intravenous immunoglobulin in autoimmunity and cancer. J Clin Immunol 2007;27:257-65.
94. Toungouz M, Denys CH, De Groote D, Dupont E. In vitro inhibition of tumour necrosis factor-alpha and interleukin-6 production by intravenous immunoglobulins. Br J Haematol 1995; 89:698-703.
95. Kieseier BC, Kiefer R, Clements JM, et al. Matrix metalloproteinase-9 and -7 are regulated in experimental autoimmune encephalomyelitis. Brain 1998;121(Pt 1):159-66.
96. Dalakas MC. Mechanisms of action of IVIG and therapeutic considerations in the treatment of acute and chronic demyelinating neuropathies. Neurology 2002;59:S13-21.
97. Senzaki H, Masutani S, Kobayashi J, et al. Circulating matrix metalloproteinases and their inhibitors in patients with Kawasaki disease. Circulation 2001;104:860-3.
98. Kekow J, Reinhold D, Pap T, Ansorge S. Intravenous immunoglobulins and transforming growth factor beta. Lancet 1998;351:184-5.
99. Clark DA, Wong K, Banwatt D, et al. CD200-dependent and nonCD200-dependent pathways of NK cell suppression by human IVIG. J Assist Reprod Genet 2008;25:67-72.
100. Blaszczyk R, Westhoff U, Grosse-Wilde H. Soluble CD4, CD8, and HLA molecules in commercial immunoglobulin preparations. Lancet 1993;341:789-90.
101. Altznauer F, von Gunten S, Spath P, Simon HU. Concurrent presence of agonistic and antagonistic anti-CD95 autoantibodies in intravenous Ig preparations. J Allergy Clin Immunol 2003;112:1185-90.
102. Vuist WM, Van Schaik IN, Van Lint M, Brand A. The growth arresting effect of human immunoglobulin for intravenous use is mediated by antibodies recognizing membrane glycolipids. J Clin Immunol 1997;17:301-10.
103. Prasad NK, Papoff G, Zeuner A, et al. Therapeutic preparations of normal polyspecific IgG (IVIg) induce apoptosis in human lymphocytes and monocytes: A novel mechanism of action of IVIG involving the Fas apoptotic pathway. J Immunol 1998;161:3781-90.
104. Viard I, Wehrli P, Bullani R, et al. Inhibition of toxic epidermal necrolysis by blockade of CD95 with human intravenous immunoglobulin. Science 1998;282:490-3.
105. Romanelli P, Schlam E, Green JB, et al. Immunohistochemical evaluation of toxic epidermal necrolysis treated with human intravenous immunoglobulin. G Ital Dermatol Venereol 2008;143:229-33.

106. Michael D, Grando SA. Novel mechanism for therapeutic action of IVIG in autoimmune blistering dermatoses. Curr Dir Autoimmun 2008;10:333-43.
107. Caccavelli L, Field AC, Betin V, et al. Normal IgG protects against acute graft-versus-host disease by targeting CD4(+)CD134(+) donor alloreactive T cells. Eur J Immunol 2001; 31:2781-90.
108. Tsujimoto H, Takeshita S, Nakatani K, et al. Intravenous immunoglobulin therapy induces neutrophil apoptosis in Kawasaki disease. Clin Immunol 2002;103:161-8.
109. Leytin V, Mykhaylov S, Starkey AF, et al. Intravenous immunoglobulin inhibits anti-glycoprotein IIb-induced platelet apoptosis in a murine model of immune thrombocytopenia. Br J Haematol 2006;133:78-82.
110. von Gunten S, Simon HU. Natural anti-Siglec autoantibodies mediate potential immunoregulatory mechanisms: Implications for the clinical use of intravenous immunoglobulins (IVIg). Autoimmun Rev 2008;7:453-6.
111. von Gunten S, Vogel M, Schaub A, et al. Intravenous immunoglobulin preparations contain anti-Siglec-8 autoantibodies. J Allergy Clin Immunol 2007;119:1005-11.
112. von Gunten S, Schaub A, Vogel M, et al. Immunologic and functional evidence for anti-Siglec-9 autoantibodies in intravenous immunoglobulin preparations. Blood 2006;108:4255-9.
113. Tsurikisawa N, Taniguchi M, Saito H, et al. Treatment of Churg-Strauss syndrome with high-dose intravenous immunoglobulin. Ann Allergy Asthma Immunol 2004;92:80-7.
114. Zhou B, Zhao H, Yang RC, Han ZC. Multi-dysfunctional pathophysiology in ITP. Crit Rev Oncol Hematol 2005;54:107-16.
115. Cooper N, Heddle NM, Haas M, et al. Intravenous (IV) anti-D and IV immunoglobulin achieve acute platelet increases by different mechanisms: Modulation of cytokine and platelet responses to IV anti-D by FcgammaRIIa and FcgammaRIIIa polymorphisms. Br J Haematol 2004;124:511-18.
116. Sewell WA, North ME, Cambronero R, et al. In vivo modulation of cytokine synthesis by intravenous immunoglobulin. Clin Exp Immunol 1999;116:509-15.
117. Aukrust P, Froland SS, Liabakk NB, et al. Release of cytokines, soluble cytokine receptors, and interleukin-1 receptor antagonist after intravenous immunoglobulin administration in vivo. Blood 1994;84:2136-43.
118. Arend WP, Leung DY. IgG induction of IL-1 receptor antagonist production by human monocytes. Immunol Rev 1994;139:71-8.
119. Arend WP, Malyak M, Guthridge CJ, Gabay C. Interleukin-1 receptor antagonist: Role in biology. Annu Rev Immunol 1998;16:27-55.
120. Iizasa H, Yoneyama H, Mukaida N, et al. Exacerbation of granuloma formation in IL-1 receptor antagonist-deficient mice with impaired dendritic cell maturation associated with Th2 cytokine production. J Immunol 2005;174: 3273-80.
121. Ibanez C, Sune P, Fierro A, et al. Modulating effects of intravenous immunoglobulins on serum cytokine levels in patients with primary hypogammaglobulinemia. BioDrugs 2005;19: 59-65.
122. Deng H, Yang X, Jin T, et al. The role of IL-12 and TNF-alpha in AIDP and AMAN. Eur J Neurol 2008;15:1100-5.
123. Sharief MK, Ingram DA, Swash M, Thompson EJ. I.v. immunoglobulin reduces circulating proinflammatory cytokines in Guillain-Barré syndrome. Neurology 1999;52:1833-8.
124. Reinhold D, Perlov E, Schrecke K, et al. Increased blood plasma concentrations of TGF-beta isoforms after treatment with intravenous immunoglobulins (i.v.IG) in patients with multiple sclerosis. J Neuroimmunol 2004; 152:191-4.
125. Dalakas MC, Illa I, Dambrosia JM, et al. A controlled trial of high-dose intravenous immune globulin infusions as treatment for dermatomyositis. N Engl J Med 1993;329:1993-2000.
126. Keskin DB, Stern JN, Fridkis-Hareli M, Razzaque Ahmed A. Cytokine profiles in pemphigus vulgaris patients treated with intravenous immunoglobulins as compared to conventional immunosuppressive therapy. Cytokine 2008; 41:315-21.
127. Kieseier BC, Tani M, Mahad D, et al. Chemokines and chemokine receptors in inflammatory demyelinating neuropathies: A central role for IP-10. Brain 2002;125:823-34.
128. Damas JK, Gullestad L, Aass H, et al. Enhanced gene expression of chemokines and their corresponding receptors in mononuclear blood cells in chronic heart failure—modulatory effect of intravenous immunoglobulin. J Am Coll Cardiol 2001;38:187-93.
129. Hirono K, Kemmotsu Y, Wittkowski H, et al. Infliximab reduces the cytokine-mediated inflammation but does not suppress cellular infiltration of the vessel wall in refractory

Kawasaki disease. Pediatr Res 2009;65:696-701.
130. Gullestad L, Aass H, Fjeld JG, et al. Immunomodulating therapy with intravenous immunoglobulin in patients with chronic heart failure. Circulation 2001;103:220-5.
131. Kishimoto C, Shioji K, Kinoshita M, et al. Treatment of acute inflammatory cardiomyopathy with intravenous immunoglobulin ameliorates left ventricular function associated with suppression of inflammatory cytokines and decreased oxidative stress. Int J Cardiol 2003; 91:173-8.
132. Stouffer GA, Sheahan RG, Lenihan DJ, et al. The current status of immune modulating therapy for myocarditis: A case of acute parvovirus myocarditis treated with intravenous immunoglobulin. Am J Med Sci 2003;326:369-74.
133. Leung DY, Cotran RS, Kurt-Jones E, et al. Endothelial cell activation and high interleukin-1 secretion in the pathogenesis of acute Kawasaki disease. Lancet 1989;2:1298-1302.
134. Achiron A, Margalit R, Hershkoviz R, et al. Intravenous immunoglobulin treatment of experimental T cell-mediated autoimmune disease. Upregulation of T cell proliferation and downregulation of tumor necrosis factor alpha secretion. J Clin Invest 1994;93:600-5.
135. Andersson U, Bjork L, Skansen-Saphir U, Andersson J. Pooled human IgG modulates cytokine production in lymphocytes and monocytes. Immunol Rev 1994;139:21-42.
136. Ruiz de Souza V, Carreno MP, Kaveri SV, et al. Selective induction of interleukin-1 receptor antagonist and interleukin-8 in human monocytes by normal polyspecific IgG (intravenous immunoglobulin). Eur J Immunol 1995;25: 1267-73.
137. Mouzaki A, Theodoropoulou M, Gianakopoulos I, et al. Expression patterns of Th1 and Th2 cytokine genes in childhood idiopathic thrombocytopenic purpura (ITP) at presentation and their modulation by intravenous immunoglobulin G (IVIg) treatment: Their role in prognosis. Blood 2002;100:1774-9.
138. Bruhns P, Samuelsson A, Pollard JW, Ravetch JV. Colony-stimulating factor-1-dependent macrophages are responsible for IVIG protection in antibody-induced autoimmune disease. Immunity 2003;18:573-81.
139. Crow AR, Song S, Semple JW, et al. A role for IL-1 receptor antagonist or other cytokines in the acute therapeutic effects of IVIg? Blood 2007;109:155-8.
140. Aubin E, Lemieux R, Bazin R. Absence of cytokine modulation following therapeutic infusion of intravenous immunoglobulin or anti-red blood cell antibodies in a mouse model of immune thrombocytopenic purpura. Br J Haematol 2007;136:837-43.
141. Basta M, Fries LF, Frank MM. High doses of intravenous Ig inhibit in vitro uptake of C4 fragments onto sensitized erythrocytes. Blood 1991;77:376-80.
142. Lutz HU, Stammler P, Bianchi V, et al. Intravenously applied IgG stimulates complement attenuation in a complement-dependent autoimmune disease at the amplifying C3 convertase level. Blood 2004;103:465-72.
143. Basta M, Van Goor F, Luccioli S, et al. F(ab)'2-mediated neutralization of C3a and C5a anaphylatoxins: A novel effector function of immunoglobulins. Nat Med 2003;9:431-8.
144. Basta M, Langlois PF, Marques M, et al. High-dose intravenous immunoglobulin modifies complement-mediated in vivo clearance. Blood 1989;74:326-33.
145. Mollnes TE, Hogasen K, De Carolis C, et al. High-dose intravenous immunoglobulin treatment activates complement in vivo. Scand J Immunol 1998;48:312-17.
146. Basta M, Illa I, Dalakas MC. Increased in vitro uptake of the complement C3b in the serum of patients with Guillain-Barré syndrome, myasthenia gravis and dermatomyositis. J Neuroimmunol 1996;71:227-9.
147. Laupland KB, Kirkpatrick AW, Delaney A. Polyclonal intravenous immunoglobulin for the treatment of severe sepsis and septic shock in critically ill adults: A systematic review and meta-analysis. Crit Care Med 2007;35:2686-92.
148. Arumugam TV, Tang SC, Lathia JD, et al. Intravenous immunoglobulin (IVIG) protects the brain against experimental stroke by preventing complement-mediated neuronal cell death. Proc Natl Acad Sci U S A 2007;104: 14104-9.
149. Persson L, Boren J, Nicoletti A, et al. Immunoglobulin treatment reduces atherosclerosis in apolipoprotein E–low-density lipoprotein recepto–mice via the complement system. Clin Exp Immunol 2005;142:441-5.
150. Rostoker G, Desvaux-Belghiti D, Pilatte Y, et al. High-dose immunoglobulin therapy for severe IgA nephropathy and Henoch-Schonlein purpura. Ann Intern Med 1994;120:476-84.

151. Basta M, Dalakas MC. High-dose intravenous immunoglobulin exerts its beneficial effect in patients with dermatomyositis by blocking endomysial deposition of activated complement fragments. J Clin Invest 1994;94:1729-35.
152. Hed J. Role of complement in immune or idiopathic thrombocytopenic purpura. Acta Paediatr Suppl 1998;424:37-40.
153. Basta M, Frank M, Fries LF. Attenuation of complement immune damage by intravenous immunoglobulins. In: Rewald E, Morell A, eds. Immunomodulation by intravenous immunoglobulin. New York: The Parthenon Publishing Group, 1993:43-55.
154. Nomura S, Miyazaki Y, Miyake T, et al. IgG inhibits the increase of platelet-associated C3 stimulated by anti-platelet antibodies. Clin Exp Immunol 1993;93:452-5.
155. Winiarski J, Kreuger A, Ejderhamn J, Holm G. High dose intravenous IgG reduces platelet associated immunoglobulins and complement in idiopathic thrombocytopenic purpura. Scand J Haematol 1983;31:342-8.
156. Simister NE, Mostov KE. An Fc receptor structurally related to MHC Class I antigens. Nature 1989;337:184-7.
157. Fateh-Moghadam A, Wick M, Besinger U, Geursen RG. High-dose intravenous gammaglobulin for myasthenia gravis. Lancet 1984;1:848-9.
158. Hammarstrom L, Abedi MR, Hassan MS, Smith CI. The SCID mouse as a model for autoimmunity. J Autoimmun 1993;6:667-74.
159. Dalakas MC, Fujii M, Li M, et al. High-dose intravenous immune globulin for stiff-person syndrome. N Engl J Med 2001;345:1870-6.
160. Israel EJ, Wilsker DF, Hayes KC, et al. Increased clearance of IgG in mice that lack beta 2-microglobulin: Possible protective role of FcRn. Immunology 1996;89:573-8.
161. Junghans RP, Anderson CL. The protection receptor for IgG catabolism is the beta2-microglobulin-containing neonatal intestinal transport receptor. Proc Natl Acad Sci U S A 1996;93:5512-16.
162. Hansen RJ, Balthasar JP. Intravenous immunoglobulin mediates an increase in anti-platelet antibody clearance via the FcRn receptor. Thromb Haemost 2002;88:898-9.
163. Akilesh S, Petkova S, Sproule TJ, et al. The MHC class I-like Fc receptor promotes humorally mediated autoimmune disease. J Clin Invest 2004;113:1328-33.
164. Li N, Zhao M, Hilario-Vargas J, et al. Complete FcRn dependence for intravenous Ig therapy in autoimmune skin blistering diseases. J Clin Invest 2005;115:3440-50.
165. Villadangos JA, Schnorrer P. Intrinsic and cooperative antigen-presenting functions of dendritic-cell subsets in vivo. Nat Rev Immunol 2007;7:543-55.
166. Banchereau J, Schuler-Thurner B, Palucka AK, Schuler G. Dendritic cells as vectors for therapy. Cell 2001;106:271-4.
167. Bayry J, Lacroix-Desmazes S, Carbonneil C, et al. Inhibition of maturation and function of dendritic cells by intravenous immunoglobulin. Blood 2003;101:758-65.
168. Bogdan C, Vodovotz Y, Nathan C. Macrophage deactivation by interleukin 10. J Exp Med 1991;174:1549-55.
169. Smed-Sorensen A, Moll M, Cheng TY, et al. IgG regulates the CD1 expression profile and lipid antigen-presenting function in human dendritic cells via FcgammaRIIa. Blood 2008;111:5037-46.
170. Shioji K, Kishimoto C, Sasayama S. Fc receptor-mediated inhibitory effect of immunoglobulin therapy on autoimmune giant cell myocarditis: Concomitant suppression of the expression of dendritic cells. Circ Res 2001;89:540-6.
171. Ohkuma K, Sasaki T, Kamei S, et al. Modulation of dendritic cell development by immunoglobulin G in control subjects and multiple sclerosis patients. Clin Exp Immunol 2007;150:397-406.
172. Kaneko Y, Nimmerjahn F, Ravetch JV. Anti-inflammatory activity of immunoglobulin G resulting from Fc sialylation. Science 2006;313:670-3.
173. Jefferis R, Lund J. Interaction sites on human IgG-Fc for FcgammaR: Current models. Immunol Lett 2002;82:57-65.
174. Takeda M, Yamada H, Iwabuchi K, et al. Administration of high-dose intact immunoglobulin has an anti-resorption effect in a mouse model of reproductive failure. Mol Hum Reprod 2007;13:807-14.
175. Anthony RM, Wermeling F, Karlsson MC, Ravetch JV. Identification of a receptor required for the anti-inflammatory activity of IVIG. Proc Natl Acad Sci U S A 2008;105:19571-8.
176. Park-Min KH, Serbina NV, Yang W, et al. FcgammaRIII-dependent inhibition of interferon-gamma responses mediates suppressive

effects of intravenous immune globulin. Immunity 2007;26:67-78.
177. Moretta L, Ferlazzo G, Bottino C, et al. Effector and regulatory events during natural killer-dendritic cell interactions. Immunol Rev 2006;214:219-28.
178. Tha-In T, Metselaar HJ, Tilanus HW, et al. Intravenous immunoglobulins suppress T-cell priming by modulating the bidirectional interaction between dendritic cells and natural killer cells. Blood 2007;110:3253-62.
179. Savill J, Dransfield I, Gregory C, Haslett C. A blast from the past: Clearance of apoptotic cells regulates immune responses. Nat Rev Immunol 2002;2:965-75.
180. Pillarisetty VG, Katz SC, Bleier JI, et al. Natural killer dendritic cells have both antigen presenting and lytic function and in response to CpG produce IFN-gamma via autocrine IL-12. J Immunol 2005;174:2612-18.
181. Akira S, Uematsu S, Takeuchi O. Pathogen recognition and innate immunity. Cell 2006;124:783-801.
182. Taieb J, Chaput N, Menard C, et al. A novel dendritic cell subset involved in tumor immunosurveillance. Nat Med 2006;12:214-19.
183. Chauvin C, Josien R. Dendritic cells as killers: Mechanistic aspects and potential roles. J Immunol 2008;181:11-16.
184. Sakaguchi S, Sakaguchi N, Asano M, et al. Immunologic self-tolerance maintained by activated T cells expressing IL-2 receptor alpha-chains (CD25). Breakdown of a single mechanism of self-tolerance causes various autoimmune diseases. J Immunol 1995;155:1151-64.
185. Vignali DA, Collison LW, Workman CJ. How regulatory T cells work. Nat Rev Immunol 2008;8:523-32.
186. Ephrem A, Chamat S, Miquel C, et al. Expansion of CD4+CD25+ regulatory T cells by intravenous immunoglobulin: A critical factor in controlling experimental autoimmune encephalomyelitis. Blood 2008;111:715-22.
187. Chi LJ, Wang HB, Zhang Y, Wang WZ. Abnormality of circulating CD4(+)CD25(+) regulatory T cell in patients with Guillain-Barré syndrome. J Neuroimmunol 2007;192:206-14.
188. Kessel A, Ammuri H, Peri R, et al. Intravenous immunoglobulin therapy affects T regulatory cells by increasing their suppressive function. J Immunol 2007;179:5571-5.
189. Barreto M, Ferreira RC, Lourenco L, et al. Low frequency of CD4+CD25+ Treg in SLE patients: A heritable trait associated with CTLA4 and TGFbeta gene variants. BMC Immunol 2009;10:5.
190. Liu B, Zhao H, Poon MC, et al. Abnormality of CD4(+)CD25(+) regulatory T cells in idiopathic thrombocytopenic purpura. Eur J Haematol 2007;78:139-43.
191. Yu J, Heck S, Patel V, et al. Defective circulating CD25 regulatory T cells in patients with chronic immune thrombocytopenic purpura. Blood 2008;112:1325-8.
192. De Groot AS, Moise L, McMurry JA, et al. Activation of natural regulatory T cells by IgG Fc-derived peptide "Tregitopes." Blood 2008;112:3303-11.
193. Anthony RM, Nimmerjahn F, Ashline DJ, et al. Recapitulation of IVIG anti-inflammatory activity with a recombinant IgG Fc. Science 2008;320:373-6.
194. Ammann AJ, Ashman RF, Buckley RH, et al. Use of intravenous gamma-globulin in antibody immunodeficiency: Results of a multicenter controlled trial. Clin Immunol Immunopathol 1982;22:60-7.
195. Buckley RH, Schiff RI. The use of intravenous immune globulin in immunodeficiency diseases. N Engl J Med 1991;325:110-17.
196. Cunningham-Rundles C, Siegal FP, Smithwick EM, et al. Efficacy of intravenous immunoglobulin in primary humoral immunodeficiency disease. Ann Intern Med 1984;101:435-9.
197. Aghamohammadi A, Moin M, Farhoudi A, et al. Efficacy of intravenous immunoglobulin on the prevention of pneumonia in patients with agammaglobulinemia. FEMS Immunol Med Microbiol 2004;40:113-18.
198. Busse PJ, Razvi S, Cunningham-Rundles C. Efficacy of intravenous immunoglobulin in the prevention of pneumonia in patients with common variable immunodeficiency. J Allergy Clin Immunol 2002;109:1001-4.
199. Martinez Garcia MA, de Rojas MD, Nauffal Manzur MD, et al. Respiratory disorders in common variable immunodeficiency. Respir Med 2001;95:191-5.
200. Roifman CM, Rao CP, Lederman HM, et al. Increased susceptibility to Mycoplasma infection in patients with hypogammaglobulinemia. Am J Med 1986;80:590-4.
201. Stroehlein JR. Treatment of *Clostridium difficile* infection. Curr Treat Options Gastroenterol 2004;7:235-9.
202. Dodel R, Hampel H, Depboylu C, et al. Human antibodies against amyloid beta peptide: A

potential treatment for Alzheimer's disease. Ann Neurol 2002;52:253-6.
203. Relkin NR, Szabo P, Adamiak B, et al. 18-Month study of intravenous immunoglobulin for treatment of mild Alzheimer disease. Neurobiol Aging 2008;30:1728-36.
204. Warrington AE, Asakura K, Bieber AJ, et al. Human monoclonal antibodies reactive to oligodendrocytes promote remyelination in a model of multiple sclerosis. Proc Natl Acad Sci U S A 2000;97:6820-5.
205. Stangel M, Compston A, Scolding NJ. Polyclonal immunoglobulins for intravenous use do not influence the behaviour of cultured oligodendrocytes. J Neuroimmunol 1999;96:228-33.
206. Gabriel CM, Gregson NA, Redford EJ, et al. Human immunoglobulin ameliorates rat experimental autoimmune neuritis. Brain 1997;120(Pt 9):1533-40.
207. Negi VS, Elluru S, Siberil S, et al. Intravenous immunoglobulin: An update on the clinical use and mechanisms of action. J Clin Immunol 2007;27:233-45.
208. Kuhlmann T, Bruck W. Immunoglobulins induce increased myelin debris clearance by mouse macrophages. Neurosci Lett 1999;275:191-4.
209. Zivadinov R, Reder AT, Filippi M, et al. Mechanisms of action of disease-modifying agents and brain volume changes in multiple sclerosis. Neurology 2008;71:136-44.
210. Spahn JD, Leung DY, Chan MT, et al. Mechanisms of glucocorticoid reduction in asthmatic subjects treated with intravenous immunoglobulin. J Allergy Clin Immunol 1999;103:421-6.
211. Lapointe BM, Herx LM, Gill V, et al. IVIg therapy in brain inflammation: Etiology-dependent differential effects on leucocyte recruitment. Brain 2004;127:2649-56.
212. Miller DH, Khan OA, Sheremata WA, et al. A controlled trial of natalizumab for relapsing multiple sclerosis. N Engl J Med 2003;348:15-23.
213. Gill V, Doig C, Knight D, et al. Targeting adhesion molecules as a potential mechanism of action for intravenous immunoglobulin. Circulation 2005;112:2031-9.
214. Turhan A, Jenab P, Bruhns P, et al. Intravenous immune globulin prevents venular vaso-occlusion in sickle cell mice by inhibiting leukocyte adhesion and the interactions between sickle erythrocytes and adherent leukocytes. Blood 2004;103:2397-400.
215. Arumugam TV, Woodruff TM, Lathia JD, et al. Neuroprotection in stroke by complement inhibition and immunoglobulin therapy. Neuroscience 2009;158:1074-89.
216. Xu C, Poirier B, Van Huyen JP, et al. Modulation of endothelial cell function by normal polyspecific human intravenous immunoglobulins: A possible mechanism of action in vascular diseases. Am J Pathol 1998;153:1257-66.
217. Jerzak M, Rechberger T, Gorski A. Intravenous immunoglobulin therapy influences T cell adhesion to extracellular matrix in women with a history of recurrent spontaneous abortions. Am J Reprod Immunol 2000;44:336-41.
218. Vassilev TL, Kazatchkine MD, Van Huyen JP, et al. Inhibition of cell adhesion by antibodies to Arg-Gly-Asp (RGD) in normal immunoglobulin for therapeutic use (intravenous immunoglobulin, IVIg). Blood 1999;93:3624-31.

4

IVIG for Hematologic Disorders

W. Beau Mitchell, MD, and James B. Bussel, MD

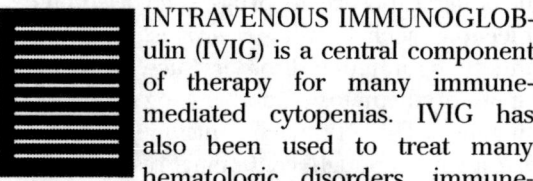INTRAVENOUS IMMUNOGLOBulin (IVIG) is a central component of therapy for many immune-mediated cytopenias. IVIG has also been used to treat many hematologic disorders, immune-mediated and otherwise, but much of what is known about the use of IVIG for hematologic diseases has been gleaned from its use in immune thrombocytopenia (ITP), where it is clearly efficacious in 80% of cases. IVIG treatment is effective for mothers and neonates at risk for fetal/neonatal ITP as well as for patients with human immunodeficiency virus (HIV)-related thrombocytopenia. IVIG therapy is also warranted in posttransfusion purpura (PTP), which is rare. Other immune cytopenias have been variably responsive to IVIG therapy: autoimmune-mediated neutropenia is generally responsive to IVIG therapy, whereas autoimmune hemolytic anemia (AIHA) is much less responsive. Evans syndrome, which is combined ITP and hemolytic anemia, can be transiently responsive to IVIG.

The mechanism of the IVIG effect in hematologic diseases has been explored most thoroughly in ITP, revealing a surprisingly wide range of potential interactions with the immunologic abnormalities and characteristics of ITP. Models of IVIG effects on the immune system have ranged from peripheral anti-idiotype blockade to central regulation of the immune response via direct interaction with dendritic cells. The major indications for IVIG in hematologic diseases will be presented in this chapter.

Immune Thrombocytopenia

ITP is an acquired autoimmune disease generally characterized by a mild-to-severe decrease in platelet number (thrombocytopenia), increased

---

W. Beau Mitchell, MD, Associate Member and Head of Laboratory of Platelet Biology, New York Blood Center, and James B. Bussel, MD, Professor, Departments of Pediatrics, Medicine, and Obstetrics and Gynecology, New York Presbyterian Hospital, Weill Cornell Medical Center, New York, New York

W.B. Mitchell has disclosed no conflicts of interest. J. Bussel has disclosed financial relationships with Amgen, Cangene, GlaxoSmithKline, Genzyme, Immunomedics, Ligand, Eisai, and Sysmex.

megakaryocyte number in the marrow, and a variable degree of bleeding from the mucus membranes and skin. The disorder results primarily from the production of autoantibodies against platelet glycoproteins, which causes both accelerated clearance of platelets from the blood and impaired platelet production in the marrow. The clear demonstration that "idiopathic" thrombocytopenia was actually "immune" came in 1951 with Harrington's famous experiments, in which he injected plasma from ITP patients into his and his colleagues' blood streams.[1]

Not all ITP is clearly the result of antibody-mediated platelet clearance, because autoantibodies are not detected in 40% of patients. Whether this results from the limitations of current detection methods or is indicative of an alternate destructive pathway is not known. However, because splenectomy and IVIG are initially effective in 80% of patients, it is presumed that at least 80% of cases are antibody mediated. Several studies have also indicated a role for T-cell-mediated cytotoxicity in at least some cases of ITP, with the clinical implication that an IVIG-insensitive mechanism leads to the thrombocytopenia in a fraction of patients with ITP.

Treatment of ITP with IVIG was one of the earliest uses—and certainly the most successful use—of IVIG for hematologic disease other than in gammaglobinopathy. The first reported use of IVIG for ITP was by Paul Imbach and colleagues from Bern, Swizerland in 1981.[2] Over the preceding several years, Imbach and colleagues—in particular, Silvio Barandun—had noted that one boy with thrombocytopenia secondary to Wiskott-Aldrich syndrome had had substantial improvement in his platelet counts after he received IVIG for his immunodeficiency. Thus, when they were faced with a child with ITP in whom all other therapies had failed and whose levels of immunoglobulins were low (in large part because of previous therapy including cyclophosphamide), they decided to try IVIG. The patient responded dramatically to the IVIG, as did the next 12 children with ITP who were treated similarly.[2] A smaller group of patients with marrow failure disorders and thrombocytopenia were also treated, but without any platelet effect. These findings were rapidly translated to adults, with substantial and dramatic platelet increases occurring in most patients.[3-5] Thus, IVIG became firmly established as a new, important treatment modality for ITP by 1983, and it quickly became a first-line agent for treatment of ITP, especially in children but also, more slowly, in adults.

Children account for about 50% of ITP patients, and in 80% to 90% of cases, their symptoms typically resolve or at least substantially improve within 1 year, regardless of therapy.[6-10] However, many adults and some children will develop chronic ITP, with their symptoms persisting beyond 1 year from diagnosis, if not indefinitely. Patients with concurrent illness, abnormal physical exam, or medication use may have secondary ITP, which accounts for approximately 20% of so-called ITP. Secondary ITP has many known causes, including exposure to drugs such as quinine, infections such as with *Helicobacter pylori*, or underlying immune disorders such as systemic lupus erythematosus and hypogammaglobulinemia. The primary inciting event is unknown, although continuing research indicates that ITP may represent the cumulative response to a diverse collection of immune insults. This diversity is reflected in the heterogeneity of the clinical picture of ITP, its pathophysiology, and in the variable responses to therapy, including IVIG. Remarkably, despite this heterogeneity, 80% of ITP patients are responsive to therapy with IVIG. Many of the identified immunologic defects of ITP are modulated in some way by IVIG, and as more of the pathophysiology of ITP is revealed, more is understood about the mechanisms of IVIG therapy.

Many potential mechanisms of action have been hypothesized for the effects of IVIG in ITP, not nearly all of which can be considered or fully discussed here. IVIG was originally thought to physically interfere with the clearance of autoantibody-coated platelets by blockade of (activating) Fc receptors on macrophages of the reticuloendothelial system. This was suggested by the need for intact IgG molecules[11,12] and strongly supported by studies that showed that IVIG interfered with the clearance of radiolabeled antibody-coated red cells.[5,13] Further work in the first half of the 1980s also demonstrated remarkable, albeit very transient, effects to increase the platelet count in patients with refractory ITP with infusion of a monoclonal antibody that inhibited ligand binding to FcRIII.[14] Furthermore, IV anti-D was tried in ITP patients, based on studies by Salama and Mueller-Eckhardt indicating that the direct antiglobulin test was often transiently positive after IVIG and other laboratory parameters (eg, bilirubin and haptoglobin) were also consistent with hemolysis.[15] The initial set of four trials with IV anti-D all showed a clear majority of Rh+, nonsplenectomized patients having an important increase in the platelet count.[15-18] The clinical effects of the monoclonal anti-FcRIII antibody and of anti-D therapy therefore strongly supported the hypothesis that IVIG worked primarily by interference with the destruction of antibody-coated platelets.

Evolution of IVIG Treatment of Immune Thrombocytopenia

The primary medical goal in therapy for ITP is to prevent life-threatening bleeding such as bleeding within the brain. These events are rare, occurring in <1% of patients,[19] and usually occur when the platelet count is below 20,000/μL. Thus, the nominal goal of therapy is to raise the platelet count above 20,000/μL as rapidly as possible. IVIG infusion most often raises the platelet count over 20,000 to 50,000/μL within 24 hours and is nearly universally effective, making it a first-line therapy for severe ITP. A high-dose of IV anti-D, 75 μg/kg, can also rapidly increase the platelet count[20] but is effective only in Rh+, DAT−, nonsplenectomized individuals and will decrease the hemoglobin by 1 to 2 g/dL, which excludes a small percentage of patients and somewhat limits its tolerability.

Imbach and colleagues treated their pediatric ITP patients with the same IVIG administration regimen that they and others were using for hypogammaglobulinemia patients in 1981— 400 mg/kg daily—but for 5 days.[2] In the same year, Schmidt and colleagues reported that high-dose IVIG resulted in increased platelet counts in four adults with ITP, confirming that both adults and children with either chronic or new-onset ITP responded to high-dose IVIG.[3] Newland and colleagues treated a larger group of adults with ITP and reported that although all 25 patients had some response, the effects were not sustained; hence, IVIG was not curative by itself.[4] Bussel and colleagues treated a group of pediatric and adult ITP patients and found that children had a better response to IVIG than adults.[5] Seven of the eight children had lasting responses to IVIG therapy, including two who went into remission, whereas only two of four adults remained responsive to IVIG. These studies established IVIG as a potent novel therapy for ITP.

Since the initial dosing of IVIG was empirically based on therapy for hypogammaglobinopathy, several dose-finding studies were reported over the next decade. Bussel and colleagues compressed the 5-day IVIG regimen into a single dose of 1 g/kg, which could be administered to children in the clinic rather than in the hospital, and treated 29 children with new-onset ITP.[21] Not only did all 29 children respond to the single dose, but, remarkably, 40% required no further therapy for ITP, and the majority needed only a single dose to dramatically increase their platelet count by the next day. This study established a new paradigm in the clinical management of children with new-onset ITP: rather than automatically being admitted to the hospital for several days, children could receive therapy in 1 day or even be treated in the clinic and sent home. Further studies to explore the lowest effective dose of IVIG for children demonstrated that 2 doses of 250 mg/kg for children <5 years old, and 2 doses of 400 mg/kg for children 5 to 12 years old, were sufficient to induce a response in many of these patients who were being treated at diagnosis.[22] In contrast to pediatric patients, adult patients did not respond as well to reduced IVIG doses. A dose-finding study of adult patients revealed that a single dose of

500 mg/kg IVIG was not sufficient to induce a platelet response.[23] Fortunately, these patients typically were responsive to higher-dose IVIG (1 g/kg).

Chronic ITP was also found to be responsive to the single-dose, 1 g/kg regimen. Bussel and colleagues treated a cohort of adults with chronic ITP with repeated infusions of 800 to 1000 mg/kg IVIG. Of the 40 patients, 16 were able to decrease or stop other therapies, and 5 had complete remission.[24] These results required up to 15 repeated infusions of IVIG but clearly demonstrated its utility in the management of chronic ITP. However, 11 patients lost their response to IVIG within 3 months, and the rest required continued maintenance. A subsequent study by Godeau and colleagues showed an equivalent effect from initial doses of either 1 g/kg or 2 g/kg IVIG on the platelet counts of adults with chronic ITP, and it confirmed the potential of repeated IVIG infusions to induce remission in some of these patients.[25] Thus, long-term use of repeated IVIG infusions can not only increase and stabilize the platelet counts of patients with chronic ITP but may be curative with multiple infusions. There is also evidence that the use of IVIG therapy at the time of diagnosis may have a mild effect to prevent the development of chronic ITP. Analysis of the clinical outcomes of nearly 2000 children in an international ITP registry showed a 1.8-fold increase in the risk of developing chronic ITP in children who did not receive IVIG therapy initially.[26]

Fetal/Neonatal Alloimmune Thrombocytopenia

The other immune cytopenia beyond ITP in which there are considerable data for the use of IVIG and for which IVIG is the treatment of choice is fetal/neonatal alloimmune thrombocytopenia (F/NAIT; see Table 4-1).[27,28] F/NAIT results when the mother produces an alloantibody against a fetal platelet antigen (eg, human platelet antigen 1, or HPA-1) that was inherited from the father. The maternal IgG antibody crosses the placenta and causes destruction of the fetal platelets. If severe, the thrombocytopenia in the fetus can result in intracranial hemorrhage (ICH) and death either in utero or shortly after birth. F/NAIT is most common in people of European ethnicity, with an incidence of 1:1000 to 1:1500 births. The disease can occur in the first pregnancy (unlike hemolytic disease of the fetus and newborn) and so may be undiagnosed until birth. The thrombocytopenia tends to be more severe with subsequent pregnancies; hence, prenatal treatment of the mother is recommended.

The exact course of therapy is complicated because recent data suggest it is important to stratify treatment for an affected fetus according to the history of the previous affected sibling, especially if the previous sibling had an ICH. In general, the current minimum therapy for an HPA-1a-affected fetus whose previous sibling did not have an ICH would be IVIG, 1 g/kg/week, from 20 to 30 weeks of gestation until delivery. The authors recommend adding prednisone, 0.5 mg/kg daily, because it is of concern that this therapy is not sufficient if the initial fetal platelet count is <10,000 to 20,000/μL, and this is not predictable without fetal sampling. Because fetal blood sampling is not currently recommended before initiation of therapy, the authors' recommendation is to provide treatment that is likely to be effective even in those patients with very low starting platelet counts—eg, IVIG, 1 g/kg/week, plus prednisone, 0.5 mg/kg/day, or IVIG, 2 infusions of 1 g/kg/week.

For affected fetuses whose previous siblings were affected by alloimmune thrombocytopenia and experienced a perinatal or third-trimester ICH, the recommended therapy is more intensive. In those mothers, IVIG, 1g/kg/week, is started at 12 weeks of gestation, and the dose would be increased and prednisone added later in pregnancy. For example, at 20 to 26 weeks of gestation, 0.5 mg/kg prednisone should be added; then a second dose of IVIG, 1g/kg/week, can be added at 30 to 32 weeks of gestation. Alternatively, therapy could be guided by fetal blood sampling and therapy increased only with demonstration of thrombocytopenia.

IVIG initially was found to be an effective treatment for alloimmune thrombocytopenia

Table 4-1. IVIG Efficacy in Auto- and AlloImmune Cytopenias*

Cytopenia	Cell Type		
	Platelets	Neutrophils	Red Cells
Fetal alloimmune	++++[†]	NA	–/+[†]
Fetal autoimmune	NA	NA	NA
Neonatal alloimmune	+++[‡]	++[‡]	+
Neonatal autoimmune	++++[†]	++	NA
Child autoimmune	++++[†]	++++[‡]	+[§]
Adult autoimmune	++++[†]	+[‖]	+[§]
HIV-TP	+++	NA	NA
Posttransfusion purpura	+++	NA	NA

*A plus or minus sign represents the range of effectiveness, from – (no effect) to ++++ (highly effective). NA (not applicable) means that intravenous immunoglobulin (IVIG) has never been tried or else tried only in 1 or 2 cases.
[†]First-line therapy—effective therapy that is either the treatment of choice or one of the treatments of choice.
[‡]An effective therapy but not a first-line therapy; IVIG is either supportive for use with the first-line therapy or is second-line therapy.
[§]A marginally effective treatment to be used in combination with other treatments in desperation or when other therapies have failed.
[‖]To be used primarily if the neutropenia is seen in conjunction with immunodeficiency, especially a form of hypogammaglobulinemia.
HIV-TP = human immunodeficiency virus-associated thrombocytopenia.

also in the neonate (Table 4-1). In 1984, Sideropoulos and Mueller-Eckhardt separately demonstrated that IVIG was effective in alloimmune thrombocytopenia.[29,30] Traditional postnatal management of thrombocytopenia in NAIT has been transfusion of washed platelets from the mother or an antigen-compatible blood donor. However, recent work has shown, surprisingly, that random-donor, mismatched platelets are also effective in NAIT and have the advantage of immediate efficacy in most cases.[31,32] A concern with using IVIG alone in the neonate is that it may require 24 to 72 hours to increase the platelet count substantially in a clinical setting in which a relatively urgent platelet increase is felt to be important. Thus, a conservative approach is to institute treatment with both platelets and IVIG to attempt to achieve a good short-term effect with random-donor platelet transfusion as well as a longer-term increase in the neonate's own platelets with the IVIG. This is especially critical if an ultrasound of the neonatal head demonstrates an ICH, in which case the need to maintain a higher platelet count for a longer time (eg, 1-4 weeks at a count >50,000-100,000/µL) probably mandates the supportive use of IVIG in addition to random and/or matched platelet transfusion.

Neonatal Immune Thrombocytopenia

Significant thrombocytopenia requiring management in neonatal immune thrombocytopenia (NITP) occurs less frequently than in F/NAIT, and there are fewer data regarding effective therapy, but the approach is straightforward. One study of 11 neonates published in

1989 suggested that IVIG was effective and that use with low-dose, short-term steroids may be better than IVIG alone.[33] There are no data regarding the use of random-donor platelet transfusion in this setting. Current recommendations are for IVIG, 1 g/kg/day, with low-dose steroids (1 mg IV every 8 hours) to be given for 1 to 3 days until there is a substantial platelet increase. Platelet counts in these cases should be followed because although the neonatal platelet count may increase with therapy, it may slowly drift down and decrease to below 20,000 to 30,000/μL, at which point more therapy would be recommended. This is in contrast to F/NAIT, in which the platelet count, if it increases after 1 to 2 weeks, generally becomes and remains normal.[27]

HIV-Associated Thrombocytopenia

Thrombocytopenia is a common occurrence during HIV infection, affecting up to 40% of patients, and up to 10% will have thrombocytopenia at presentation. HIV-associated thrombocytopenia (HIV-TP) presents analogously to ITP and, like ITP, carries a small risk of ICH. The risk of developing HIV-TP increases with decreasing CD4 cell count. There are many potential causes of thrombocytopenia in HIV patients, and diagnosis of HIV-TP requires exclusion of other causes such as infection and thrombotic thrombocytopenic purpura (TTP). The primary pathophysiology of HIV-TP is direct HIV infection of marrow precursor cells, resulting in the production of platelet and megakaryocyte antibodies. Both megakaryocytes and platelets are destroyed, and erythropoietin levels are increased, unlike the effects of ITP. The thrombocytopenia is responsive to IVIG, 1 g/kg daily for 2 days as in ITP (although IV anti-D is more effective in most patients), but the most effective therapy is therapy against HIV itself. Platelet counts will typically recover when the viral load is reduced. Thus, IVIG is recommended in combination with antiretroviral therapy for active bleeding or impending hemostatic challenge.

Posttransfusion Purpura

PTP is a very rare posttransfusion syndrome seen primarily in women over the age of 60, characterized by severe thrombocytopenia in the week following a transfusion. Patients with PTP are sensitized to a platelet epitope, usually HPA-1, through pregnancy or a prior transfusion. Upon transfusion with HPA-1-expressing platelets, patients have an anamnestic response resulting in immune clearance of the transfused platelets, accompanied by destruction of their own platelets through one of several hypothesized but not proven mechanisms. The thrombocytopenia can be severe, mandating immediate treatment, but is usually responsive to IVIG, 1 g/kg for 2 days.

Autoimmune Neutropenia

IVIG at doses of 2 g/kg (1 g/kg for 2 days) has also been used for autoimmune neutropenia (AIN; see Table 4-1). The first patient reported had combined variable immune deficiency (CVID) with AIN and received standard 400-mg/kg dosing of IVIG.[34] Subsequently, a series of children with AIN were treated,[35,36] culminating in a series of 20 patients, including those in earlier reports.[37] Seventeen of 20 had dramatic responses wherein the absolute neutrophil count (ANC) rose from <300/μL to >1000/μL within 2 to 3 days. Infections ongoing at the time of treatment, such as skin abscesses, pneumonia, or chronic otitis media, cleared promptly. In several children, abscesses that had been heavily pretreated with antibiotics would often ameliorate overnight, even though the ANC would not increase substantially for 48 hours. This suggested that the initial responding neutrophils had entered the abscess and thus were not detectable in the peripheral blood, as is believed to occur following the use of chemotherapy. Studies demonstrated[38] that granulocyte colony-stimulating factor (G-CSF) levels in AIN were "normal," thus corroborating anecdotal clinical information that G-CSF treatment could also be used if any treatment was required and drawing a parallel with the normal thrombopoietin (TPO) levels found in ITP and the use of thrombopoietic agents.

AIN is typically diagnosed in infants of 3 to 18 months of age and spontaneously improves by 24 months in <80% to 90% of cases.[39] AIN in older children and adults may respond transiently to IVIG but does not typically improve in the same way. Cases of AIN in CVID may improve with persistent high-dose IVIG and (it may be speculated) with rituximab.[40] Neutropenia seen with X-linked hyper-IgM syndrome also typically responds to IVIG, which, as with CVID, is normally given to these patients, albeit at a lower dose (400 mg/kg every 4 weeks).[41,42] Other neutropenias not mediated by antibody (eg, those seen with Felty syndrome) do not respond to IVIG.[43]

Evans Syndrome

In 1951, Evans described a cohort of patients with AIHA who also had thrombocytopenia and a "thrombocyte agglutinating factor," which suggested that the thrombocytopenia was autoimmune as well.[44] Thus, Evans syndrome is the simultaneous (or sequential) occurrence of AIHA and ITP. It is clear now that Evans syndrome encompasses a wide range of autoimmune defects that share a final common phenotype of combined AIHA and ITP. This syndrome has a chronic relapsing course and poor response to any therapy, including IVIG. Reported treatment modalities are essentially a combination of therapy for AIHA and ITP and demonstrate a very high rate of relapse.[45] Current recommendations are to use IVIG for the thrombocytopenia symptoms. Case series using IVIG in combination with corticosteroids show a response in 25% to 70% of patients, with most relapsing.[46] However, some patients could be maintained on an intermittent IVIG regimen. Rituximab and mycophenalate mofetil may be more efficacious in this disorder.

Autoimmune Hemolytic Anemia

AIHA is caused by autoantibodies to red cell antigens, resulting in red cell destruction. It is the autoimmune cytopenia that is least responsive to IVIG. One large series that summarized 37 cases from published reports and 36 cases from the authors' experiences found that the response rate was surprisingly low.[47] Of interest, hepatomegaly was a positive prognostic factor for IVIG treatment, and splenomegaly was a negative prognostic factor; in addition, 6 of 11 children responded. Because response in this study allowed other ongoing treatments (eg, prednisone) and required an increase of hemoglobin of only 2 g/dL within 10 days, the <40% response rate suggests that, in general, IVIG is not an optimal first-line treatment for this indication, although it may be used in combination therapy for life-threatening AIHA.

Other Hematologic Diseases

In other hematologic diseases, IVIG has been used primarily to treat the hypogammaglobulinemia secondary to the disease process rather than to modulate the hematologic disease itself. For example, after hematopoietic stem cell transplant, IVIG may be given to prevent or treat infections such as cytomegalovirus.[48] Other than in anecdotal cases, IVIG has not demonstrated any important utility in TTP or posttransplant lymphoproliferative disease. Neonatal alloimmune neutropenia could presumably be treated with IVIG but is very infrequently diagnosed and infrequently symptomatic, and G-CSF would be the first choice of therapy in the vanishingly rare instances when treatment is required. In contrast to its role in fetal alloimmune thrombocytopenia, IVIG administered to the pregnant mother affected with Rh disease has little effect. Studies have, however, suggested that IVIG administered in the neonatal period for either Rh or ABO incompatibility may ameliorate the disease process because it clearly reduces bilirubin levels—by a clinically important, albeit numerically small, amount.[49]

Toxicity

The most common toxicities of IVIG in ITP are headache and fever with chills. Headaches occur in over half of patients and may occasionally be severe, depending on infusion rate, dose, and individual susceptibility.[50,51] A few patients developed aseptic meningitis, which subsequently resolved.[52] Fever and chills, sometimes with abdominal pain and nausea, also occur but are more common in patients receiving IVIG for hypogammaglobulinemia. Both the headaches and fever/chills may be ameliorated by using concomitant oral or IV steroids.

True anaphylaxis occurs very rarely; in patients with underlying hypogammaglobulinemia this may be caused by the presence of anti-IgA, and these rare patients may continue to be treated with IgA-depleted IVIG.

Venous and arterial thrombosis resulting in pulmonary embolus, myocardial infarction, and stroke have been reported both during and after IVIG infusion.[53] Thrombosis is more commonly seen in adults and those with underlying thrombotic risk factors but has also been reported in children.[54] The etiology likely includes both the increase in blood viscosity following IVIG infusion and the sudden increase in young and hemostatically active circulating platelets.

Acute renal failure has been reported after IVIG infusion, related to the high sucrose content in some older IVIG formulations.[55] This complication is seen primarily in diabetic and elderly patients with underlying risks for renal toxicity.

Other toxicities related to IVIG use include fluid overload, hypertension, and complications related to the actual infusion, which may be treated symptomatically.

Conclusions

IVIG is an effective and versatile tool for treating some, but not all, immune cytopenias and is most efficacious against various forms of thrombocytopenia. It is a highly successful therapy for ITP, as shown in a high percentage of patients of all ages with both acute and chronic ITP, and is effective therapy for F/NAIT, either for the mother or for the neonate. IVIG is also effective for HIV-TP, although antiretrovirals are the therapy of choice for that disorder. ITP is generally but not exclusively the end result of autoantibody-coated platelet removal by macrophages of the reticuloendothelium. The varying degrees of defective thrombopoiesis in the marrow and central immune defects in both T regulatory cells and immunomodulatory dendritic cells could explain the heterogeneity of response to IVIG and other therapies. IVIG is not as effective against AIHA or Evans syndrome, possibly reflecting that the pathophysiology of those cytopenias differs substantially from that of ITP.

Recent advances represent a paradigm shift in understanding the mechanisms of IVIG therapy in immune disorders, which is remarkable for a drug that has been in use for over 30 years. Evidence from mouse models of autoimmune disease suggests that IVIG imparts its therapeutic effect through the interaction of the Fc portion of a small fraction of IgG molecules bearing a specific glycan moiety with activating FcRs on dendritic cells, which in turn up-regulate the inhibitory FcRIIB receptors on leukocytes. These findings have raised the possibility of a new generation of IVIG-based therapies; new therapeutics might be based either on IVIG that is highly enriched for this specific sialylated Fc or on completely recombinant sialylated Fc molecules. Other recent research has identified the dendritic cell receptor, DC-sign, as a putative target for the sialylated Fc molecules. These findings, if translatable to humans, also reveal novel therapeutic possibilities to recapitulate the anti-inflammatory effects of IVIG. Significantly, these lines of research demonstrate that there is much to learn about both the underlying immune defects in the immune cytopenias and the mechanisms by which IVIG ameliorates them. As has been the case for three decades, efforts to understand the mechanisms of IVIG continue to provide insight into the central immune regulatory defects that lead to the peripheral destruction of blood cells.

References

1. Harrington WJ, Minnich V, Hollingsworth JW, Moore CV. Demonstration of a thrombocytopenic factor in the blood of patients with thrombocytopenic purpura. J Lab Clin Med 1951;38:1-10.
2. Imbach P, Barandun S, d'Apuzzo V, et al. High-dose intravenous gammaglobulin for idiopathic thrombocytopenic purpura in childhood. Lancet 1981;1:1228-31.
3. Schmidt RE, Budde U, Schafer G, Stroehmann I. High-dose intravenous gammaglobulin for idiopathic thrombocytopenic purpura. Lancet 1981;2:475-6.
4. Newland AC, Treleaven JG, Minchinton RM, Waters AH. High-dose intravenous IgG in adults with autoimmune thrombocytopenia. Lancet 1983;1:84-7.
5. Bussel JB, Kimberly RP, Inman RD, et al. Intravenous gammaglobulin treatment of chronic idiopathic thrombocytopenic purpura. Blood 1983;62:480-6.
6. Cines DB, Bussel JB, Liebman HA, Luning Prak ET. The ITP syndrome: Pathogenic and clinical diversity. Blood 2009;113:6511-21.
7. Kuhne T, Buchanan GR, Zimmerman S, et al. A prospective comparative study of 2540 infants and children with newly diagnosed idiopathic thrombocytopenic purpura (ITP) from the intercontinental childhood ITP study group. J Pediatr 2003;143:605-8.
8. Imbach P, Kühne T, Müller D, et al. Childhood ITP: 12 months follow-up data from the prospective registry I of the Intercontinental Childhood ITP Study Group (ICIS). Pediatr Blood Cancer 2006;46:351-6.
9. Feudjo-Tepie MA, Robinson NJ, Bennett D. Prevalence of diagnosed chronic immune thrombocytopenic purpura in the US: Analysis of a large US claim database: A rebuttal. J Thromb Haemost 2008;6:711-12.
10. Daou S, Federici L, Zimmer J, et al. Idiopathic thrombocytopenic purpura in elderly patients: A study of 47 cases from a single reference center. Eur J Intern Med Oct 2008;19:447-51.
11. Burdach SE, Evers KG, Geursen RG. Treatment of acute idiopathic thrombocytopenic purpura of childhood with intravenous immunoglobulin G: Comparative efficacy of 7S and 5S preparations. J Pediatr 1986;109:770-5.
12. Tovo PA, Miniero R, Fiandino G, et al. Fc-depleted vs intact intravenous immunoglobulin in chronic ITP. J Pediatr 1984;105:676-7.
13. Fehr J, Hofmann V, Kappeler U. Transient reversal of thrombocytopenia in idiopathic thrombocytopenic purpura by high-dose intravenous gamma globulin. N Engl J Med 1982;306:1254-8.
14. Clarkson SB, Bussel JB, Kimberly RP, et al. Treatment of refractory immune thrombocytopenic purpura with an anti-Fc gamma-receptor antibody. N Engl J Med 1986;314:1236-9.
15. Salama A, Mueller-Eckhardt C, Kiefel V. Effect of intravenous immunoglobulin in immune thrombocytopenia. Lancet 1983;2:193-5.
16. Salama A, Kiefel V, Mueller-Eckhardt C. Effect of IgG anti-Rho(D) in adult patients with chronic autoimmune thrombocytopenia. Am J Hematol 1986;22:241-50.
17. Becker T, Kuenzlen E, Salama A, et al. Treatment of childhood idiopathic thrombocytopenic purpura with Rhesus antibodies (anti-D). Eur J Pediatr 1986;145:166-9.
18. Salama A, Kiefel V, Amberg R, Mueller-Eckhardt C. Treatment of autoimmune thrombocytopenic purpura with rhesus antibodies [anti-RhO(D)]. Blut 1984;49:29-35.
19. Psaila B, Petrovic A, Page LK, et al. Intracranial hemorrhage (ICH) in children with immune thrombocytopenia (ITP): Study of 40 cases. Blood 2009;114:4777-83.
20. Tarantino MD, Young G, Bertolone SJ, et al. Single dose of anti-D immune globulin at 75 microg/kg is as effective as intravenous immune globulin at rapidly raising the platelet count in newly diagnosed immune thrombocytopenic purpura in children. J Pediatr 2006;148:489-94.
21. Bussel JB, Goldman A, Imbach P, et al. Treatment of acute idiopathic thrombocytopenia of childhood with intravenous infusions of gammaglobulin. J Pediatr 1985;106:886-90.
22. Warrier I, Bussel JB, Valdez L, et al. Safety and efficacy of low-dose intravenous immune globulin (IVIG) treatment for infants and children with immune thrombocytopenic purpura. Low-Dose IVIG Study Group. J Pediatr Hematol Oncol 1997;19:197-201.
23. Godeau B, Caulier MT, Decuypere L, et al. Intravenous immunoglobulin for adults with autoimmune thrombocytopenic purpura: Results of a randomized trial comparing 0.5 and 1 g/kg b.w. Br J Haematol 1999;107:716-19.

24. Bussel JB, Pham LC, Aledort L, Nachman R. Maintenance treatment of adults with chronic refractory immune thrombocytopenic purpura using repeated intravenous infusions of gammaglobulin. Blood 1988;72:121-7.
25. Godeau B, Lesage S, Divine M, et al. Treatment of adult chronic autoimmune thrombocytopenic purpura with repeated high-dose intravenous immunoglobulin. Blood 1993;82:1415-21.
26. Tamminga R, Berchtold W, Bruin M, et al. Possible lower rate of chronic ITP after IVIG for acute childhood ITP: An analysis from Registry I of the Intercontinental Cooperative ITP Study Group (ICIS). Br J Haematol 2009;146:180-4.
27. Bussel J. Diagnosis and management of the fetus and neonate with alloimmune thrombocytopenia. J Thromb Haemost 2009;7(Suppl 1):253-7.
28. Murphy MF, Bussel JB. Advances in the management of alloimmune thrombocytopenia. Br J Haematol 2007;136:366-78.
29. Mueller-Eckhardt C, Kiefel V, Grubert A. High-dose IgG treatment for neonatal alloimmune thrombocytopenia. Blut 1989;59:145-6.
30. Sidiropoulos D, Straume B. The treatment of neonatal isoimmune thrombocytopenia with intravenous immunoglobin (IgG i.v.). Blut 1984;48:383-6.
31. Kiefel V, Bassler D, Kroll H, et al. Antigen-positive platelet transfusion in neonatal alloimmune thrombocytopenia (NAIT). Blood 2006;107:3761-3.
32. Bussel JB, Zacharoulis S, Kramer K, et al. Clinical and diagnostic comparison of neonatal alloimmune thrombocytopenia to non-immune cases of thrombocytopenia. Pediatr Blood Cancer 2005;45:176-83.
33. Blanchette V, Andrew M, Perlman M, et al. Neonatal autoimmune thrombocytopenia: Role of high-dose intravenous immunoglobulin G therapy. Blut 1989;59:139-44.
34. Pollack S, Cunningham-Rundles C, Smithwick EM, et al. High-dose intravenous gamma globulin for autoimmune neutropenia (letter). N Engl J Med 1982;307:253.
35. Bussel J, Lalezari P, Fikrig S. Intravenous treatment with gamma-globulin of autoimmune neutropenia of infancy. J Pediatr 1988;112:298-301.
36. Bussel J, Lalezari P, Hilgartner M, et al. Reversal of neutropenia with intravenous gamma-globulin in autoimmune neutropenia of infancy. Blood 1983;62:398-400.
37. Dunkel IJ, Bussel JB. New developments in the treatment of neutropenia. Am J Dis Child 1993;147:994-1000.
38. Corbacioglu S, Bux J, Konig A, et al. Serum granulocyte colony-stimulating factor levels are not increased in patients with autoimmune neutropenia of infancy. J Pediatr 2000;137:96-9.
39. Bux J, Behrens G, Jaeger G, Welte K. Diagnosis and clinical course of autoimmune neutropenia in infancy: Analysis of 240 cases. Blood 1998;91:181-6.
40. Chapel H, Cunningham-Rundles C. Update in understanding common variable immunodeficiency disorders (CVIDs) and the management of patients with these conditions. Br J Haematol 2009;145:709-27.
41. Winkelstein JA, Marino MC, Ochs H, et al. The X-linked hyper-IgM syndrome: Clinical and immunologic features of 79 patients. Medicine 2003;82:373-84.
42. Jacov L, Teresa E-B, Carolin T, et al. Clinical spectrum of X-linked hyper-IgM syndrome. J Pediatr 1997;131:47-54.
43. Breedveld FC, Brand A, van Aken WG. High dose intravenous gamma globulin for Felty's syndrome. J Rheumatol 1985;12:700-2.
44. Evans RS, Takahashi K, Duane RT, et al. Primary thrombocytopenic purpura and acquired hemolytic anemia: Evidence for a common etiology. AMA Arch Intern Med 1951;87:48-65.
45. Scaradavou A, Bussel J. Evans syndrome: Results of a pilot study utilizing a multiagent treatment protocol. J Pediatr Hematol Oncol 1995;17:290-5.
46. Anderson D, Ali K, Blanchette V, et al. Guidelines on the use of intravenous immune globulin for hematologic conditions. Transfus Med Rev 2007;21(2 Suppl 1):S9-56.
47. Flores G, Cunningham-Rundles C, Newland AC, Bussel JB. Efficacy of intravenous immunoglobulin in the treatment of autoimmune hemolytic anemia: Results in 73 patients. Am J Hematol 1993;44:237-42.
48. Raanani P, Gafter-Gvili A, Paul M, et al. Immunoglobulin prophylaxis in hematopoietic stem cell transplantation: Systematic review and meta-analysis. J Clin Oncol 2009;27:770-81.
49. Miqdad AM, Abdelbasit OB, Shaheed MM, et al. Intravenous immunoglobulin G (IVIG) therapy for significant hyperbilirubinemia in ABO hemolytic disease of the newborn. J Matern Fetal Neonatal Med 2004;16:163-6.

50. Schiavotto C, Ruggeri M, Rodeghiero F. Adverse reactions after high-dose intravenous immunoglobulin: Incidence in 83 patients treated for idiopathic thrombocytopenic purpura (ITP) and review of the literature. Haematologica 1993;78(6 Suppl 2):35-40.
51. Dashti-Khavidaki S, Aghamohammadi A, Farshadi F, et al. Adverse reactions of prophylactic intravenous immunoglobulin; a 13-year experience with 3004 infusions in Iranian patients with primary immunodeficiency diseases. J Investig Allergol Clin Immunol 2009;19:139-45.
52. Bussel J, Cunningham-Rundles C, Feldman C, Horowitz B. Transmission of viral infection by preparations of intravenous immunoglobulin. Plasma Ther Transfus Technol 1989;9:193-205.
53. Paran D, Herishanu Y, Elkayam O, et al. Venous and arterial thrombosis following administration of intravenous immunoglobulins. Blood Coagul Fibrinolysis 2005;16:313-18.
54. Pui-Ying Iroh Tam MRSG. Fatal case of bilateral internal jugular vein thrombosis following IVIg infusion in an adolescent girl treated for ITP. Am J Hematol 2008;83:323-5.
55. Chapman SA, Gilkerson KL, Davin TD, Pritzker MR. Acute renal failure and intravenous immune globulin: Occurs with sucrose-stabilized, but not with D-sorbitol-stabilized, formulation. Ann Pharmacother 2004;38:2059-67.

5

Clinical Use of IVIG in Neurology

Marinos C. Dalakas, MD

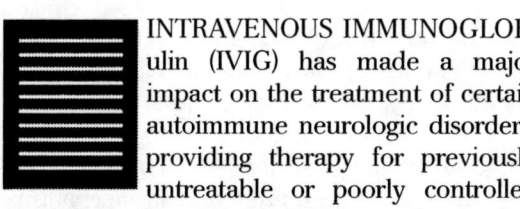

INTRAVENOUS IMMUNOGLOBulin (IVIG) has made a major impact on the treatment of certain autoimmune neurologic disorders, providing therapy for previously untreatable or poorly controlled conditions. Controlled trials have shown that IVIG is effective as first-line therapy in patients with Guillain-Barré syndrome (GBS), chronic inflammatory demyelinating polyneuropathy (CIDP), and multifocal motor neuropathy (MMN), and as second-line therapy in dermatomyositis (DM), myasthenia gravis (MG), Lambert-Eaton myasthenic syndrome (LEMS), and stiff-person syndrome (SPS). In paraproteinemic IgM anti-myelin-associated-glycoprotein (anti-MAG) demyelinating polyneuropathies and inclusion body myositis (IBM), the benefit of IVIG is variable, marginal, and not statistically significant. In spite of its undisputed efficacy, IVIG has gained approval by the Food and Drug Administration (FDA) only for CIDP, for which a large controlled study has recently shown effectiveness in maintaining remission and preventing axonal loss in the early and chronic management of the disease. Emerging molecular markers appear promising in identifying responders from nonresponders, especially in patients with CIDP. IVIG exerts multiple actions on the immunoregulatory network that operate in concert with each other; for each of the aforementioned autoimmune neuromuscular diseases, there appears to be a predominant mechanism of action that relates to the underlying immunopathogenetic cause of the respective disorder.

IVIG has a remarkably good safety record for long-term administration in a large number of neurologic patients worldwide. Mild infusion-rate-related reactions such as headaches, myalgia, and fever are the most common; aseptic meningitis, skin rash, thromboembolic events, and renal tubular necrosis are rare events.

In spite of the progress made, future studies are still required to resolve the following issues:
- To find the appropriate dose and frequency of infusions that maintain a response.

Marinos C. Dalakas, MD, Professor of Neurology, Imperial College, London, United Kingdom
The author has disclosed no conflicts of interest.

- To address pharmacoeconomics, comparing the high cost of IVIG to the cost of the other therapies which, although less expensive, may cause more significant long-term side effects.
- To identify, with molecular biomarkers, the patients more likely to respond.
- To examine the merits of combining IVIG with other immunosuppressive drugs, especially monoclonal antibodies against B or T cells.
- To evaluate the effectiveness of IVIG in conditions for which its efficacy is not proven, especially for some neuroinflammatory/neurodegenerative disorders.

Introduction

During the last two decades, the use of IVIG has changed dramatically the approach to treatment of autoimmune neuromuscular disorders and has dominated immunotherapeutic drugs. Its relative safety for long-term therapy and undisputable efficacy based on class I evidence derived from randomized trials have had a major impact on the quality of life of patients with a number of these disorders, some of which were previously unresponsive, or insufficiently responsive, to available immunotherapies.[1-3] In some disorders, IVIG is as effective as plasma exchange (PE) or steroids but safer and easier to administer; in others, it is superior to all existing drugs; and in still others such as MMN, it is the only effective therapy.[1,3,4] On the basis of controlled clinical trials, IVIG has been effective in various acute and chronic demyelinating neuropathies, neuromuscular transmission defects, inflammatory myopathies, and SPS and is providing promise in treating various neuroinflammatory or even neurodegenerative disorders.[1-3,5]

The success in treating effectively and safely such immunologically diverse disorders and the resultant enthusiasm has led clinicians to use the drug more liberally even in diseases where the data are weak and not evidence based, causing logistical problems regarding supply, drug reimbursement, and long-term safety.[6,7] Because all indications for IVIG in neurology (except for CIDP, using one proprietary IVIG product) are still "off label," these issues have generated considerable skepticism and scrutiny from insurance carriers, health-care organizations, and government agencies.

This review will present the evidence-based indications for IVIG in autoimmune neuromuscular diseases; summarize practical guidelines for the practicing neurologists on how best to make judicious decisions in the use of the drug; summarize some of the known mechanisms of action based on work carried out in neurologic disorders; and address some promising new applications from early clinical studies that may have an impact on the future of neurologic therapeutics.

Mechanisms of Action of IVIG in Autoimmune Neurologic Disorders: General Issues

The mechanisms of action of IVIG are discussed extensively in this book. There is overwhelming evidence that multiple actions of IVIG often operate in concert with each other. For each neuromuscular disorder, however, there appears to be a predominant mechanism dictated by the underlying immunopathogenetic cause of the respective disorder.[6] Among the main mechanisms of action of IVIG,[8] those relevant to its efficacy in autoimmune neuromuscular disorders include those described below.

Effect on Autoantibodies

The IgG molecules within IVIG contain antibodies with a wide range of idiotypic and anti-idiotypic specificities that may neutralize pathogenic autoantibodies and prevent their interaction with the autoantigen. This effect has been shown experimentally, using extracted F(ab')$_2$ fragments of IVIG bound to and neutralizing autoantibodies, such as anti-DNA, anti-acetylcholine receptor (AChR), anti-thyroglobulin, anti-GM1, and others.[9-12] The idiotypic/anti-idiotypic effect has been shown also in patients with acute GBS whose serum contains various IgG glycolipid antibodies. In an in-vitro nerve-muscle preparation, the F(ab')$_2$ portion of IVIG neutralized the "blocking" effect exerted by the serum of acute GBS patients on the quantal release.[13,14] The effects of IVIG on autoantibodies may be relevant in explaining the effect of IVIG in antibody-mediated autoimmune neuromuscular diseases such as MG, LEMS, SPS, and the antibody-mediated demyelinating neuropathies (GBS, CIDP, MMN).

Inhibition of Complement Binding and Prevention of Membranolytic Attack Complex (MAC) Formation

The effect of IVIG on complement binding has been demonstrated in vitro, in animal models, and in patients who received IVIG. In early studies, IVIG was shown to prevent death in guinea pigs from the complement-dependent Forssman shock by inhibiting the uptake of complement C3 and C4 fragments to the endothelial cells.[15] In patients with DM, which is a complement-dependent microangiopathy mediated by activation of C3 and deposition of MAC on the endomysial capillaries,[6,15-17] IVIG is not only clinically effective, as discussed later,[18] but it also inhibits complement uptake and intercepts the formation and deposition of MAC on the endomysial capillaries.[19] Post-IVIG serum, but not postplacebo serum, inhibits the uptake of C3b and C4b fragments by sensitized in-vitro targets, probably as a result of formation of covalent or noncovalent complexes between C3 and specific receptor sites within the infused IgG molecules.[19] Such an inhibition limits the available C3 molecules for further incorporation into the C5 convertase assembly, thereby preventing the formation and in-situ deposition of MAC, as confirmed in the repeated muscle biopsy specimens of patients with dermatomyositis treated with IVIG.[2,6,18-20] The effect of IVIG on complement, as proven in dermatomyositis, is directly relevant to GBS, CIDP, and MG, where the complement pathway is activated[21] and complement fragments are fixed in the targeted tissues.[1,6] Indeed, IVIG has been shown to protect anti-ganglioside antibody-mediated cytotoxicity implicated in the pathogenesis of GBS and other autoimmune neuropathies by displacing complement C3 fragments fixed on the sciatic nerve.[22]

Modulation or Blockade of Fc Receptors on Macrophages

The IgG molecules bind through their Fc region to Fc receptors on macrophages and, via intracellular signaling, mediate inflammation or immune effector functions.[8,23] The ratio of the expression of inhibitory to activating Fc receptors determines the final immune response; overexpression of activating Fc receptor I (FcRI) and FcRIII favor activation, whereas overexpression of inhibitory FcRIIB infers inhibition of phagocytosis and antibody-dependent cell-mediated cytotoxicity.[8,23] IVIG up-regulates the inhibitory FcRIIB and modulates the FcRIIB/FcRIII ratio on macrophages.[23] In GBS and CIDP, blockade of activating Fc receptors on the macrophages could inhibit the macrophage-mediated phagocytosis of antigen-bearing target cells and might counter macrophage-mediated demyelination.[20,24,25] An increase in the number of monocytes bearing the FcRIIB inhibitory receptors and an increase in the FcRIIB/FcRIII ratio on monocytes has been noted 1 week after IVIG treatment in GBS and CIDP patients who started to improve, suggesting that such inhibitory signaling may be clinically relevant.[26]

Suppression of Pathogenic Cytokines and Other Immunoregulatory Molecules

In-vitro and in-vivo studies have shown that IVIG causes a dose-dependent downregulation of tissue expression or reduction in the circulating levels of cytokines and adhesion molecules, such as interleukin (IL)-1; tumor necrosis factor alpha (TNF); IL-1; transforming growth factor beta (TGF) and TGF mRNA; major histocompatibility complex Class I (MHC-I); intracellular adhesion molecule-1 (ICAM-1) on the endothelial cells; and lymphocyte function-associated antigen 1 (LFA-1) on activated T cells.[27-31] The latter has been convincingly shown in the repeated muscle biopsies of patients with DM who improved after IVIG therapy[18] and on the lymphocytes of GBS patients 1 week after infusion with IVIG.[26] Because up-regulation of cytokines and adhesion molecules is critical in almost all of the autoimmune neuromuscular diseases in which IVIG appears to be effective,[4,24] its down-regulatory effect on these molecules is probably pathogenetically relevant. Whether such an effect is a downstream event related to upstream effects on the primary immune process of the disease remains unclear.

Possible Effect on Remyelination

Treatment with IVIG suppresses experimental allergic encephalomyelitis and experimental allergic neuritis,[32] probably via a combined effect on the immunoregulatory network mentioned above. Whether it also enhances remyelination by an effect directly on the myelin sheath, as has been suggested,[33] remains to be determined.

Kinetics of Infused IVIG

Kinetic studies performed at the author's facility in patients with autoimmune neurologic disorders revealed that, after an intravenous infusion of 2 g/kg IVIG, the serum IgG level increases fivefold, but it declines by 50% in 72 hours and returns to the pretreatment level after 21 to 28 days.[24,25,34] The marked initial decrease reflects extravascular redistribution. The half-life of IVIG is approximately 18 to 32 days, which is similar to that of native immunoglobulin. During the first 48 hours of the infusion when the serum IgG level is high, IgG enters the cerebrospinal fluid, where its concentration increases as much as twofold, returning to normal within a week.[24,25,34] This may be of relevance to neurologic therapeutics because the infused IVIG should enter freely at the end plate and the dorsal root level, which lack the blood-cerebrospinal fluid (CSF) barrier, and may bathe the distal nerve terminals and nerve roots; whether it exerts a local effect on those areas, complementing its general immunomodulatory effect on the immune network described above, remains unclear.

Status of IVIG in Autoimmune Neuromuscular Disorders: Evidence from Controlled Clinical Trials

Guillain-Barré Syndrome

GBS is an acute demyelinating polyneuropathy that peaks within 2 weeks of onset and causes severe weakness or paralysis of the limbs and respiratory muscles. Although the target antigen is still unknown, humoral and cellular immune mechanisms are implicated, as evidenced by activation of complement and deposition of MAC on the myelin sheath, the presence of circulating antiganglioside or glycolipid antibodies, an increase of T-cell activation products and cytokines, and invasion of the myelin sheath by sensitized macrophages.[35-39]

Up to about a decade ago, during the first week of the illness, the recommended therapy for patients with GBS who have severe disease and require assistance to walk has been plasmapheresis. This practice has been based on controlled clinical trials that showed that plasmapheresis hastens recovery in as many as 52% of patients, compared to 38% of patients receiving sham apheresis.[40,41] Since then, this practice has changed based on at least two randomized controlled trials that have shown that IVIG has comparable effects. The first randomized trial concluded that up to 52.7% of 74 patients receiving IVIG, compared to 34% of 73 patients undergoing plasmapheresis, had functional improvement of one grade or more after 4 weeks.[42] This conclusion was strengthened with a second, larger trial that compared, in parallel, the efficacy of IVIG therapy alone (5-day regimen of 0.4 g/kg/day), plasmapheresis alone, and plasmapheresis followed by IVIG therapy. After 4 weeks of therapy and 48 weeks of follow-up, no statistically significant difference was seen among the three treatments in outcome measures, including time to unaided walking and discontinuation of ventilation.[43] The study confirmed that although each treatment is beneficial, combining IVIG with PE produces no incremental response. A pilot study of GBS patients that combined IVIG and 500 mg intravenous methylprednisone showed that the combination was better than IVIG therapy alone.[44] However, a randomized controlled trial showed no benefit of steroids.[45] In atypical GBS (such as the Miller-Fisher variant,[46] acute dysautonomia, or other variants), IVIG appears to be efficacious, but controlled studies have not been conducted.

Dosing

Insight into the optimal IVIG dosing in GBS was provided by another study comparing 1.2 g/kg IVIG given in 3 days and 2.4 g/kg given in 6 days.[47] The study showed that the time to walking with assistance was shorter in the 6-day group (84 vs 131) and significantly shorter in ventilated patients. Also, the proportion of patients who recovered full muscular strength at 1 year was greater in the 6-day group. As previously reviewed,[6] this study concluded that a full dose of at least 2 g/kg of IVIG is more beneficial in GBS patients who need ventilatory assistance.

Need for a Second IVIG Infusion

A common clinical dilemma in managing patients with GBS is whether a second IVIG infusion may add more benefit when, 3 weeks after the first infusion, improvement either has not occurred or is deemed inadequate. There is a clinical inclination to attempt a second IVIG infusion, but the available data are not adequate to support such practice.[6] The reported improvement of a few patients following a second infusion 3 to 4 weeks later[48] requires confirmation with a controlled study to assess whether the reported benefit is the result of IVIG rather than of the natural course of the disease. After almost 10 years of trying to conduct such a study, funding became possible only recently and a controlled study is expected to begin in 2010 in the Netherlands.

Early Relapses

In some patients with GBS, early relapse may occur after the initial beneficial response either with plasmapheresis or with IVIG therapy. On the basis of the two large controlled trials, it is clear that relapses occur almost equally in patients treated first with plasmapheresis and those treated first with IVIG therapy.[42,43,49] Another retrospective study by Romano and coworkers in 1998 also showed no increased relapses in 54 patients treated with IVIG as opposed to plasmapheresis.[50] Changing from one treatment to another is not recommended; instead, staying with the chosen treatments supplemented with supportive care is most appropriate. An associated medical condition appears to correlate best with an increased risk of relapses, whereas earlier initiation of treatment is associated with a lesser chance for relapse.[50]

Markers of Response to Therapy with IVIG

Correlation of Responsiveness to GM1 Antibodies, *Campylobacter Jejuni* Infection, and Motor Predominance. In patients with the predominantly axonal form of GBS (the acute motor or motor-sensory axonal neuropathy), the disease is most often associated with *Campylobacter jejuni* infection and GM1 antibodies. Although it was thought that these patients may not recover well, studies of Chinese cases do not show differences in the degree of recovery between the axonal and demyelinating types of disease.[51,52] A subgroup of such patients may even respond better to IVIG than to plasmapheresis.[49] Further, some patients with IgG anti-GM1 may recover faster than the GM1-negative patients.[53] In general, it seems that the presence of anti-GM1 antibodies in GBS patients is not a marker of poor recovery. Instead, the degree of axonal degeneration—especially proximally, or perhaps infection with *Campylobacter jejuni*[53]—appears to be associated with less favorable outcome. Analysis from the multicenter trial has shown that the outcomes in response to IVIG or plasmapheresis is the same in all subsets of GBS, including patients with the demyelinating or axonal forms, patients with inexcitable nerves, and patients with pure motor forms, regardless of an antecedent *Campylobacter*-related diarrhea.[43] More recent data, however, indicate that age, preceding diarrhea, and GBS disability score at 2 weeks after entry were factors associated with poor outcome.[54] This is an important observation because it identifies the subsets of patients that might benefit from early re-treatment with IVIG or with new immunomodulating agents.

Correlation with Serum IgG Levels. Recently, the pharmacokinetics of IVIG in relation to clinical outcome were examined in 174 patients with GBS treated with IVIG.[55] It was found that the increase in serum IgG (delta IgG) 2 weeks after IVIG treatment varied considerably between patients (mean = 7.8 g/L; standard deviation = 5.6 g/L). Patients with a low delta IgG recovered significantly more slowly, and fewer reached the ability to walk unaided at 6 months (log-rank p <0.001). In multivariate analysis adjusted for other known prognostic factors, a low delta IgG was independently associated with poor outcome (p = 0.022). It therefore seems that patients with a small increase in serum IgG level after IVIG may have a poor outcome; if confirmed, this is important because such patients may benefit from a higher dosage or second course of IVIG early in the disease course. One explanation for the lesser increase of IgG level is probably a redistribution of infused IgGs into the extravascular space owing to endothelial cell dysfunction, which is more profound in patients with severe disease. Comparison of similar kinetics in other disorders will solidify the specificity of this finding and help predict unresponsiveness to IVIG therapy.

IVIG in Childhood Guillain-Barré Syndrome

The easy access of IVIG and its administration without the need to place a central line has made IVIG the treatment of choice in children with GBS, even though its effectiveness in this population has been based on uncontrolled trials or small series of patients.[56-58] Nine such children treated with IVIG (1 g/kg body weight/day for 2 days) recovered more rapidly compared to 9 others not treated. In another study, IVIG shortened the recovery of moderately-afflicted children compared to the more severely affected ones who did not differ from historic controls.[57] In a large cumulative study from two centers involving 75 children, IVIG was effective, with a faster rate of recovery in the patients who received a total dose in 2 days as opposed to 5 days,[56] supporting further the view that a 2-day infusion may be more effective than a 5-day infusion, as discussed below. A beneficial effect of IVIG in speeding recovery and reducing morbidity in childhood GBS was also suggested by a retrospective record review of 37 patients treated with IVIG compared to 67 historical controls.[58] Undoubtedly, IVIG remains the treatment of choice in childhood GBS even though large, controlled studies are not available and may not be performed.

Chronic Inflammatory Demyelinating Polyneuropathy

CIDP is a distinct acquired demyelinating polyneuropathy characterized by the slow onset (over weeks to months) of weakness, areflexia, and impaired sensation. The immunopathologic alternations in CIDP, although fragmentary, are considered similar to GBS.[37,59] Molecular mimicry, antiglycolipid antibodies, T-cell sensitization, myelin invasion by activated macrophages, and activation of complement are the main immunopathologic features of the disease.[37,59-61] However, unlike GBS, which is a monophasic disease, CIDP requires long-term therapy to maintain improvement. Steroids have long been considered the first choice for treating CIDP—hence its designation as a "steroid-responsive neuropathy." Evidence from controlled studies, however, has shown that plasmapheresis and IVIG are also effective and their efficacy is similar or even superior to steroids.[6]

A randomized, controlled, crossover study compared a 6-week course of oral prednisolone (tapered from 60 to 10 mg/day) with a 2-day course of IVIG (1 g/kg/day) for the treatment of CIDP.[62] Treatment was switched after a 4-

week washout period. Both treatments produced significant improvements from disability after 2 weeks, although there was slightly more improvement with IVIG in the two treatment periods. Also observed were improvements favoring IVIG in the time to walk 10 meters after 2 weeks and in disability grade after 6 weeks. IVIG was also equal to PE in a single-blind, controlled, crossover study of CIDP patients assigned to a 6-week course of PE or IVIG, 0.2 to 0.4 g/kg given weekly.[63] Improvements in neurologic disability that occurred with IVIG were similar to those with placebo in a parallel controlled study.[64]

The position of IVIG in the hierarchy of CIDP treatment was investigated in a 3-year placebo-controlled study of IVIG in treatment-naive patients.[65] Patients received an infusion of IVIG, 1 g/kg/day, or placebo on days 1, 2, and 21. Differences in muscle strength favoring IVIG were seen as early as day 10, and this trend increased over time. At day 42, muscle strength had improved significantly more with IVIG than with placebo ($p = 0.006$), and functional performance was also significantly better ($p = 0.019$). These findings support IVIG as first-line therapy in the early inflammatory phase of CIDP, a strategy that could ameliorate the significant axonal degeneration that typically accompanies disease progression.

A number of disease-associated variants of CIDP have been identified.[66,67] Although IVIG seems to be effective in these forms, formal controlled trials have not been conducted. Some reports indicate that 12% to 18% of patients with diabetes meet the electrophysiologic criteria for CIDP, and the risk of CIDP is 11 times greater in those with type 2 diabetes than in those without diabetes.[68] According to anecdotal reports, 20% to 80% of patients with demyelinating polyneuropathy in the setting of diabetes respond to IVIG treatment, but the response rate depends on how the disease is defined. Clearly, a controlled study is needed to establish the potential role and efficacy of IVIG in diabetes-associated CIDP.

Maintenance Therapy

The IVIG-triggered improvement generally begins after a mean period of 9 days and reaches maximum improvement after 3 to 4 weeks. Repeated treatments every 3 to 6 weeks, usually with 1 g/kg, are needed to maintain response. It should be noted that sometimes a number of patients who initially respond to IVIG may show a less consistent response in subsequent infusions; such patients should be identified early to supplement their therapy with other agents. In general, CIDP may be more difficult to treat if axonal changes have become extensive, regardless of the regimen used.

The ICE Study: Long-Term Therapy and FDA-Approval of IVIG in CIDP

The most important study in the use of IVIG, not only in CIDP but in neurology in general, was the IVIG CIDP Efficacy (ICE) trial.[69] This was the largest trial ever conducted, involving 117 CIDP patients randomized to IVIG (Gammunex, Talecris Biotherapeutics, Research Triangle Park, NC) or placebo given every 3 weeks for 24 weeks (primary end point). Patients who showed an improvement at 24 weeks were re-randomized in a blinded 24-week extension. The study confirmed that 54% of those receiving Gammunex, compared to 21% receiving placebo, improved their disability scores and maintained them up to 24 weeks ($p = 0.0002$). Results were similar in the extension phase for another 24 weeks. A strong and positive effect on quality of life was also noted[70]; some electrophysiologic measurements also improved.[71] The study not only confirmed the short-term efficacy of IVIG in CIDP but also established the long-term benefit and safety of maintenance therapy. The study led to the first FDA-approved indication of this IVIG product in CIDP and the first for any neurologic disease.

Starting Therapy

The choice of initiating therapy with prednisone, IVIG, or plasmapheresis (all effective in controlled trials) is judged against cost, long-term side effects, patient age, venous access, disease severity, and concurrent illnesses. If steroids are contraindicated, have produced unacceptable side effects, or become ineffective, IVIG therapy is preferable because it is easier to administer than plasmapheresis. It remains unclear, however, why some patients respond predominantly to IVIG, others to prednisone, and still others to plasmapheresis. Combination therapy may be at times appropriate.

Cost remains a significant factor in determining how to start therapy, especially in certain countries. The ICE study has provided the tool to initiate treatment with IVIG as this product is now an FDA-approved indication and reimbursement is secured. IVIG is seemingly much more costly than prednisone, but patients treated and maintained on long-term steroids to avoid the high-cost of IVIG usually experience the irreversible steroid side effects (osteoporosis, cataracts, diabetes, hypertension, obesity). These along with the seemingly incomplete response, frequent doctor visits, time lost from work, and quality of life issues may finally prove the cost is competitive with that of IVIG. Pharmacoeconomic assessments, as done for one small study,[72] are needed to determine the most economical long-term management approach for CIDP.

Predictors of Response and New Molecular Markers

Factors proposed to be associated with a better response to IVIG include 1) disease duration of less than 1 year, 2) progression of weakness until treatment, 3) absence of discrepancy in weakness between arms and legs, 4) areflexia of the arms, and 5) slowing of motor conduction velocities of the median nerve (all signs of ongoing, generalized, and recent-onset demyelination). The chances for a favorable response to IVIG are up to 90% if all the above five parameters are met.[73] In another study, patients with acutely relapsing CIDP were more likely (71%) to respond to IVIG.[64] It is the author's experience that patients with less severe axonal changes improve much better; hence, the need to initiate therapy early.

An association analysis with single nucleotide polymorphisms (SNPs) and haplotype studies was recently performed in 100 Japanese patients categorized as responders or nonresponders to IVIG therapy.[74] Two separate SNPs, corresponding to transient axonal glycoprotein 1 (TAG-1) and C-type lectin domain family 10, member A (CLEC10A), showed strong significant differences between responders and nonresponders. Haplotype analysis of a series of expanded SNPs, from TAG-1 or CLEC10A, showed that only TAG-1 included a significant haplotype within 1 linkage disequilibrium block, which accommodates IVIG responsiveness. This interesting study is the first to show that TAG-1 is a crucial molecule involved in IVIG responsiveness in Japanese patients with CIDP and opens the way to explore whether responsiveness to IVIG is dependent on genetic determinants.

Another marker recently explored in CIDP was the expression of the inhibitory FcRIIB on B cells.[75] The FcRIIB on B cells transduces inhibitory signals on B cells and prevents their transformation into IgG-producing plasma cells; as a result, mice lacking FcRIIB develop autoimmune diseases. Patients with CIDP were found to have lower FcRIIB on naive B cells and failed to up-regulate or maintain FcRIIB as the disease progressed.[75] Of interest, FcRIIB protein expression was up-regulated on monocytes and B cells after clinically effective IVIG therapy, suggesting that the effect of IVIG on FcRIIB may be a factor predicting the patients more likely to respond to IVIG. These results are arguably very preliminary but of potential significance if confirmed in a large number of patients studied prospectively.

IVIG in Children with CIDP

Although controlled studies have not yet been performed, IVIG may also be efficacious in childhood CIDP.[76,58] Multiple courses of IVIG appear to secure continuous efficacy.[77] The author's facility has found the need to combine alternate-day prednisone with IVIG in difficult cases, which met with considerable success and minimal toxicity. Treatment can at times be discontinued, and in that sense, childhood CIDP may have a more favorable outcome than CIDP in adults, provided treatment starts very early before axonal degeneration takes place.

Multifocal Motor Neuropathy

MMN presents with a slow-onset weakness and muscular atrophy, usually in the distal upper extremities, with areflexia and preserved sensation. The disease is characterized by conduction block of the motor axons and, in many patients, by the presence of antibodies to the GM1 ganglioside. Unlike CIDP, MMN does not respond to steroids or plasmapheresis. However, based on controlled trials and several open-label studies, MMN responds remarkably well to IVIG therapy.[78-86] The improvement usually begins after 7 to 10 days, as in CIDP, and predictably lasts for 4 to 6 weeks, at which time a new infusion is required either with 2 g/kg or 1 g/kg. The author has noticed that even chronic cases of MMN with already significant loss of motor axons can respond to a certain degree. As symptoms diminish, the electrophysiologic conduction block may resolve.[85]

Therapy with IVIG is currently the treatment of choice in MMN. However, some patients may not respond adequately after a period of time, probably because of further progression of the underlying disease and axonal degeneration.[86,87] In these circumstances, anti-CD20 (rituximab) or intravenous cyclophosphamide, as much as 1 g/m^2 body surface area, may be helpful.[88,89] Long-term maintenance therapy with IVIG was investigated in 11 MMN patients followed for 4 to 8 years.[86,87] Patients initially received IVIG, 0.4 g/kg/day, for 5 days followed by one 0.4-g/kg infusion every week for 1 year and as needed in subsequent years, with a mean dose of 7 to 48 g/week. Muscle strength improved significantly within 3 weeks of IVIG treatment but declined slightly and significantly during the follow-up period. It is interesting that electrophysiologic changes consistent with improvement (remyelination or reinnervation) and worsening (demyelination or axon loss) occurred simultaneously in different nerves. Conduction block also disappeared in some nerve segments but appeared in others. These results contrast with those from Vucic et al,[90] who were able to maintain response when the monthly infusions of IVIG were kept high, up to 2 g/kg monthly (instead of less than 1 g/kg as in the Dutch study). Although the optimal maintenance dose still remains empirical, the latter study suggests that IVIG, at the full maintenance dose, has the potential to arrest disease progression and prevent axonal degeneration.[90] Patients with amyotrophic lateral sclerosis (ALS), which sometimes resembles MMN, do not respond to IVIG. In a study of 9 patients with ALS, IVIG treatment failed to change the course of the disease.[91]

Paraproteinemic Demyelinating Polyneuropathies

Demyelinating polyneuropathies associated with IgG or IgA monoclonal gammopathies respond to IVIG therapy in ways similar to CIDP. Patients with IgM monoclonal gammopathy and demyelinating polyneuropathy, however, form a distinct subset. More than 50% of these patients have antibodies against MAG and sphingoglycolipids and compose a more uniform group, which is clinically characterized by a predominantly sensory ataxic or a sensorimotor neuropathy. Because patients with anti-MAG neuropathies respond poorly to therapies, a double-blind controlled study with IVIG was performed.[92] The study was prompted after the improvement observed in 2 patients treated with IVIG in an open-label fashion.[93]

Eleven patients were randomized to IVIG or placebo, given monthly for 3 months in a double-blind study; after a washout period, they crossed over to the alternate therapy. The trial showed modest, but not significantly different, benefits. After IVIG treatment, strength improved in only 2 of 11 patients and declined after placebo; in one other patient, only the sensory scores improved.[92] Antibody titers to MAG/SGPG or gangliosides did not change appreciably. A second trial, conducted in Europe, also showed modest benefits that were statistically significant only in the secondary end points.[94] Because elevated IgM may cause high serum viscosity, which can be further increased with IVIG as discussed below, caution is needed when IVIG is infused in such patients to avoid triggering thromboembolic events. Because the disease responds to rituximab, based on a controlled study,[89] rituximab is becoming the treatment of choice for the IgM-anti-MAG neuropathy.

Other Neuropathies

Other peripheral neuropathies in which there are reports of the efficacy of IVIG include diabetic amyotrophy, vasculitic peripheral neuropathy, and painful sensory neuropathy associated with Sjögren's syndrome. The evidence for these conditions has been insufficient, however, to earn a recommendation for the use of IVIG from national or international guidelines.[95]

Myasthenia Gravis

MG is characterized by fluctuating weakness or fatigability of the extraocular, bulbar, respiratory, and limb muscles. Diplopia, dysphagia, and dysathria are common. Myasthenia is the prototypic autoimmune disease for the following reasons[96,97]:
1. Two antigens, the acetylcholine receptor (AChR) or muscle-specific tyronsine kinase (MuSK), are known and can be detected and measured in the patients' serum.
2. The patient's IgG binds to the AChRs at the postsynaptic region and, by fixing complement or cross-linking, results in internalization or degradation of the AChRs and simplification of the postsynaptic junctional folds.
3. IgG antibodies are pathogenic because they transmit the disease to experimental animals and cause destruction of AChRs in cultured myotubes.
4. Immunization of healthy animals with AChRs leads to MG that can be subsequently passed to other animals with purified IgG.
5. Removal of the pathogenic autoantibodies results in clinical improvement.

Patients with MG respond fairly well to the available therapies, such as anticholinesterases, thymectomy, steroids, azathioprine, cyclosporine, and plasmapheresis. The need for another effective immunomodulating therapy without long-term side effects has prompted experimentation with high-dose IVIG.

As reviewed previously,[98,99] IVIG is likely to be successful in MG patients either during acute exacerbations or as a means of managing difficult cases during the chronic phases of the disease. However, the published series on the use of IVIG, although promising for the treatment of exacerbations, have not been adequately designed to provide evidence-based answers regarding the use of IVIG in the chronic management of the disease or as a steroid-sparing agent.[98,100]

Between 1986 and 2001, a number of patients have been enrolled in small, uncontrolled studies that showed that the majority of patients (sometimes as high as 78%) respond to IVIG. However, these studies, again, had been small and uncontrolled; the studied patients were heterogeneous regarding disease severity and duration; the effect of other treatments used concurrently with IVIG had not been factored in; and the means of assessing efficacy had been heterogeneous. Some of these concerns have been resolved with the randomized trials discussed below, but others remain unsettled.

The first randomized study compared the efficacy and tolerance of two doses of IVIG to PE in MG exacerbations.[101] A total of 87 patients were randomized to receive either three courses of PE or 0.4 g/kg/day of IVIG for 3 or 5 days. The study demonstrated similar efficacy, measured by variation in myasthenic muscular score, in both the PE and IVIG groups; the anti-AChR antibody titers fell by about two-thirds in both groups. Interestingly, the 3-day IVIG regimen was slightly superior to the 5-day regimen, although methodologic deficiencies limit a rigorous comparison. A second, large, controlled study, conducted by the same group, randomized 173 patients to 1 g/kg IVIG for 1 day or to 2 g/kg for 2 days.[102] At day 15, the myasthenic scores improved equally in both groups, leading to the conclusion that IVIG is efficacious in MG but that there is no difference between 2 g/kg vs 1 g/kg.

A recent trial compared IVIG to placebo in MG patients who had "worsening weakness," defined as increasing symptoms or signs severe enough (as judged by both the patient and the physician) to warrant a change in therapy.[103] Fifty-one AChR-positive patients were randomized to receive either 2 g/kg IVIG or the equivalent volume of dextrose 5% over 2 days. The main end point was the change in quantitative MG scores (QMGSs) from baseline (day 0) to day 14. A post-hoc analysis of the IVIG treatment effect was performed by stratifying the patients according to their baseline severity: mild, moderate, or severe. On day 14, the mean change in QMGS was -2.5 in the IVIG group and -0.9 in the placebo group (p = 0.047). On day 28, these values were -3 in the IVIG group and -1.2 in the placebo group (p = 0.055). For the mild MG cases, the mean change in QMGS on day 14 was similar in the two groups: -0.7 in the IVIG group and -1.1 in the placebo group. The only significant difference was noted for the moderate to severe MG group where these values were -4.1 in the IVIG group and -0.7 in the placebo group (p = 0.01); that treatment effect was maintained at day 28.

This study, has several limitations. First, the effect was modest, as patients improved by 2.54 QMG units compared to 0.89 in the placebo; considering that individual QMGSs usually vary up to 2.6 units, this effect might not have been clinically significant. Second, the effect did not reach the 3.5 units cited as clinically significant and used to calculate the sample size. Third, it was statistically significant (by more than 4.1 points) only in a small number of patients with severe MG, suggesting that the study lost power because of including patients with less severe disease. Fourth, the definition of "worsening weakness" was rather subjective.

Two additional randomized, controlled studies[104,105] have addressed the efficacy of IVIG for the treatment of moderate to severe but stable MG, one comparing IVIG to plasma exchange and the other to placebo. Neither showed a significant difference.

From these data, along with other published series and the author's own observations, several conclusions can be drawn, as recently discussed.[98,99] First, the majority of patients with MG exacerbations can respond to IVIG therapy. The improvement is seen early, beginning after a mean period of 3 to 10 days and lasting for a mean period of 30 days. Second, IVIG appears to be as effective as plasmapheresis, but for myasthenic crises plasmapheresis is superior. Third, the role of IVIG in the chronic management of MG has not yet been established. The numbers of confounding factors involved in deciding the best therapy for MG at a given state of the disease demand carefully designed studies, clear objectives, accurate assessment of efficacy, and precise control of the concomitant immunosuppressive drugs.

The following questions remain unanswered regarding the use of IVIG in the chronic management of MG[99]:

1. Is IVIG effective in patients with mild-to-severe but stable MG not adequately controlled with immunosuppressive drugs? If so, when should it be used in relationship to the other drugs, and is it cost effective?
2. Does IVIG have a role as a steroid-sparing drug?
3. Is the effect of IVIG temporary, or does it have a long-term benefit?
4. Is IVIG effective in a crisis, and is it as good as plasmapheresis?
5. Is there a synergistic effect of IVIG with the other drugs used in the treatment of the disease?
6. What is the mechanism of action of IVIG in MG, and does it have an effect on AChR antibody titers, immunoregulatory T cells, or other immune factors?
7. Is IVIG effective in seronegative MG or in MuSk-positive patients?

Until further controlled trials are conducted, IVIG may be justified in lieu of plasmapheresis 1) for acutely worsening disease to prevent or minimize impending bulbar or respiratory failure, 2) to prepare a weak patient for thymectomy, and 3) as an adjuvant to immunosuppressive therapies and periodically (every 1 to 3 months) to minimize the long-term side effects or stabilize a patient until immunosuppressants, such as azathioprine or cyclosporin, become effective.[2]

Lambert-Eaton Myasthenic Syndrome

Patients with LEMS have a presynaptic neuromuscular junction defect that results in proximal muscle weakness, oculomotor signs, and autonomic dysfunction. The symptoms are caused by antibodies against presynaptic voltage-gated calcium channels, resulting in decreased acetylcholine release. Patients respond to diaminopyridine, steroids, and azathioprine. Even though IVIG is rarely needed, a controlled study has been conducted comparing IVIG to placebo. The IVIG-randomized patients showed a statistically significant increase in muscle strength compared to placebo, which peaked at 2 to 4 weeks and declined by 8 weeks. The effectiveness of IVIG was associated with a statistically significant reduction of antibodies against voltage-gated calcium channels.[106] IVIG is useful in difficult cases of LEMS, especially when steroids and azathioprine are not very effective or cause significant side effects.

Inflammatory Myopathies

The main subsets in the group of inflammatory myopathies include DM, polymyositis, and IBM. IVIG has been tried in all three of them, but controlled trials have been performed only in DM and IBM.

Dermatomyositis

DM is an acquired myopathy causing proximal muscle weakness and a violaceous rash on the face and extremities. Early deposition of MAC on the endomysial capillaries leads to capillary destruction, muscle ischemia, and inflammation. Cytokines and adhesion molecules participate in the trafficking of sensitized lymphocytes and macrophages from intramuscular blood vessels to muscle fibers.[16,17] The disease responds to steroids but often becomes steroid resistant. Azathioprine, methotrexate, and cyclosporine offer modest benefit but rarely cause a remission.

Effects of Treatment. Administration of IVIG to patients with DM is effective and can produce striking clinical and histopathologic improvements. In a double-blind, placebo-controlled study, 15 patients with treatment-resistant DM received IVIG, 2.0 g/kg, or placebo once a month for 3 months, with the option of crossing over to the alternative therapy for 3 more months.[18] At the end of the first 3-month treatment phase, IVIG-treated patients experienced a significant improvement in Medical Research Council scores ($p < 0.018$) and neuromuscular symptoms ($p < 0.035$) compared with those receiving placebo. Marked improvements were also noted in the active violaceous rash or the chronic scaly eruptions.[18] In subsequent open-label infusions, the benefit of IVIG has been documented in a large number of patients treated by the author's facility or under its supervision and by several investigators throughout the world.[107,108] Repeat open muscle biopsies on patients who clinically improved have shown marked improvement in the muscle cytoarchitecture, including muscle fiber diameter, revascularization with increased number of capillaries per fiber, and reduction of inflammation and connective tissue.[18] Immunopathologically, it was shown that IVIG inhibits the deposition of MAC on the endomysial capillaries by intercepting the incorporation of C3 into the C5 convertase assembly, down-regulates the expression of the ICAM-1 on the endomysial capillaries and the MHC-I antigen on muscle fibers, and reduces the expression of TGFβ_1 protein and mRNA in connective tissue.[19,107,18,28] IVIG also modified certain immunoregulatory and structural genes in the muscles of DM patients who responded to IVIG therapy, as determined by gene array studies.

Most notable about those genes was the expression of the chemokine Mig/CXCL9 gene, which was up-regulated in the repeated muscle biopsies after IVIG treatment only in DM patients who improved but not in IBM patients who did not respond.[109] Additionally, the expression of the anosmin-1/KAL-1 gene, which encodes a protein involved in fibrosis, was reduced after IVIG therapy only in improved DM muscles but not in IBM. These molecules probably represent proteins associated with tissue remodeling and need to be further explored as potential markers of response to IVIG.

Maintenance and Chronic Use. An improvement in strength becomes noticeable after 15 days and peaks after 1 month, but it does not usually last more than 4 to 8 weeks; repeated infusions are therefore required periodically to maintain the response. Some patients may additionally require low-dose steroids or rituximab, which seems to be a promising agent for some patients.[107] Because DM initially responds to steroids, IVIG therapy is best reserved as second-line add-on therapy for patients who are not adequately controlled with a combination of steroids and methotrexate or azathioprine, and for patients who are immunodeficient or in whom steroids are contraindicated.[110]

Inclusion Body Myositis

IBM is the most common acquired inflammatory myopathy in patients above the age of 50 years. The condition presents with selective atrophy of forearm flexor muscles, frequent falls, atrophy of the quadricep muscles, and dysphagia. Immunopathologically, IBM is identical to polymyositis, characterized by sensitized, antigen-driven cytotoxic T cells that invade MHC-I-expressing muscle fibers.[16,17] What makes IBM unique, however, is the presence of vacuolated fibers that contain amyloid deposits and the resistance of the disease to most immunosuppressive medications.

The efficacy of IVIG was tested in 19 patients with IBM in a study designed similarly to the previously mentioned DM trial.[107,111] In the IVIG-treated group, there was an increase in muscle scores compared to placebo, but the differences were not statistically significant, perhaps because the study lacked sufficient power.[111] Nonetheless, significant regional differences occurred in IVIG-treated patients, especially in the swallowing function, which improved significantly in patients receiving IVIG compared with those receiving placebo (p <0.05).

The mild benefits noted in certain muscle groups prompted a larger study aimed to investigate the potential synergistic effect of IVIG with prednisone.[112] Thirty-six patients were randomized to IVIG, 2 g/kg, or placebo once a month for 3 months. Before infusions, all patients received prednisone (tapered from 60 mg/day). After 3 months of treatment, there was no significant difference in muscle strength score between the IVIG-plus-prednisone group and the placebo-plus-prednisone group. A third trial showed similar results.[113] In spite of these negative results, a few patients may show transient signs of improvement which, although minor and difficult to capture with the methods used, can be at times clinically significant for the patients' activities and lifestyles, at least for a period of time. When life-threatening dysphagia is apparent, IVIG is a treatment option in view of the positive results noted above.[114]

Stiff-Person Syndrome

SPS is a disabling central nervous system disorder characterized by muscle rigidity, episodic muscle spasms, and high titers of antibodies against glutamic acid decarboxylase, the rate-limiting enzyme for synthesis of gamma-aminobutyric acid (GABA). Various other autoantibodies (eg, anti-amphiphysin) are also present.[115]

Drugs that enhance GABA neurotransmission, such as diazepam, provide only mild-to-modest relief of clinical symptoms[115]; however, treatment with IVIG confers substantial benefit, as documented in a placebo-controlled crossover study in 16 patients administered IVIG, 2 g/kg, or placebo once a month for 3 months.[112] Efficacy was assessed with the use of an objective distribution-of-stiffness index and heightened-sensitivity scale. Among patients initially treated with IVIG, stiffness scores decreased significantly (p = 0.02) and heightened-sensitivity scores declined markedly, but they rebounded during placebo administration; the opposite pattern occurred among those treated with placebo first. Eleven patients who received IVIG were able to walk more easily or without assistance and to perform work-related or household tasks; their frequency of falls decreased. The study convincingly showed that IVIG is effective as supplementary therapy in patients with SPS.[110]

Multiple Sclerosis

In multiple sclerosis (MS), the most common neuroimmunologic disorder, IVIG would be expected to be successful,[116] but the results have been disappointing. On the basis of a number of controlled studies, IVIG is not effective in patients with progressive forms or those with fixed deficits. Some encouraging results in the relapsing-remitting cases were overshadowed by the less-than-optimal design of the conducted trials, the noninclusion magnetic resonance imaging (MRI) parameters, the small number of treated patients, and the overpowering results of the interferons trials, which had been based on a large number of patients. Perhaps the only indication of IVIG in MS may be to treat relapses occurring during the postpartum period in breast-feeding women and in rare patients who had a relapse during pregnancy and failed to respond to intravenous steroids.[117,118]

Novel and Promising Applications

In the central nervous system (CNS), chronic inflammatory conditions can lead to a chronic degenerative state, mediated mostly via cytokines, in what is called "neuroinflammation." There has been significant interest in exploring, via controlled studies, the role of IVIG in these conditions, most notably Alzheimer disease (AD), post-polio syndrome, tissue fibrosis, autoimmune sleep disorders, and chronic pain syndrome associated with reflex sympathetic dystrophy.[119] The most significant efforts are summarized below.

Alzheimer Disease

One of the pathologic hallmarks of AD is the extracellular accumulation of amyloid-beta (Aβ) peptides in the senile plaques, along with activation of microglia and up-regulation of cytokines such as TGFβ. Because IVIG has been shown to contain autoantibodies against Aβ amyloid and is known to suppress cytokines, it was considered as a novel therapeutic approach for the treatment of AD.

In an open-label study of eight patients with mild AD, IVIG increased the level of plasma anti-Aβ titers, which was associated with an increase in Aβ peptide levels in the serum and a decrease in Aβ peptide levels in the CSF. Cognitive function improved in six of eight patients after 6 months of IVIG therapy.[120] These encouraging results led to a Phase II study performed in three groups of eight patients with mild-to-moderate AD who were randomly assigned to groups receiving 0.4 g IVIG/kg/month, 0.8 g IVIG/kg/month, or placebo. The levels of anti-Aβ antibodies and of Aβ 40/42 peptides were quantified in plasma and CSF before and after therapy. Cognitive and behavioral assessments and activities of daily living scales were performed before and after 3, 6, and 9 months of infusions. IVIG infusions increased anti-Aβ and Aβ 40/42 peptides in plasma and decreased Aβ 40/42 peptides in CSF compared with values before treatment.[95] Cerebral glucose uptake, measured by positron emission tomography (PET) scanning after 18-fluorodeoxyglucose injection before and 6 months after infusion therapy, showed stable metabolic activity in the IVIG-treated patients but a reduction in the placebo-treated group.[95] The results seem encouraging but require a controlled study, which is now under way in a large number of patients.

Post-Polio Syndrome

This is a chronic degenerative condition that develops many years after an initial attack of acute paralytic poliomyelitis infection. It is thought to be caused by attrition of the surviving motor neurons.[121] Because lymphocytic infiltrates have been observed in the patients' spinal cords even many years later,[22] along with up-regulated cytokines in the CSF, the possibility of a persistent smoldering inflammatory response has been proposed as having a role in the patients' symptomatology. Accordingly, the role of IVIG in the patients' weakness and fatigue was explored in a controlled study performed in 135 patients. The study showed some benefits in physical activity scores, compared to placebo, but they were of unclear clinical importance; a down-regulation of cytokines was also noted after IVIG.[123] These results have not been reconfirmed.

Treatment Considerations Using IVIG in Neurology

Dose

The therapeutic dose of IVIG is empirically set at 2 g/kg. Although past practice has been to divide the total dose for infusion into five daily doses of 400 mg/kg each, the preference now is to divide the total dose into two daily doses of 1 g/kg each, especially in younger patients who have normal renal and cardiovascular function.[1] In the author's experience, the 2-day infusion is not associated with more adverse reactions than the 5-day infusion, and it is preferable except for patients with major cardiovascular risks. Considering the drug's rapid diffusion to the extravascular space, achieving a high concentration of IVIG within 2 days may enhance its efficacy. Experimental studies, both in vitro and in vivo, suggest a superior effect on cytokine neutralization, Fc receptor manipulation,[124] and inhibition of C3 fragments[15] when IVIG concentrations equivalent to 2 g/kg are given in a bolus infusion rather than in divided doses. In children with Kawasaki syndrome, a single, large, 2-g/kg dose of IVIG given in a 10-hour infusion was more effective than four daily infusions of 400 mg/kg each.[125] A similar experience was noted in children with GBS.[56] The new ICE trial in CIDP was also conducted with a 2-day infusion with an excellent safety and tolerance profile.

Adverse Reactions and Risk Factors

In general, adverse reactions to IVIG therapy are usually minor and occur in no more than 10% of the patients with neurologic disorders. Mild-to-moderate headache, which responds to nonsteroidal anti-inflammatory medications, is common. Chills, myalgia, or chest discomfort may develop in the first hour of the infusion and usually abate when the infusion is stopped for 30 minutes and resumed at a slower rate. Postinfusion fatigue, fever, or nausea may occur and last for up to 24 hours. The cause of these reactions is unclear, but activation of complement by aggregated immunoglobulin molecules or various stabilizing agents in the IVIG preparation have been implicated.[1,126] A slow rate of infusion is advisable in patients with a compromised cardiovascular system or congestive heart failure to avoid rapid fluid overload.

Serum Viscosity and Thromboembolic Events

IVIG therapy causes an increase in serum viscosity, up to 0.5 centipoise (cp); in patients with high-normal or slightly elevated serum viscosity, such as those with cryoglobulinemia, hypercholesterolemia, or hypergammaglobulinemia, the viscosity level increases even further.[127] Serum viscosity greater than 2.5 cp (normal = 1.2 to 1.8 cp) increases the risk of thromboembolic events and may be one of the factors responsible for rare cases of stroke, pulmonary embolism, or myocardial infarction noted after IVIG treatment.[127-133] Patients with recent deep vein thrombosis or immobilized patients who are at higher risk of having a subclinical thrombosis may be more prone to develop a thromboembolic event after IVIG. In such patients, prudence in justifying the use of IVIG, screening the legs with an ultrasound for subclinical clots, and a very slow infusion rate are recommended. Whether low-dose heparin or antiplatelet agents can prevent thromboembolic events in such patients is uncertain. A reversible cerebral vasospasm has also been noted.[134]

Migraine Headache

In patients with a history of migraine, IVIG therapy may trigger a migraine attack, which can be prevented by pretreatment with propranolol.[135] The occurrence of aseptic meningitis, discussed below, is also high in migrainous patients.[136] IVIG therapy has been associated with a stroke in a young woman with a history of migraine.[131]

Aseptic Meningitis

Aseptic meningitis develops in some patients treated with IVIG. Its occurrence is unrelated to the proprietary product, the rate of infusion, or the underlying disease.[136-138] Prophylaxis with intravenous steroids is often ineffective. The symptoms respond to strong analgesia and subside in 24 to 48 hours. Additional diagnostic testing is rarely necessary.[137,138]

Skin Reactions

Skin reactions to IVIG therapy, although rare, can develop 2 to 5 days after the infusions and may last up to 30 days. They include urticaria, lichenoid cutaneous lesions, pruritus of the palms, and petechiae of the extremities.[1,137] Skin reactions, associated with various lots of IVIG, have occurred in 7 of the 120 patients initially treated at the author's facility.[1,137]

Severe Anaphylactic Reaction

Severe anaphylactic reaction has been reported in patients with an absence or severe deficiency of IgA who also have IgA antibodies. Selective IgA deficiency is common (prevalence is ~1:1000) but asymptomatic. About 29% of individuals with this reaction have IgA antibodies, which does not necessarily predict the development of adverse reactions.[139] Theoretically, when these patients receive IVIG, the small amount of IgA present with the IVIG may lead to an anaphylactic reaction caused by formation of macromolecular complexes between the infused IgA and circulating anti-IgA. The reaction is rare and has not been seen in the author's facility, nor has it been reported, in neurologic patients; it may occur in patients with common variable immunodeficiency.[140]

Renal Tubular Necrosis

Acute renal tubular necrosis, mostly reversible, occurs rarely with IVIG therapy in patients who have preexisting kidney disease and volume depletion, especially the elderly and those with diabetes or poor hydration.[141] It is usually reversible, but rare fatalities have been noted.[142,143] Serum creatinine may rise 1 to 10 days after the infusion but returns to baseline within 2 to 60 days of discontinuation.[143] This complication has often, but not exclusively, been associated with the high concentration of sucrose in some proprietary IVIG products.[142] Osmotically-induced tubular injury and vacuolization are the common histopathologic findings on renal biopsy.[143] Identical osmotic tubular nephrosis is caused by intravenous solutions containing a concentration of hypertonic sucrose similar to that of IVIG.[142] Diluting the IVIG preparation, slowing the rate of infusion, or selecting products with low osmolality minimizes the risk. In patients with preexisting kidney disease, if there is no alternate therapy to IVIG treatment, close monitoring of creatinine and blood urea nitrogen are essential.

Spurious Results on Serologic Tests

After IVIG therapy, the erythrocyte sedimentation rate increases sixfold or more,[144] probably as the result of enhanced rouleux formation and reduced surface area caused by the infused gamma globulin.[1] This increase can persist for 2 to 3 weeks and should not be considered a sign of a developing vasculitis. The author has also observed hyponatremia, with sodium concentrations as low as 130 mg/L (normal = 135-145 mg/L) after IVIG therapy but not after placebo use.[144] Hyponatremia appears to be related to the assay method used to measure Na$^+$ because additional dilution of the sample is required, owing to the high serum protein concentration that follows IVIG infusion.

References

1. Dalakas MC. Intravenous immunoglobulin in the treatment of autoimmune neuromuscular diseases: Present status and practical therapeutic guidelines. Muscle Nerve 1999;22:1479-97.
2. Dalakas MC. Intravenous immunoglobulin in autoimmune neuromuscular diseases. JAMA 2004;291:2367-75.
3. Dalakas MC, Spath PJ, eds. Intravenous immunoglobulins in the third millennium. Lancaster, UK: Parthenon Publishing, 2004.
4. Stangel M, Hartung HP, Marx P, Gold R. Intravenous immunoglobulin treatment of neurological autoimmune diseases. J Neurol Sci 1998;153:203-14.
5. Dalakas MC. Interplay between inflammation and degeneration: Using inclusion body myositis to study neuroinflammation (editorial). Ann Neurol 2008;64:1-3.
6. Dalakas MC. The use of intravenous immunoglobulin in the treatment of autoimmune neurological disorders: Evidence-based indications and safety profile. Pharmacol Ther 2004;102:177-93.
7. Gold R, Stangel M, Dalakas MC. Drug insight: Use of intravenous immunoglobulin in neurology: Practical issues and therapeutic considerations. Nature Clin Pract Neurol 2007;3:36-44.
8. Kazatchkine MD, Kaveri SV. Immunomodulation of autoimmune and inflammatory diseases with intravenous immune globulin. N Engl J Med 2001;345:747-55.
9. Dietrich G, Kazatchkine MD. Normal immunoglobulin G (IgG) for therapeutic use (intravenous Ig) contains anti-idiotypic specificities against an immunodominant, disease-associated, cross-reactive idiotype of human anti-thyroglobulin autoantibodies. J Clin Invest 1990;85:620-9.
10. Kaveri S, Prasad N, Vassilev T, et al. Modulation of autoimmune responses by intravenous immunoglobulin. Mult Scler 1997;3:121-8.
11. Kazatchkine MD, Dietrich G, Hurez V, et al. V region-mediated selection of autoreactive repertoires by intravenous immunoglobulin. Immunol Rev 1994;139:79-107.
12. Malik U. Oleksowicz L, Latov N, Cardo LJ. Intravenous [gamma]-globulin inhibits binding of anti-GM1 to its target antigen. Ann Neurol 1996;39:136-9.
13. Buchwald B, Ahangari R, Weishaupt A, Toyka KV. Intravenous immunoglobulins neutralize blocking antibodies in Guillain-Barré syndrome. Ann Neurol 2002;51:673-80.
14. Dalakas MC. Blockade of blocking antibodies in Guillain-Barré syndromes: "Unblocking" the mystery of action of intravenous immunoglobulin. Ann Neurol 2002;51:667-9.
15. Basta M, Kirshbom P, Frank MM, Fries LF. Mechanisms of therapeutic effect of high-dose intravenous immunoglobulin. J Clin Invest 1989;84:1974-81.
16. Dalakas MC. Polymyositis, dermatomyositis and inclusion-body myositis. N Engl J Med 1991;325:1487-98.
17. Dalakas MC, Hohlfeld R. Polymyositis and dermatomyositis. Lancet 2003;362:971-82.
18. Dalakas MC, Illa I, Dambrosia JM, et al. A controlled trial of high-dose intravenous immunoglobulin infusions as treatment for dermatomyositis. N Engl J Med 1993;329:1993-2000.
19. Basta M, Dalakas MC. High-dose intravenous immunoglobulin exerts its beneficial effect in patients with dermatomyositis by blocking endomysial deposition of activated complement fragments. J Clin Invest 1994;94:1729-35.
20. Dalakas MC. Mechanism of action of intravenous immunoglobulin and therapeutic considerations in the treatment of autoimmune neurologic diseases. Neurology 1998;51(Suppl):S2-S8.
21. Basta M, Illa I, Dalakas MC. Increased in vitro uptake of the complement C3b in the serum of patients with Guillain Barré syndrome, myasthenia gravis and dermatomyositis. J Neuroimmunol 1996;71:227-9.
22. Zhang G, Lopez PH, Li CY, et al. Anti-ganglioside antibody-mediated neuronal cytotoxicity and its protection by intravenous immunoglobulin: Implications for immune neuropathies. Brain 2004;127:1085-100.
23. Samuelsson A, Towers TL, Ravetch JV. Anti-inflammatory activity of IVIG mediated through the inhibitory Fc receptor. Science 2001;291:484-6.

24. Dalakas MC. Intravenous immunoglobulin therapy for neurological diseases. Ann Intern Med 1997;126:721-30.
25. Dalakas MC. Mechanisms of action of IVIG and therapeutic considerations in the treatment of acute and chronic demyelinating neuropathies. Neurology 2002;59(Suppl 6):S13-21.
26. Creange A, Gregson NA, Hughes RA. Intravenous immunoglobulin modulates lymphocyte CD54 and monocyte FcgammaRII expression in patients with chronic inflammatory neuropathies. J Neuroimmunol 2003;135:91-5.
27. Svenson M, Hansen MB, Bendtzen K. Binding of cytokines to pharmaceutically prepared human immunoglobulin. J Clin Invest 1993;92:2533-9.
28. Amemiya K, Semino-Mora C, Granger RP, Dalakas MC. Downregulation of TGF-β1 mRNA and protein in the muscles of patients with inflammatory myopathies after treatment with high-dose intravenous immunoglobulin. Clin Immunol 2000;94:99-104.
29. Rigal D, Vermot-Desroches C, Heitz S, et al. Effect of IVIG in peripheral blood B, NK, and T cell subpopulations in women with recurrent spontaneous abortions: Specific effect on LFA-1 and CD56 molecules. Clin Immunol Immunopathol 1994;71:309-14.
30. Abe Y, Horiuchi A, Miyake M, Kimura S. Anticytokine nature of natural human immunoglobulin: One possible mechanism of the clinical effect of intravenous immunoglobulin therapy. Immunol Rev 1994;139:5-19.
31. Ankrust P, Muller F, Svenson M, et al. Administration of intravenous immunoglobulin (IVIg) in vivo downregulatory effects on the IL-1 system. Clin Exp Immunol 1999;115:136-43.
32. Gabriel CM, Gregson NA, Redford EJ, et al. Human immunoglobulin ameliorates rat experimental allergic neuritis. Brain 1997;120:1533-40.
33. 33. van Engelson BGM, Miller DJ, Pavelko KD, et al. Promotion of remyelination by polyclonal immunoglobulin in Theiler's virus-induced demyelination and in multiple sclerosis. J Neurol Neuros Psych 1994;57(Suppl):65-8.
34. Sekul EA, Cupler EJ, Dalakas MC. Aseptic meningitis associated with high-dose intravenous immunoglobulin therapy: Frequency and risk factors. Ann Intern Med 1994;121:259-62.
35. Hahn AF. Guillain-Barré syndrome. Lancet 1998;352:635-41.
36. Hartung HP, Pollard JD, Harvey GK, Toyka KV. Immunopathogenesis and treatment of the Guillain-Barré syndrome—Part II. Muscle Nerve 1995;18:154-64.
37. Gold R, Dalakas MC, Toyka KV. Immunotherapy in autoimmune neuromuscular disorders. Lancet Neurology 2003;2:22-32.
38. Hafer-Macko C, Hsieh ST, Li CY, et al. Acute motor axonal neuropathy: An antibody-mediated attack on axolemma. Ann Neurol 1996;40:635-44.
39. Hafer-Macko CE, Sheikh KA, Li CY, et al. Immune attack on the Schwann cell surface in acute inflammatory demyelinating polyneuropathy. Ann Neurol 1996;39:625-35.
40. French Cooperative Group on Plasma Exchange in Guillain-Barré Syndrome. Efficiency of plasma exchange in Guillain-Barré syndrome: Role of replacement fluids. Ann Neurol 1987;22:753-61.
41. Guillain-Barré Study Group. Plasmapheresis and acute Guillain-Barré syndrome. Neurology 1985;35:1096-104.
42. van der Meche FGA, Schmitz PIM. A randomized trial comparing intravenous immune globulin and plasma exchange in Guillain-Barré syndrome. Dutch Guillain-Barré Study Group. N Engl J Med 1992;326:1123-9.
43. Plasma Exchange/Sandoglobulin Guillain-Barré Syndrome Trial Group. Randomized trial of plasma exchange, intravenous immunoglobulin, and plasma exchange followed by intravenous immunoglobulin in Guillain-Barré syndrome. Lancet 1997;349:225-30.
44. Dutch Guillain-Barré Study Group. Treatment of Guillain-Barré syndrome with high-dose immune globulins combined with methylprednisolone: A pilot study. Ann Neurol 1994;35:749-52.
45. van Koningsveld R, Schmitz PIM, van der Meché FG, et al. Effect of methylprednisolone when added to standard treatment with intravenous immunoglobulin for Guillain-Barré syndrome: Randomized trial. Lancet 2004;363:192-6.
46. Arakawa Y, Yoshimura M, Kobayashi S, Ichihashi K. The use of intravenous immunoglobulin in Miller-Fisher syndrome. Brain Dev 1993;15:231-3.
47. Raphael JC, Chevret S, Harboun M, Jars-Guincestre MC. Intravenous immune globulins in patients with Guillain-Barré syndrome and contraindications to plasma exchange: 3 days

versus 6 days. J Neurol Neurosurg Psychiatry 2001;71:235-8.
48. Farcas P, Avnun L, Frisher S, et al. Efficacy of repeated intravenous immunoglobulin in severe unresponsive Guillain-Barré syndrome. Lancet 1997;350:1747.
49. Visser LH, van der Meché FG, Meulstee J, van Doorn PA. Risk factors for treatment related clinical fluctuations in Guillain-Barré syndrome. Dutch Guillain-Barré Study Group. J Neurol Neurosurg Psychiatry 1998;64:242-4.
50. Romano JG, Rotta FT, Potter P, et al. Relapses in the Guillain-Barré syndrome after treatment with intravenous immune globulin or plasma exchange. Muscle Nerve 1998;21:1327-30.
51. Ho TW, Hsieh ST, Nachamkin I, et al. Motor nerve terminal degeneration provides a potential mechanism for rapid recovery in acute motor axonal neuropathy after Campylobacter infection. Neurology 1997;48:695-700.
52. Kuwabara S, Asahina M, Koga M, et al. Two patterns of clinical recovery in Guillain-Barré syndrome with IgG anti-GM1 antibody. Neurology 1998;51:1656-60.
53. Rees JH, Gregson NA, Hughes RAC. Antiganglioside antibodies in Guillain Barré syndrome and their relationship to Campylobacter jejuni infection. Ann Neurol 1995;38:809-16.
54. van Koningsveld R, Steyerberg EW, Hughes RA, et al. A clinical prognostic scoring system for Guillain-Barré syndrome. Lancet Neurol 2007;6:589-94.
55. Kuitwaard K, de Gelder J, Tio-Gillen AP, et al. Pharmacokinetics of intravenous immunoglobulin and outcome in Guillain-Barré syndrome. Ann Neurol 2009;66:597-603.
56. Kanra G, Uzon A, Vajsar J, et al. Intravenous immunoglobulin treatment in children with Guillain-Barré syndrome. Eur J Paediatr Neurol 1997;1:7-12.
57. Reisin RC, Pociecha J, Rodriguez E, et al. Severe Guillain-Barré syndrome in childhood treated with human immune globulin. Pediatr Neurol 1996;14:308-12.
58. Kornberg AJ. Clinical experience with intravenous immunoglobulin for treatment of pediatric Guillain-Barré syndrome and chronic inflammatory demyelinating polyradiculoneuropathy. In: Dalakas MC, Spath PJ, eds. Intravenous immunoglobulin in the third millennium. Lancaster, UK: Parthenon Publishers, 2004.
59. Kieseier BC, Dalakas MC, Hartung HP. Immune mechanisms in chronic inflammatory demyelinating neuropathy. Neurology 2002; 59(Suppl 6):S7-12.
60. Yuki N. Infectious origins of, and molecular mimicry in, Guillain-Barré and Fisher syndromes. Lancet Infect Dis 2001;1:29-37.
61. Weiss MD, Luciano CA, Semino-Mora C, et al. Molecular mimicry in chronic inflammatory demyelinating polyneuropathy and melanoma. Neurology 1998;51:1738-41.
62. Hughes R, Bensa S, Willison H, et al. Randomized controlled trial of intravenous immunoglobulin versus oral prednisolone in chronic inflammatory demyelinating polyradiculoneuropathy. Ann Neurol 2001;50:195-201.
63. Dyck PJ, Litchy WJ, Kratz KM, et al. A plasma exchange versus immune globulin infusion trial in chronic inflammatory demyelinating polyradiculoneuropathy. Ann Neurol 1994;36: 838-45.
64. Hahn AF, Bolton CF, Zochodne D, Feasby TE. Intravenous immunoglobulin treatment in chronic inflammatory demyelinating polyneuropathy. A double-blind, placebo-controlled, cross-over study. Brain 1996;119:1067-77.
65. Mendell JR, Barohn RJ, Freimer ML, et al. Randomized controlled trial of IVIG in untreated chronic inflammatory demyelinating polyradiculoneuropathy. Neurology 2001;56:445-9.
66. Dalakas MC. Advances in chronic inflammatory demyelinating polyneuropathy: Disease variants and inflammatory response mediators and modifiers. Curr Opin Neurol 1999;12: 403-9.
67. Saperstein DS, Katz JS, Amato AA, Barohn RJ. Clinical spectrum of chronic acquired demyelinating polyneuropathies. Muscle Nerve 2001; 24:311-24.
68. Sharma KR, Cross J, Farronay O, et al. Demyelinating neuropathy in diabetes mellitus. Arch Neurol 2002;59:758-65.
69. Hughes RA, Donofrio P, Bril V, et al. Intravenous immune globulin (10% caprylate-chromatography purified) for the treatment of chronic inflammatory demyelinating polyradiculoneuropathy (ICE study): A randomised placebo-controlled trial. Lancet Neurol 2008;7:136-44. Erratum in: Lancet Neurol 2008;7:771.
70. Merkies IS, Bril V, Dalakas MC, et al. Health-related quality-of-life improvements in CIDP with immune globulin IV 10%: The ICE study. Neurology 2009;72:1337-44.
71. Bril V, Katzberg H, Donofrio P, et al. Electrophysiology in chronic inflammatory demyeli-

nating polyneuropathy with IGIV. Muscle Nerve 2009;39:448-55.
72. McCrone P, Chisholm D, Knapp M, et al. Cost-utility analysis of intravenous immunoglobulin and polyradiculoneuropathies (CIDP). Eur J Neurol 2003;10:687-94.
73. Vermeulen M, van Doorn PA, Brand A, et al. Intravenous immunoglobulin treatment in patients with chronic inflammatory demyelinating polyneuropathy: A double blind, placebo controlled study. J Neurol Neurosurg Psychiatry 1993;56:36-9.
74. Iijima M, Tomita M, Morozumi S, et al. Single nucleotide polymorphism of TAG-1 influences IVIG responsiveness of Japanese patients with CIDP. Neurology 2009;73:1348-52.
75. Tackenberg B, Jelcic I, Baerenwaldt A, et al. Impaired inhibitory Fcgamma receptor IIB expression on B cells in chronic inflammatory demyelinating polyneuropathy. Proc Natl Acad Sci U S A 2009;106:4788-92.
76. Nevo V, Pestronk A, Kornberg AJ, et al. Childhood chronic inflammatory demyelinating neuropathies: Clinical course and long-term follow-up. Neurology 1996;47:98-102.
77. Simmons Z, Wald JJ, Albers JW. Chronic inflammatory demyelinating polyradiculoneuropathy in children: II. Long-term follow-up, with comparison to adults. Muscle Nerve 1997;20:1569-75.
78. Azulay JP, Blin O, Pouget J, et al. Intravenous immunoglobulin treatment in patients with motor neuron syndromes associated with anti-GM1 antibodies. Neurology 1994;44:429-32.
79. Bouche P, Moulonguet A, Younes-Chennoufi AB, et al. Multifocal motor neuropathy with conduction block: A study of 24 patients. J Neurol Neurosurg Psychiatry 1995;59:38-44.
80. Chaudhry V, Corse AM, Cornblath DR, et al. Multifocal motor neuropathy: Response to human immune globulin. Ann Neurol 1993;33:237-42.
81. Leger JM, Younes-Chennoufi AB, Chassande B, et al. Human immunoglobulin treatment of multifocal motor neuropathy and polyneuropathy associated with monoclonal gammopathy. J Neurol Neurosurg Psychiatry 1994;57S:46-9.
82. Nobile-Orazio E, Meucci N, Barbieri S, et al. High-dose immunoglobulin therapy in multifocal motor neuropathy. Neurology 1993;43:537-44.
83. Van den Berg LH, Franssen H, Wokke JHJ. The long term effect of intravenous immunoglobulin treatment in multifocal motor neuropathy. Brain 1998;121:421-8.
84. Van den Berg LH, Kerkhoff H, Oey PL, et al. Treatment of multifocal motor neuropathy with high dose intravenous immunoglobulins: A double blind, placebo controlled study. J Neurol Neurosurg Psychiatry 1995;59:248-52.
85. Federico P, Zochodne DW, Hahn AF, et al. Multifocal motor neuropathy improved by IVIG: Randomized, double-blind, placebo-controlled study. Neurology 2000;55:1256-62.
86. Van den Berg-Vos RM, Franssen H, Wokke JH, Van den Berg LH. Multifocal motor neuropathy: Long-term clinical and electrophysiological assessment of intravenous immunoglobulin maintenance treatment. Brain 2002;125:1875-86.
87. Terenghi F, Cappellari A, Bersano A, et al. How long is IVIG effective in multifocal motor neuropathy? Neurology 2004;62:666-8.
88. Elliott JL, Pestronk A. Progression of multifocal motor demyelinating neuropathy during apparently successful treatment with human immunoglobulin. Neurology 1994;44:967-8.
89. Dalakas MC, Rakocevic G, Salajegheh M, et al. Placebo-controlled trial of rituximab in IgM anti-myelin-associated glycoprotein antibody demyelinating neuropathy. Ann Neurol 2009;65:286-93.
90. Vucic S, Black KR, Chong PS, Cros D. Multifocal motor neuropathy: Decrease in conduction blocks and reinnervation with long-term IVIG. Neurology 2004;63:1264-9.
91. Dalakas MC, Stein DP, Otero C, et al. Effect of high-dose intravenous immunoglobulin on amyotrophic lateral sclerosis and multifocal motor neuropathy. Arch Neurol 1994;51:861-4.
92. Dalakas MC, Quarles RH, Farrer RG, et al. A controlled study of intravenous immunoglobulin in demyelinating neuropathy with IgM gammopathy. Ann Neurol 1996;40:792-5.
93. Cook D, Dalakas MC, Galdi A, et al. High-dose intravenous immunoglobulin in the treatment of demyelinating neuropathy associated with monoclonal gammopathy. Neurology 1990;40:212-14.
94. 94. Comi G, Roveri L, Swan A, et al. A randomized controlled trial of intravenous immunoglobulin in IgM paraprotein associated demyelinating neuropathy. J Neurol 2002;249:1370-7.
95. Hughes RA, Dalakas MC, Cornblath DR, et al. Clinical applications of intravenous immu-

noglobulins in neurology. Clin Exp Immunol 2009;158(Suppl 1):34-42.
96. Drachman DB. Myasthenia gravis. N Engl J Med 1994;330:1797-810.
97. Hoch W, McConville J, Helms S, et al. Autoantibodies to the receptor tyrosine kinase MuSK in patients with myasthenia gravis without acetylcholine receptor antibodies. Nat Med 2001;7:365-8.
98. Dalakas MC. Experience with IVIG in the treatment of patients with myasthenia gravis. Neurolog 1997;48(Suppl 5):S64-S69.
99. Dalakas MC. IVIG Therapy in myasthenia gravis and mechanism of immunosuppression. In: Christados P, ed. Myasthenia gravis: Disease mechanisms and immune interventions. Deer Park, NY: Linus Publications, 2010:89-102.
100. Gajdos P, Chevret S, Toyka K. Intravenous immunoglobulin for myasthenia gravis. Cochrane Database Syst Rev 2008 Jan 23;(1): CD002277.
101. Gajdos PH, Chevret S, Clair B, et al. Clinical trial of plasma exchange and high-dose intravenous immunoglobulin in myasthenia gravis. Ann Neurol 1997;41:789-96.
102. Gadjos P. Intravenous immunoglobulin for myasthenia gravis. In: Dalakas MC, Spath PJ, eds. Intravenous immunoglobulins in the third millennium. Lancaster, UK: Parthenon Publishing, 2004:203-5.
103. Zinman L, Ng E, Bril V. IV immunoglobulin in patients with myasthenia gravis: A randomized controlled trial. Neurology 2007;68:837-41.
104. Ronager J, Ravnborg M, Hermansen I, Vorstrup S. Immunoglobulin treatment versus plasma exchange in patients with chronic moderate to severe myasthenia gravis. Artif Organs 2001; 25:967-73.
105. Wolf HM, Eibl MM. Immunomodulatory effect of immunoglobulins. Clin Exp Rheumatol 1996;14(Suppl 15):S17-25.
106. Bain PG, Motomura M, Newsom-Davis J, et al. Effects of intravenous immunoglobulin (IVIG) treatment on muscle weakness and calcium channel autoantibodies in the Lambert-Eaton myasthenic syndrome. Neurology 1996;47: 678-83.
107. Dalakas MC. Controlled studies with high-dose intravenous immunoglobulin in the treatment of dermatomyositis, inclusion body myositis and polymyositis. Neurology 1998;51(Suppl): S37-45.
108. Mastaglia FL, Phillips BA, Zilko PJ. Immunoglobulin therapy in inflammatory myopathies. J Neurol Neurosurg Psychiatry 1998;65:107-110.
109. Raju R, Dalakas MC. Gene expression profile in the muscles of patients with inflammatory myopathies: Effect of therapy with IVIG and biologic validation of clinical relevant genes. Brain 2005;128:1887-96.
110. Dalakas MC. IVIG in patients with anti-GAD antibody associated neurological diseases and patients with inflammatory myopathies: Effects on clinicopathologic features and immunoregulatory genes. Clin Rev Allergy Immunol 2005; 29:255-69.
111. Dalakas MC, Sonies B, Dambrosia J, et al. Treatment of inclusion body myositis with IVIG: A double-blind, placebo-controlled study. Neurology 1997;48:712-16.
112. Dalakas MC, Fujii M, Li M, et al. High-dose intravenous immune globulin for stiff-person syndrome. N Engl J Med 2001;345:1870-6.
113. Walter MC, Lochmuller H, Toepfer M, et al. High-dose immunoglobulin therapy in sporadic inclusion body myositis: A double-blind, placebo-controlled study. J Neurol 2000;247:22-8.
114. Cherin P, Pelletier S, Teixeira A, et al. Intravenous immunoglobulin for dysphagia of inclusion body myositis. Neurology 2002;58:326.
115. Dalakas MC, Fujii M, Li M, McElroy B. The clinical spectrum of anti-GAD antibody-positive patients with stiff-person syndrome. Neurology 2000;55:1531-5.
116. Dalakas MC. Inhibiting leucocyte recruitment to the brain by IVIG. Is it relevant to the treatment of demyelinating CNS disorders (editorial)? Brain 2004;127:2569-71.
117. Achiron A, Kishner I, Dolev M, et al. Effect of intravenous immunoglobulin treatment on pregnancy and postpartum-related relapses in multiple sclerosis. J Neurol 2004;251:1133-7.
118. Stangel M, Gold R. Intravenous immunoglobulins in MS. Int MS J 2005;12:4, 5-10.
119. Dalakas MC. Role of IVIG in autoimmune, neuroinflammatory and neurodegenerative disorders of the central nervous system: Present and future prospects. J Neurol 2006;253 (Suppl 5):v25-v32.
120. Dodel RC, Du Y, Depboylu C, et al. Intravenous immunoglobulins containing antibodies against beta-amyloid for the treatment of Alzheimer's disease. J Neurol Neurosurg Psychiatry 2004;75:1472-4.

121. Dalakas MC. Post-polio syndrome 12 years later: How it all started. Ann N Y Acad Sci 1995;753:11-18.
122. Pezeshkpoor GH, Dalakas MC. Long-term changes in the spinal cords of patients with old poliomyelitis. Arch Neurol 1988;45:505-8.
123. Gonzalez H, Sunnerhagen KS, Sjöberg I, et al. Intravenous immunoglobulin for post-polio syndrome: A randomised controlled trial. Lancet Neurol 2006;5:493-500.
124. Kurlander RJ, Hall J. Comparison of intravenous gammaglobulin and a monoclonal anti-Fc receptor antibody as inhibitors of immune clearance in vivo in mice. J Clin Invest 1986; 77, 2010-18.
125. Newburger JW, Takahashi M, Berser AS, et al. A single intravenous infusion of gamma globulin as compared with four infusions in the treatment of acute Kawasaki syndrome. N Engl J Med 1991;324:1633-9.
126. Dwyer JM. Manipulating the immune system with immune globulin. N Engl J Med 1992; 326:107-16.
127. Dalakas MC. High-dose intravenous immunoglobulin and serum viscosity: Risk of precipitating thromboembolic events. Neurology 1994; 44:223-6.
128. Hague RA, Eden DB, Yap PL, et al. Hyperviscosity in HIV infected children: A potential hazard during intravenous immunoglobulin therapy. Blut 1990;61:66-7.
129. Schiff RJ. Transmission of viral infections through intravenous immune globulin. N Engl J Med 1994;331:1649-50.
130. Silbert PL, Knezevic WV, Bridge DT. Cerebral infarction complicating intravenous immunoglobulin therapy for polyneuritis cranialis. Neurology 1992;42:257-8.
131. Steg RE, Lefkowitz DM. Cerebral infarction following intravenous immunoglobulin therapy for myasthenia gravis. Neurology 1994;44: 1180-1.
132. Woodruff RK, Griff AP, Firkin FL, Smith IL. Fatal thrombic events during treatment of autoimmune thrombocytopenia with intravenous immunoglobulin in elderly patients. Lancet 1986;2:217-18.
133. Dalakas MC, Clark WM. Strokes, thromboembolic events, and IVIG: Rare incidents blemish an excellent safety record. Neurology 2003; 60:1736-7.
134. Voltz RV, Rosen F, Yousry T, et al. Reversible encephalopathy with cerebral vasospasm in a GBS patient treated with IV immunoglobulin. Neurology 1996;46:250-1.
135. Constantinescu CS, Chang AP, McClusky LF. Recurrent migraine and intravenous immune globulin therapy. N Engl J Med 1993;329: 583-4.
136. Sekul EA, Cupler EJ, Dalakas MC. Aseptic meningitis associated with high-dose intravenous immunoglobulin therapy: Frequency and risk factors. Ann Intern Med 1994;121:259-62.
137. Dalakas MC. Meningitis and skin reactions after intravenous immunoglobulin therapy. Ann Intern Med 1997;127:1130.
138. Dalakas MC. Aseptic meningitis and intravenous immunoglobulin. Ann Intern Med 1995; 122:316-7.
139. Burks AW, Sampson HA, Buckley RH. Anaphylactic reactions after gamma globulin administration in patients with hypogammaglobulinemia. N Engl J Med 1986;314:560-4.
140. Björkander J, Hammarström L, Smith E, et al. Immunoglobulin prophylaxis in patients with antibody deficiency syndromes and anti-IgA antibodies. J Clin Immunol 1987;7:8-15.
141. Ellie E, Combe C, Ferrer X. High-dose intravenous immune globulin and acute renal failure. N Engl J Med 1992;327:1032-3.
142. Ahsan N, Palmer BF, Wheeler D, et al. Intravenous immunoglobulin-induced osmotic nephrosis. Arch Intern Med 1994;154:1985-7.
143. Ahsan N. Intravenous immunoglobulin induced-nephropathy: A complication of IVIG therapy. J Nephrol 1998;11:157-61.
144. Koffman BM, Dalakas MC. Effect of high-dose intravenous immunoglobulin on serum chemistry, hematology and lymphocyte subpopulations: Assessments based on controlled treatment trials in patients with neurological diseases. Muscle Nerve 1997;20:1102-7.

6

Clinical Use of IVIG in Infectious Diseases and Inflammatory Response Syndromes

Kevin B. Laupland, MD, MSc, FRCPC

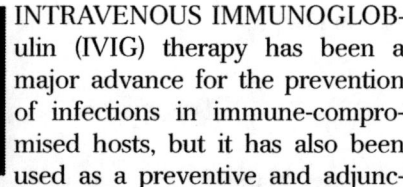

INTRAVENOUS IMMUNOGLOBulin (IVIG) therapy has been a major advance for the prevention of infections in immune-compromised hosts, but it has also been used as a preventive and adjunctive therapy for infections and infection-associated inflammatory conditions in patients without preexisting immune deficiencies. Commercial preparations of IVIG contain antibodies with high activity against a broad range of viruses and bacteria pathogens and their toxins.[1] Although IVIG may theoretically exert a therapeutic benefit in patients without preexisting immune deficiencies by direct anti-antigen effects among specific infection-naive patients, it may also have a number of favorable effects on blood rheology, the microvasculature and immune modulatory effects not limited to enhancement of opsonic activity, prevention of excessive complement activation, and promotion of antibody-dependent cytotoxicity.[1-4] Because of these numerous theoretical benefits, IVIG has been used broadly for "off-label" indications for prevention and treatment of infections.[5-7] However, despite the intrinsic appeal for using this agent, its high cost, limitations in supply, and the potential for side effects has required rationing of its use.

This chapter aims to review the use of standard polyclonal IVIG for the prevention and treatment of infections and infection-associated

---

Kevin B. Laupland, MD, MSc, FRCPC, Associate Professor, Departments of Medicine, Critical Care Medicine, Pathology and Laboratory Medicine, and Community Health Sciences, University of Calgary, Calgary, Alberta, Canada

The author has disclosed no conflicts of interest.

inflammation in patients without preexisting immune impairment. It will focus on standard polyclonal IVIG and will therefore not review specific hyperimmune immunoglobulin preparations.

Prevention in Neonates

Newborns normally have low levels of endogenous immunoglobulins (Ig) A and M and, when premature, have deficiencies in maternal IgG because this immunoglobulin crosses the placenta to the fetus after approximately 32 weeks gestation.[8] Supplemental IVIG has therefore been proposed as a preventive therapy for infection in high-risk neonates. Ohlsson and Lacy conducted a systematic review and meta-analysis of randomized and quasi-randomized controlled trials assessing IVIG as a preventive measure for infection in preterm (<37 weeks gestation) and/or low-birth-weight (<2500 g) infants on behalf of the Cochrane Collaboration.[9] Nineteen studies involving a total of 4986 subjects were included. They observed significant overall pooled reductions both for sepsis [relative risk (RR) = 0.85; 95% confidence interval (95% CI) = 0.74-0.98] and for any serious infection (RR = 0.82; 95% CI = 0.74-0.92) for IVIG use as compared to placebo or usual care. Significant between-study heterogeneity existed for both of these outcomes. It is important to note that no statistically significant differences were observed between IVIG and control for all cause mortality, infection-associated death, or incidence of serious complications of necrotizing enterocolitis, bronchopulmonary dysplasia, or intraventricular hemorrhage or for length of hospital stay. Although statistically significant reductions in sepsis and serious infections occurred with IVIG prophylaxis, other important outcomes were not different between IVIG and control patients. As a result, the routine use of IVIG to prevent infections in preterm and low-birth-weight neonates cannot be supported.

Prevention in Critically Ill and High-Risk Surgical Patients

Although not usually classified as a specific immune-compromised state, critical illness is associated with immune system anergy, reduced antibody levels, and an associated increased risk for invasive infections. By virtue of its potent anti-antigen and immune modulatory effects, IVIG has been studied as a measure to prevent complicating infections in high-risk surgical and critically ill patients. A number of randomized clinical trials have been conducted over recent decades,[10] and these are summarized in Table 6-1.[11-20] Of note, one additional trial has apparently found a positive effect of adjuvant treatment of mediastinitis after cardiac surgery,[21] although actual results have yet to be published in the peer-reviewed literature. The available evidence evaluating IVIG as a preventive therapy in high-risk surgical and critically ill patients indicates variable but generally significant effects on reducing the incidence of infections and attenuation of postoperative inflammation. However, it does not appear to have a detectable effect on reducing mortality. The overall risk-benefit and cost-effectiveness of IVIG prophylaxis in this setting has yet to be established, and thus its routine use cannot not be currently recommended.

Treatment

Neonatal Sepsis

Based on a similar rationale as for the use of IVIG in the prevention of infection in high-risk neonates, Ohlsson and Lacy also performed a systematic review and meta-analysis of IVIG as a therapy for suspected or proven infection in newborns.[22] They searched for randomized and quasi-randomized trials evaluating IVIG as compared to control for treatment of infection in newborns less than 28 days old. A total of 529 subjects were enrolled in nine trials. Methodologic limitations were numerous and included small sample size (studies ranged from 22 to 82 subjects) and use of a wide range of

Table 6-1. Randomized Clinical Trials of IVIG for Prophylaxis of Infection and Severe Systemic Inflammatory Response Syndromes in Critically Ill and High-Risk Surgical Patients

Setting	Treatments Tested	Patients	Outcomes	Limitations	First Author, Year, Reference
Trauma patients ventilated in ICU >24 hours	36 g IVIG vs 0.03% albumin	150	Decreased overall incidence of infection and antibiotic use in IVIG group	Blinding not well described	Glinz, 1985[11]
Major trauma and surgery ICU patients	40 g IVIG vs 5% dextrose	40	No difference in rates of sepsis or mortality; fewer positive blood cultures in second week of observation	Small numbers; incidence of nonseptic infections not reported; not blinded	Mao, 1989[12]
Severely burned children and adults	IVIG or placebo twice weekly for 5 weeks	50	No difference in infection incidence or mortality	Small numbers	Waymack, 1989[13]
Colorectal surgery patients at high risk for sepsis	12-15 g IVIG each on days 1 and 5 vs usual care	80	Significantly fewer infections in IVIG group	Open label	Cafiero, 1992[14]
Surgical ICUs	IVIG or hyperimmune LPS IVIG, 400 mg/kg, or 25% albumin	329	Reduced infection incidence with standard IVIG; shorter ICU stay	Intention to treat analysis not available	Intravenous Immunoglobulin Collaborative Study Group, 1992[15]
Children with severe head trauma	400 mg/kg IVIG vs 5% albumin	33	No difference in infections incidence, length of stay, or mortality	Small numbers; intention to treat analysis not available; randomization process not described	Gooding, 1993[16]

(Continued)

Table 6-1. Randomized Clinical Trials of IVIG for Prophylaxis of Infection and Severe Systemic Inflammatory Response Syndromes in Critically Ill and High-Risk Surgical Patients (Continued)

Setting	Treatments Tested	Patients	Outcomes	Limitations	First Author, Year, Reference
Postoperative open heart surgery patients with cutaneous anergy preoperatively	20 g IGM-IgA-enriched IVIG vs saline	40	Infection incidence much lower with IVIG	Selected population (40 of 515); open label; small numbers	Kress, 1999[17]
Severe trauma patients admitted to ICU	1 g/kg IVIG vs 1 g/kg albumin	39	No difference in overall infection rates, ICU length of stay, or antibiotic use	Small numbers	Douzinas, 2000[18]
Cardiac surgery patients	65 g IgM-enriched IVIG vs control	41	Significant reduction in signs of inflammation but not cytokine levels with IVIG	Small size; nonsevere disease; randomization, blinding processes not described	Friedrich, 2002[19]
Postoperative cardiac surgery patients with inflammatory response syndrome	Total 0.9 g/kg IVIG vs equivolume 0.1% albumin over 2 days	244	No difference in severity of illness or inflammatory markers during first 5 days or mortality at day 28	Selected population (244 of 6984)	Werdan, 2008[20]

ICU = intensive care unit; LPS = lipopolysaccharide.

IVIG doses and preparations. Only 5 trials had blinded randomization, only 4 studies were reported as intention to treat, and it was unclear in many cases as to whether all cause mortality was reported. In six studies involving 318 cases, IVIG treatment reduced mortality associated with suspected infection (RR = 0.63; 95% CI = 0.40-1.00). The authors also conducted a second analysis of 7 trials with 262 subjects that evaluated IVIG as compared to control but restricted assessment to subjects with subsequently proven infection. In this case, treatment with IVIG significantly reduced mortality (RR = 0.55; 95% CI = 0.31-0.98). However, given that treatment is usually initiated with suspicion of infection that may later be proven or not, the clinical value of this second analysis may be questioned.

Given the borderline statistical significance of suspected infections, cost considerations, and major methodologic limitations of these studies, IVIG cannot be routinely recommended for the treatment of infections in neonates. The International Neonatal Immunotherapy Study, which is a large (3493 subjects), multicenter, randomized trial evaluating IVIG therapy for suspected or proven sepsis, has recently been closed to further enrollment, and results are expected to be published in 2010.[23] It is hoped that this trial will support a definitive recommendation surrounding the use of IVIG as an adjunctive therapy for neonatal sepsis.

Severe Sepsis and Septic Shock in Adults

Severe sepsis and septic shock are clinical conditions characterized by serious infection associated with systemic inflammation. While numerous definitions exist, the most widely accepted and used definitions are those developed through an expert consensus in 1991.[24] Case-fatality rates are among the highest observed of any other acute illness, with severe sepsis and septic shock in adults resulting in death in approximately 30% and 50% of cases, respectively.[25-28] Despite initial results suggesting benefit for a number of adjunctive therapies, subsequent studies have questioned these and the therapeutic armamentarium has remained frustratingly limited.[29]

Numerous clinical trials evaluating IVIG adjunctive therapy for sepsis have been conducted over the past two decades and have been the subject of multiple meta-analyses.[30-35] Although these meta-analyses have varied in age range, other inclusion criteria, and the appraisal of methodology, they have all shown a clinically and statistically significant overall mortality benefit. However, conclusions by the authors and accompanying editorials have been inconsistent,[36,37] and methodologic quality has had an important influence on the interpretation of effect size in these trials. Studies conducted in adults with severe disease have averaged 50 subjects per study, and only three (four, depending on definition) trials have had more than 100 patients randomized.[34,35] In addition, only two-thirds have reported adequate allocation concealment methods, and less than one-half were adequately blinded. Recent, larger, more rigorously designed trials have demonstrated much less effect than older, smaller, less-well-designed studies. In addition, greater effect has been seen with those that use higher doses (≥1 g/kg) of IVIG and, potentially, with IgM and IgA-enriched preparations. The most important consideration of the effect of IVIG therapy in adults with sepsis is that one carefully designed, large study (representing nearly one-half of all adults studied to date) reported by Werdan et al showed no overall significant mortality difference with IVIG therapy and has had a major influence on the pooled effect attributable to IVIG therapy.[38] In sum, although IVIG has shown potential great promise, there remains clinical equipoise as to whether IVIG reduces the mortality of severe sepsis and septic shock in adults. Although it may be considered in individual cases, its routine use cannot be currently supported.

Toxic Shock Syndromes

The toxic shock syndromes (TSS) represent a subgroup of patients with septic shock as discussed in the previous section, but because of their clinical features and unique pathophysiology, they merit separate consideration.[39] Staphylococcal TSS is caused by *Staphyloccocus aureus* and is characterized by hypotension, fever, rash, desquamation, and evidence of multiorgan dysfunction. Although initially associated with use of superabsorbent tampons, non-menstrually associated cases may occur. Streptococcal TSS is caused by *Streptococcus pyogenes* and is characterized by isolation of this organism (usually from a normally sterile body site), hypotension, and multisystem impairment. It frequently occurs in association with rapidly progressive necrotizing soft tissue infection. Although the epidemiology and clinical features of these two etiologies of TSS are distinct, they share in common a presumed superantigen-mediated pathogenesis. Because IVIG contains antibodies to these exotoxins, has potent immune-modulating effects, and neutralizes superantigen activity, its use as a therapy in TSS has been proposed and widely adopted in many jurisdictions.[40,41]

The empiric clinical data supporting the use of IVIG in TSS is sparse and largely based on theoretical and retrospective observational data.[42] Patients with TSS or even invasive *S. aureus* or *S. pyogenes* infections have represented a minimal number in the overall randomized clinical trials evaluating IVIG in septic shock to date.[30-35] Only one clinical trial has directly assessed the use of IVIG for the treatment of streptococcal TSS. In this study reported by Darenburg et al, 21 patients were randomized to either 2 g/kg IVIG or albumin control.[43] Although markers of inflammation were reduced and fewer patients died with IVIG therapy, the numbers were too small to draw any conclusions. Despite the lack of empiric clinical evidence, based on the theoretical grounds, clinical observations, and the results of only one small clinical trial, there is a firm belief among many clinicians for a benefit for IVIG therapy in TSS, and it is considered a standard of care by many.[41]

Necrotizing Pneumonia and Soft Tissue Infections Caused by MRSA

The recent years have witnessed the worldwide emergence of community-associated methicillin-resistant *S. aureus* (MRSA) as a cause of serious infections, including necrotizing lung, skin, and soft tissue infections. Although the pathogenesis of these severe infections is a matter of debate, a toxin-mediated etiology is suggested, and in particular the Panton-Valentine leukocidin (PVL) has been implicated.[44] Gauduchon and colleagues assessed a French commercial IVIG preparation and found that it contained specific anti-PVL antibodies and that it neutralized pore formation and the cytopathic effect of both PVL and *S. aureus* culture supernatants.[45]

Other staphylococcal-specific polyclonal antibody preparations are under evaluation and suggest a role for manipulation of humoral immunity in the management of severe staphylococcal disease.[46] In severe cases of MRSA infection the results of past clinical trials may suggest a benefit and that these patients may be a specific subgroup that derives particular benefit. However, there is no specific empiric evidence, and an individualized approach is needed.

Clostridium Difficile-Associated Disease

Clostridium difficile-associated disease (CDAD) involves a spectrum of diarrheal diseases, including pseudomembranous colitis, and arises from exotoxins produced by *C. difficile*. Although often a mild diarrheal illness that resolves with specific antimicrobial therapy, total colectomy may be required in severe cases, and death may occur. Anecdotal case reports and series have suggested a benefit to adjunctive IVIG for this disease, and the observation that patients who develop pseudomembranous colitis have lesser responses to *C. difficile* toxins A and B has provided a rationale for its potential benefit.[47] Juang et al conducted a retrospective cohort study of 18 patients with severe CDAD disease treated with IVIG (single dose of 200-300 mg/kg) and then matched these patients to 18 controls not treated with IVIG.[48] Standard antibiotic therapy was administered to all patients. No differences in the rate of colectomies, length of stay, and all cause mortality were observed. This study was limited particularly because of its small size, retrospective design, and low dose of IVIG. However, given the lack of documented benefit, the use of IVIG in CDAD should be considered experimental.

Viral Infections

Because IVIG is prepared from large pools of plasma from thousands of donors, it has a broad range of activity against commonly circulating viral agents and contains antibodies to routinely vaccinated viral antigens in that population.[1] Although IVIG could conceivably be used for pretravel hepatitis A prevention and postexposure prophylaxis for hepatitis B and varicella-zoster virus infection, vaccination for these viruses is the primary means of prevention, and hyperimmune globulin that contains higher titers of antibody is recommended in the postexposure setting.[7,49] Similarly, while polyclonal IVIG has significant titers to tetanus and diphtheria toxins and could conceivably be used therapeutically, hyperimmune human or equine-derived immunoglobulins are the preferred standard therapy. Goldsmith et al tested eight American and two European licensed IVIG products for anti-vaccinia antibody activity.[50] Although they found significant activity with these preparations, they were not as potent as vaccinia hyperimmune globulin. In the 1950s, immune globulin was shown to reduce the risk of infection and complications when given to patients after they had been exposed to poliovirus infection.[51] Though not formally tested, preparations of IVIG made from donor pools from populations with high rates of poliovirus immunization may have similar effect.

Myocarditis

Robinson and colleagues recently reported on a systematic review through the Cochrane group on use of IVIG in the treatment of virus-infection-associated myocarditis.[52] They searched for trials comparing 1 g/kg IVIG with control for the management of acute (<6 months) presumed or documented viral myocarditis with associated reduced cardiac function. The one relevant study identified included 62 adults with acute myocarditis that were randomized to receive 2 g/kg IVIG or 0.1% albumin control.[53] The primary outcome was change in left ventricular ejection fraction at 6 and 12 months after randomization. Increases in left ventricular ejection fraction were similar in both groups (mean difference = 0.00; 95% CI = −0.07-0.07 at 6 months; and mean difference = 0.01; 95% CI = −0.06-0.08 at 12 months). Functional capacity was similar in both groups, and the requirement for cardiac transplant, placement of a left ventricular assist device, and mortality were low and comparable in both groups. Although this study was relatively small, it indicates a lack of benefit and does not support the use of IVIG in acute viral myocarditis.

Flaviviral Infection

The *Flavivirus* genus includes a number of important human infections not limited to yellow fever, St Louis encephalitis, Japanese encephalitis, West Nile encephalitis, and dengue fever. There are anecdotal reports suggesting benefit of IVIG in several of these infections, but further evidence to guide the use of IVIG is limited to dengue and West Nile virus (WNV) infection.[54-62] Most severe cases of dengue infection are associated with thrombocytopenia caused by anti-platelet IgG, and high-dose IVIG has therefore been evaluated as therapy for this complication. Dimaano et al conducted a randomized, controlled study comparing 0.4 g/kg/day IVIG for 3 days with standard therapy in 31 patients with dengue hemorrhagic fever.[54] Treatment with IVIG did not have any effect in the recovery of platelet counts. These data do not therefore support the use of IVIG in acute dengue infection.

Experimental animal studies and anecdotal case reports in humans suggest a potential benefit for IVIG use in WNV infection, particularly in its early stages.[55-60,62] Although WNV is typically a mild illness in the normal host, it may rarely (<1%) cause severe manifestations such as meningitis, encephalitis, and acute flaccid paralysis, and these are more frequently observed in immune-suppressed and chronically ill patients. Ben-Nathan and colleagues examined the prophylactic and therapeutic efficacy of human IVIG for treatment of a mouse WNV model.[58] Mice were protected in a dose- and time-dependent fashion by IVIG obtained from healthy Israeli blood donors containing WNV-specific antibodies but not by IVIG prepared from American donors that lacked these antibodies, suggesting a potential preventive and therapeutic role for IVIG preparations containing WNV-specific antibody.[58] It is important to note that since this time, WNV has become endemic in the United States, and more recent IVIG preparations from that country contain significant anti-WNV titers.[56] Ben-Nathan and colleagues also have more recently found a greater protective effect with a higher-titer WNV IVIG preparation.[62] Although case reports and these animal-based experiments suggest a potential role for IVIG in the management of severe WNV virus infection, human experimental data are lacking, and until such data are available its use will need to be based on an individualized clinical decision.[55,57,59,60] In such cases, IVIG preparations obtained from donor pools with high levels of immunity to WNV or those with documented high titers of anti-WNV should be used.

Other Viral Infections

Although a rare complication in immune-competent patients, parvovirus B19 infection with associated red cell aplasia is described in numerous anecdotal reports and recommendations for treatment.[6,63,64] Argentine hemorrhagic fever is a severe viral illness caused by a rodent-borne Junin virus. Immune plasma was found to improve outcome in a randomized controlled trial involving 188 patients conducted in Argentina in the 1970s.[65] Whether IVIG specifically prepared from pools of plasma from donors in endemic regions would be of benefit remains to be tested in this condition.[66] Although experimental evidence is limited, one echovirus outbreak investigation suggested that IVIG may attenuate the severity of disease, and there are also anecdotal reports with other enterovirus infections.[67,68]

Summary and Conclusion

Despite a strong theoretical rationale and often dramatic anecdotal clinical observations and experiences suggesting benefit in a wide range of infections in patients without preexisting immune compromise, there is generally a lack of empiric evidence to support the use of IVIG as an adjunctive therapy for infections in the nonimmunocompromised host. Although clinical trials indicate that IVIG reduces the risk of nosocomial infection in neonates and most likely in high-risk adults, it has not thus far been shown to reduce mortality, and its routine use is not justified in any age group. Clinical equipoise exists for the use of IVIG as an adjunctive therapy for severe infections and infection-associated inflammation. The results of a large, recently completed trial evaluating this therapy in neonates are awaited. While lacking specific clinical trial evidence, the use of IVIG as an adjunctive therapy for severe necrotizing MRSA infections and both streptococcal and staphylococcal TSS is common and considered a standard of care in many regions. No evidence supports the routine use of IVIG in the management of CDAD, dengue hemorrhagic fever, or viral myocarditis. Although laboratory studies and anecdotal reports suggest benefit for the use of high-titer anti-WNV IVIG, clinical trials of IVIG therapy in WNV infection in humans are needed.

References

1. Krause I, Wu R, Sherer Y, et al. In vitro antiviral and antibacterial activity of commercial intravenous immunoglobulin preparations—a potential role for adjuvant intravenous immunoglobulin therapy in infectious diseases. Transfus Med 2002;12:133-9.
2. Werdan K. Intravenous immunoglobulin for prophylaxis and therapy of sepsis. Curr Opin Crit Care 2001;7:354-61.
3. Jolles S, Sewell WA, Misbah SA. Clinical uses of intravenous immunoglobulin. Clin Exp Immunol 2005;142:1-11.
4. Madl C, Koppensteiner R, Wendelin B, et al. Effect of immunoglobulin administration on blood rheology in patients with septic shock. Circ Shock 1993;40:264-7.
5. Leong H, Stachnik J, Bonk ME, Matuszewski KA. Unlabeled uses of intravenous immune globulin. Am J Health Syst Pharm 2008;65: 1815-24.
6. Orange JS, Hossny EM, Weiler CR, et al. Use of intravenous immunoglobulin in human disease: A review of evidence by members of the Primary Immunodeficiency Committee of the

American Academy of Allergy, Asthma and Immunology. J Allergy Clin Immunol 2006; 117:S525-53.
7. Hemming VG. Use of intravenous immunoglobulins for prophylaxis or treatment of infectious diseases. Clin Diagn Lab Immunol 2001; 8:859-63.
8. Keller MA, Stiehm ER. Passive immunity in prevention and treatment of infectious diseases. Clin Microbiol Rev 2000;13:602-14.
9. Ohlsson A, Lacy JB. Intravenous immunoglobulin for preventing infection in preterm and/or low-birth-weight infants. Cochrane Database Syst Rev 2009(2):CD000361.
10. Laupland KB. Polyclonal intravenous immunoglobulin for the prophylaxis and treatment of infection in critically ill adults. Can J Infect Dis 2002;13:100-6.
11. Glinz W, Grob PJ, Nydegger UE, et al. Polyvalent immunoglobulins for prophylaxis of bacterial infections in patients following multiple trauma. A randomized, placebo-controlled study. Intensive Care Med 1985;11:288-94.
12. Mao P, Enrichens F, Olivero G, et al. Early administration of intravenous immunoglobulins in the prevention of surgical and post-traumatic sepsis: A double-blind randomized clinical trial. Surg Res Comm 1989;5:93-8.
13. Waymack JP, Jenkins ME, Alexander JW, et al. A prospective trial of prophylactic intravenous immune globulin for the prevention of infections in severely burned patients. Burns 1989;15:71-6.
14. Cafiero F, Gipponi M, Bonalumi U, et al. Prophylaxis of infection with intravenous immunoglobulins plus antibiotic for patients at risk for sepsis undergoing surgery for colorectal cancer: Results of a randomized, multicenter clinical trial. Surgery 1992;112:24-31.
15. Prophylactic intravenous administration of standard immune globulin as compared with core-lipopolysaccharide immune globulin in patients at high risk of postsurgical infection. The Intravenous Immunoglobulin Collaborative Study Group. N Engl J Med 1992;327:234-40.
16. Gooding AM, Bastian JF, Peterson BM, Wilson NW. Safety and efficacy of intravenous immunoglobulin prophylaxis in pediatric head trauma patients: A double-blind controlled trial. J Crit Care 1993;8:212-16.
17. Kress HG, Scheidewig C, Schmidt H, Silber R. Reduced incidence of postoperative infection after intravenous administration of an immunoglobulin A- and immunoglobulin M-enriched preparation in anergic patients undergoing cardiac surgery. Crit Care Med 1999;27:1281-7.
18. Douzinas EE, Pitaridis MT, Louris G, et al. Prevention of infection in multiple trauma patients by high-dose intravenous immunoglobulins. Crit Care Med 2000;28:8-15.
19. Friedrich I, Silber RE, Baumann B, et al. IgM-enriched immunoglobulin preparation for immunoprophylaxis in cardiac surgery. Eur J Med Res 2002;7:544-9.
20. Werdan K, Pilz G, Muller-Werdan U, et al. Immunoglobulin G treatment of postcardiac surgery patients with score-identified severe systemic inflammatory response syndrome—the ESSICS study. Crit Care Med 2008;36:716-23.
21. Marggraf G, Neugebauer EA. A multicentre randomised placebo-controlled double-blind study on adjuvant treatment of mediastinitis with immunoglobulins (Pentaglobin) after cardiac surgery (ATMI): Outline and preliminary study protocol for discussion. The ATMI Study Group. Eur J Surg Suppl 1999:26-32.
22. Ohlsson A, Lacy JB. Intravenous immunoglobulin for suspected or subsequently proven infection in neonates. Cochrane Database Syst Rev 2009(2):CD001239.
23. National Perinatal Epidemiology Unit. INIS: International Neonatal Immunotherapy Study. Oxford, UK: University of Oxford, 2009. [Available at: http://www.npeu.ox.ac.uk/inis (accessed February 22, 2010).]
24. American College of Chest Physicians/Society of Critical Care Medicine Consensus Conference: Definitions for sepsis and organ failure and guidelines for the use of innovative therapies in sepsis. Crit Care Med 1992;20:864-74.
25. Laupland KB, Zygun DA, Doig CJ, et al. One-year mortality of bloodstream infection-associated sepsis and septic shock among patients presenting to a regional critical care system. Intensive Care Med 2005;31:213-19.
26. Finfer S, Bellomo R, Lipman J, et al. Adult-population incidence of severe sepsis in Australian and New Zealand intensive care units. Intensive Care Med 2004;30:589-96.
27. Vincent JL, Sakr Y, Sprung CL, et al. Sepsis in European intensive care units: Results of the SOAP study. Crit Care Med 2006;34:344-53.
28. Engel C, Brunkhorst FM, Bone HG, et al. Epidemiology of sepsis in Germany: Results from

a national prospective multicenter study. Intensive Care Med 2007;33:606-18.
29. Dellinger RP, Levy MM, Carlet JM, et al. Surviving Sepsis Campaign: International guidelines for management of severe sepsis and septic shock: 2008. Crit Care Med 2008;36:296-327.
30. Alejandria MM, Lansang MA, Dans LF, Mantaring JB. Intravenous immunoglobulin for treating sepsis and septic shock. Cochrane Database Syst Rev 2002(1):CD001090.
31. Pildal J, Gotzsche PC. Polyclonal immunoglobulin for treatment of bacterial sepsis: A systematic review. Clin Infect Dis 2004;39:38-46.
32. Neilson AR, Burchardi H, Schneider H. Cost-effectiveness of immunoglobulin M-enriched immunoglobulin (Pentaglobin) in the treatment of severe sepsis and septic shock. J Crit Care 2005;20:239-49.
33. Turgeon AF, Hutton B, Fergusson DA, et al. Meta-analysis: Intravenous immunoglobulin in critically ill adult patients with sepsis. Ann Intern Med 2007;146:193-203.
34. Laupland KB, Kirkpatrick AW, Delaney A. Polyclonal intravenous immunoglobulin for the treatment of severe sepsis and septic shock in critically ill adults: A systematic review and meta-analysis. Crit Care Med 2007;35:2686-92.
35. Kreymann KG, de Heer G, Nierhaus A, Kluge S. Use of polyclonal immunoglobulins as adjunctive therapy for sepsis or septic shock. Crit Care Med 2007;35:2677-85.
36. Werdan K. Mirror, mirror on the wall, which is the fairest meta-analysis of all? Crit Care Med 2007;35:2852-4.
37. Neugebauer EA. To use or not to use? Polyclonal intravenous immunoglobulins for the treatment of sepsis and septic shock. Crit Care Med 2007;35:2855-6.
38. Werdan K, Pilz G, Bujdoso O, et al. Score-based immunoglobulin G therapy of patients with sepsis: The SBITS study. Crit Care Med 2007;35:2693-701.
39. Laupland KB, Davies HD. Toxic shock syndromes. In: Rello J, Kollef M, Diaz E, Rodriguez A, eds. Infectious diseases in critical care. 2nd ed. Berlin: Springer-Verlag, 2007:263-70.
40. Sriskandan S, Ferguson M, Elliot V, et al. Human intravenous immunoglobulin for experimental streptococcal toxic shock: Bacterial clearance and modulation of inflammation. J Antimicrob Chemother 2006;58:117-24.
41. Laupland KB, Boucher P, Rotstein C, et al. Intravenous immunoglobulin for severe infections: A survey of Canadian specialists. J Crit Care 2004;19:75-81.
42. Kaul R, McGeer A, Norrby-Teglund A, et al. Intravenous immunoglobulin therapy for streptococcal toxic shock syndrome—a comparative observational study. The Canadian Streptococcal Study Group. Clin Infect Dis 1999;28:800-7.
43. Darenberg J, Ihendyane N, Sjolin J, et al. Intravenous immunoglobulin G therapy in streptococcal toxic shock syndrome: A European randomized, double-blind, placebo-controlled trial. Clin Infect Dis 2003;37:333-40.
44. Yanagisawa C, Hanaki H, Natae T, Sunakawa K. Neutralization of staphylococcal exotoxins in vitro by human-origin intravenous immunoglobulin. J Infect Chemother 2007;13:368-72.
45. Gauduchon V, Cozon G, Vandenesch F, et al. Neutralization of Staphylococcus aureus Panton Valentine leukocidin by intravenous immunoglobulin in vitro. J Infect Dis 2004;189:346-53.
46. Rupp ME, Holley HP Jr, Lutz J, et al. Phase II, randomized, multicenter, double-blind, placebo-controlled trial of a polyclonal anti-Staphylococcus aureus capsular polysaccharide immune globulin in treatment of Staphylococcus aureus bacteremia. Antimicrob Agents Chemother 2007;51:4249-54.
47. Halsey J. Current and future treatment modalities for *Clostridium difficile*-associated disease. Am J Health Syst Pharm 2008;65:705-15.
48. Juang P, Skledar SJ, Zgheib NK, et al. Clinical outcomes of intravenous immune globulin in severe *Clostridium difficile*-associated diarrhea. Am J Infect Control 2007;35:131-7.
49. Desjardin JA, Snydman DR. Antiviral immunotherapy: A review of current status. BioDrugs 1998;9:487-507.
50. Goldsmith JC, Eller N, Mikolajczyk M, et al. Intravenous immunoglobulin products contain neutralizing antibodies to vaccinia. Vox Sang 2004;86:125-9.
51. Hammon W, Coriell LL, Stokes J. Evaluation of Red Cross gamma gloulin as a prophylactic agent for poliomyositis. 1. Plan of controlled field tests and results of the 1951 pilot study in Utah. JAMA 1952;150:739-60.
52. Robinson J, Hartling L, Vandermeer B, et al. Intravenous immunoglobulin for presumed viral myocarditis in children and adults.

Cochrane Database Syst Rev 2005(1): CD004370.
53. McNamara DM, Holubkov R, Starling RC, et al. Controlled trial of intravenous immune globulin in recent-onset dilated cardiomyopathy. Circulation 2001;103:2254-9.
54. Dimaano EM, Saito M, Honda S, et al. Lack of efficacy of high-dose intravenous immunoglobulin treatment of severe thrombocytopenia in patients with secondary dengue virus infection. Am J Trop Med Hyg 2007;77:1135-8.
55. Saquib R, Randall H, Chandrakantan A, et al. West Nile virus encephalitis in a renal transplant recipient: The role of intravenous immunoglobulin. Am J Kidney Dis 2008;52:e19-21.
56. Planitzer CB, Modrof J, Kreil TR. West Nile virus neutralization by US plasma-derived immunoglobulin products. J Infect Dis 2007; 196:435-40.
57. Rager-Zisman B, Ben-Nathan D. Efficacy of prophylactic and therapeutic human immunoglobulin on West Nile virus infection. Isr Med Assoc J 2003;5:691.
58. Ben-Nathan D, Lustig S, Tam G, et al. Prophylactic and therapeutic efficacy of human intravenous immunoglobulin in treating West Nile virus infection in mice. J Infect Dis 2003; 188:5-12.
59. Shimoni Z, Niven MJ, Pitlick S, Bulvik S. Treatment of West Nile virus encephalitis with intravenous immunoglobulin. Emerg Infect Dis 2001;7:759.
60. Haley M, Retter AS, Fowler D, et al. The role for intravenous immunoglobulin in the treatment of West Nile virus encephalitis. Clin Infect Dis 2003;37:e88-90.
61. Caramello P, Canta F, Balbiano R, et al. Role of intravenous immunoglobulin administration in Japanese encephalitis. Clin Infect Dis 2006;43: 1620-1.
62. Ben-Nathan D, Gershoni-Yahalom O, Samina I, et al. Using high titer West Nile intravenous immunoglobulin from selected Israeli donors for treatment of West Nile virus infection. BMC Infect Dis 2009;9:18.
63. Herzog-Tzarfati K, Shiloah E, Koren-Michowitz M, et al. Successful treatment of prolonged agranulocytosis caused by acute parvovirus B19 infection with intravenous immunoglobulins. Eur J Intern Med 2006;17:439-40.
64. Mouthon L, Lortholary O. Intravenous immunoglobulins in infectious diseases: Where do we stand? Clin Microbiol Infect 2003;9:333-8.
65. Maiztegui JI, Fernandez NJ, de Damilano AJ. Efficacy of immune plasma in treatment of Argentine haemorrhagic fever and association between treatment and a late neurological syndrome. Lancet 1979;2:1216-17.
66. Enria DA, Briggiler AM, Sanchez Z. Treatment of Argentine hemorrhagic fever. Antiviral Res 2008;78:132-9.
67. Pasic S, Jankovic B, Abinun M, Kanjuh B. Intravenous immunoglobulin prophylaxis in an echovirus 6 and echovirus 4 nursery outbreak. Pediatr Infect Dis J 1997;16:718-20.
68. Dwyer JM. The clinical use of intravenous gammaglobulin. Dev Biol Stand 1987;67:281-7.

7

Use of IVIG in Other Disorders

John Freedman, MD, FRCPC, and M. Bernadette Garvey, MD, FRCPC

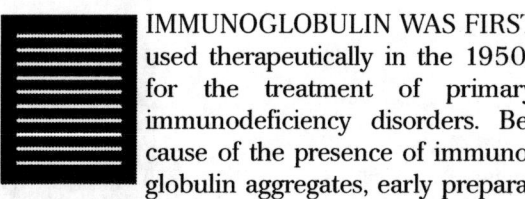IMMUNOGLOBULIN WAS FIRST used therapeutically in the 1950s for the treatment of primary immunodeficiency disorders. Because of the presence of immunoglobulin aggregates, early preparations could be given only intramuscularly or by subcutaneous infusion, limiting the size of the dose. In the late 1970s, highly purified monomeric suspensions of immunoglobulin became available that could be tolerated intravenously at larger doses. In addition to its use as replacement therapy, intravenous immunoglobulin (IVIG) can interrupt the pathologic immune responses that cause a wide range of human diseases. The immunomodulatory effects of IVIG are likely caused by several mechanisms that may act in concert. These mechanisms, which are not fully understood, include neutralization of autoantibodies, inhibition of complement binding and activation, effects mediated by Fc receptor (FcR) binding, enhanced clearance of pathogenic autoantibodies via saturation of the FcRn salvage pathway, suppression of pathogenic cytokines, neutralization of super-antigens, and down-regulation of T- or B-cell function. The following review is intended as a guide (see Table 7-1) for assessing the effectiveness of IVIG therapy in individual patients and whether to continue or cease IVIG therapy. Undoubtedly, indications will change as new data become available.

In many countries, IVIG is presently accepted for the treatment of primary humoral immunodeficiencies, chronic lymphocytic leukemia, immunodeficiency syndrome in children, multiple myeloma, allogeneic marrow transplantation, Guillain-Barré syndrome, Kawasaki disease, and immune thrombocytopenic purpura. IVIG has, however, been evaluated in a number of other conditions that are thought to result from an aberrant immunologic response. Some of the reports are purely anecdotal, but others have been well designed

---

John Freedman, MD, FRCPC, Director, Transfusion Medicine, and M. Bernadette Garvey, MD, FRCPC, Consultant Hematologist, Division of Hematology, St. Michael's Hospital, Toronto, Ontario, Canada

The authors have disclosed no conflicts of interest.

Table 7-1. Guidelines for IVIG Use*

Category	Beneficial	Evidence	Recommedation
Kawasaki disease	yes	Ia	A
Kidney transplantation: HLA sensitization	yes	Ib	B
Toxic epidermal necrolysis, Stevens-Johnson syndrome	probably	IIa	B
Dermatomyositis, polymysitis	probably	IIa	B
Autoimmune uveitis	probably	IIa	B
Stiff-person syndrome	probably	Ib	A
Pemphigus, pemphigoid	maybe	III	C
Chronic urticaria	maybe	Ib	C
Vasculitides and ANCA antibody syndromes	maybe	III	D
Systemic lupus erythematosus	maybe	III	D
Acute myocarditis	maybe	III	C
PANDAS	maybe	Ib	B
Autoimmune liver disease	maybe	III	D
Severe rheumatoid arthritis	maybe	IIb	B
Graves ophthalmopathy	maybe	Ib	A
Autoimmune diabetes mellitus	maybe	IIb	B
Kidney transplantation: rejection	maybe	Ib	B
Heart transplantation	maybe	IIb	D
Asthma: severe, persistent, high-dose steroid-dependent	maybe	Ib	A
Asthma: non-steroid-dependent	no	Ib	A
Lung transplantation	no	III	D
Liver transplantation	no	IV	D
Atopic dermatitis	no	IIa	B
Inclusion body myositis	no	IIb	B
Recurrent spontaneous abortions	no	Ia	A
Antiphospholipid antibody syndrome in pregnancy	no	III	D
Alzheimer disease	no	III	D
Dilated cardiomyopathy	no	Ib	A
Chronic fatigue syndrome	no	Ib	A
Cystic fibrosis	no	Ib	A

*See Table 7-2 for a description of evidence and recommendation levels.
ANCA = antineutrophil cytoplasmic antibodies; PANDAS = pediatric autoimmune neuropsychiatric disorder associated with streptococcus.

and make a definitive statement regarding the use of IVIG in these conditions. Many of these diseases have few or no therapeutic alternatives and warrant consideration of IVIG therapy on the basis of the available evidence (Table 7-2). For some disorders, IVIG is considered only as second-line therapy when standard therapies have proven ineffective, have become intolerable, or are contraindicated. Many of these conditions are rare, and as a result, the evidence of benefit is often inconclusive. Other conditions are more prevalent, but evidence of benefit is either conflicting or uncertain, requiring more research; for these in particular, collecting effectiveness data is important.

Rheumatologic Diseases

Inflammatory Myopathies

The inflammatory myopathies are a group of three discrete disorders: skeletal muscle dermatomyositis, polymyositis, and inclusion body myositis. The pathogenesis of the inflammatory myopathies appears to be immune mediated.[2] Optimal therapeutic regimens for dermatomyositis are unclear, and treatment remains empiric, usually including corticosteroids and immunosuppressive therapies. High-dose IVIG therapy has been reported to be efficacious in dermatomyositis in both controlled and open-label studies.[3-5] A Cochrane systematic review[6] identified one randomized controlled trial (RCT) using IVIG in adult-onset disease. In this double-blind placebo-controlled RCT,[3] 9 of 12 refractory patients given IVIG had major improvement, 2 had mild improvement, and 1 patient had no improvement. Of the 11 patients given placebo, 3 had mild improvement, 3 showed no change, and 5 had a worsening of their condition. IVIG may be of particular benefit early in the disease or for the patient who is in the intensive care unit or who has immediately life-threatening manifestations of the disease (intubated because of respiratory muscle weakness or unable to swallow because of severe esophageal involvement and on enteral feeds). Although it can be concluded that IVIG results in significant short-term improvement in

Table 7-2. Categorization of Evidence and Bases of Recommendation[1]

Levels of evidence (evidence from:)

Ia	Meta-analysis of randomized controlled trials
Ib	At least one randomized controlled study
IIa	At least one well-designed controlled study without randomization
IIb	At least one other type of well-designed quasi-experimental study
III	Nonexperimental descriptive studies (eg, comparative, correlation, or case-control studies
IV	Expert committee reports, expert opinions, or clinical experience of respected authorities, or a combination

Strength/grade of recommendation

A	Based on level I evidence
B	Based on level II evidence or extrapolated from level I evidence
C	Based on level III evidence or extrapolated from level I or II evidence
D	Based on level IV evidence or extrapolated from level I, II, or III evidence

muscle strength and activities of daily living in dermatomyositis that is refractory to steroids and/or immunosuppressants, the use of IVIG in long-term treatment (>3 months) has not been studied and further trials are needed to determine sustainability and safety of IVIG.

For juvenile dermatomyositis, several case studies that provide some evidence for the effectiveness of IVIG in pediatric practice[7-11] have been reviewed.[12] In all cases, patients reported improved muscle strength and skin changes if IVIG was used early in the course. In a report of nine children with refractory juvenile dermatomyositis, IVIG added to the therapeutic regimens gave clinical improvement in all, and in six, steroid maintenance dose could be reduced.[5]

Thus, IVIG may be considered appropriate in patients where other treatment options have failed or are inappropriate or in aggressive disease requiring hospitalization with involvement of the respiratory and bulbar musculature (level IIa evidence, grade B recommendation—see Table 7-2). In inclusion body myositis, controlled trials[13,14] failed to demonstrate objective improvement in those treated with IVIG, and, despite some suggested benefit in open studies,[15] there are no controlled trials in polymyositis.[6]

Rheumatoid Arthritis

The benefit of IVIG therapy after double-filtration plasmapheresis has been evaluated in 29 patients with rheumatoid arthritis. IVIG was most effective in patients whose serum IgG levels after infusion increased to 1000 to 1800 mg/dL.[16] Case reports and open-label trials with high-dose IVIG have suggested some benefit for patients with rheumatoid arthritis,[17,18] but in a randomized, double-blind, placebo-controlled trial of 20 patients with refractory rheumatoid arthritis, no benefit of very low-dose (5 mg/kg per 3 weeks) IVIG was seen.[19] The role of IVIG in systemic juvenile idiopathic arthritis (sJIA) is controversial.[20] In an open-label study of 27 patients with sJIA, IVIG was associated with a significant reduction in systemic symptoms and a steroid-sparing effect.

IVIG may have a role in management, but immunosuppression is the preferred treatment.[21]

Sclerosis-Scleroderma

The role of IVIG in systemic sclerosis-scleroderma has been anecdotally suggested but remains unclear.[22]

Systemic Lupus Erythematosus

In a retrospective study of 59 patients with systemic lupus erythematosus (SLE), IVIG therapy resulted in clinical improvement in 65% of the patients treated, but the response was transient in each case.[23] In case reports, high-dose IVIG has been associated with disease resolution in patients with lupus affecting specific organs, including the kidneys,[24,25] nerves,[26] myocardium,[27] marrow,[28] and multiple organs.[29] There are no randomized studies to support the use of IVIG to treat juvenile SLE. For cases of autoimmune congenital heart block (neonatal lupus), IVIG therapy may be indicated during pregnancy when there is a history of autoimmune congenital heart block in at least one previous pregnancy and maternal SS-A and/or SS-B antibodies are present. With the limited anecdotal experience and the potential prothromboembolic effects of IVIG, caution is advised in the therapeutic application of IVIG in SLE and other autoimmune disease.[18] Furthermore, reports of IVIG-associated azotemia in SLE are an additional cause for concern.[30]

Antineutrophil Cytoplasmic Antibody-Associated Systemic Necrotizing Vasculitides

Antineutrophil cytoplasmic antibody (ANCA)-associated systemic necrotizing vasculitides are life-threatening immune-mediated inflammatory diseases that include four clinical syndromes: Wegener granulomatosis, microscopic polyangiitis, Churg-Strauss syndrome, and ANCA-positive idiopathic rapidly progressive glomerulonephritis. There is one prospective, randomized, double-blind, placebo-controlled multicenter study in ANCA-associated systemic vasculitis.[31] Thirty-four patients were randomly assigned to receive IVIG (2 g/kg; n = 17) or placebo (n = 17) daily. The authors concluded that a single course of high-dose IVIG reduces disease activity where active vasculitis persists despite conventional therapy. However, the benefit of IVIG was not maintained beyond 3 months, and there are a number of concerns relating to the reliability and clinical relevance of this trial. For example, it is unclear why there was a 2-week observation period before randomization; insufficient detail was provided on individual patients, making it difficult to determine what change in score would be considered clinically relevant; the impact of the open label use of chlorpheniramine at the discretion of the treating physicians is unknown; and data were lacking on mortality and severe adverse events. The effect of IVIG on end-organ damage and the potential immunosuppressant/steroid sparing effect of IVIG are also unclear from this trial. Hence, the net effect of IVIG therapy for adjuvant therapy in ANCA-associated systemic vasculitis remains unclear. In one open-label trial, IVIG induced remission in 15 of 16 systemic vasculitis patients, which was sustained in 8 but only transient in 7.[32] IVIG thus appears to have a limited role as one of several therapeutic options in relapsing disease.[33] If it is to be used, it should be restricted to the control of vasculitic activity in the rare cases of ANCA-positive systemic necrotizing vasculitis failing to respond to corticosteroids and immunosuppression where the disorder is of recent onset.[34]

Antiphospholipid Antibody Syndrome

Several reports support a beneficial role for IVIG in antiphospholipid antibody syndrome (APS). Most reports focus on the use of IVIG in the obstetric complications of APS, and patient series have demonstrated that the use of IVIG resulted in successful pregnancy outcome in patients with APS with recurrent abortions. IVIG also benefited patients with APS undergoing in-vitro fertilization.[35] However, a meta-analysis of several modes of therapy (heparin, aspirin, glucocorticosteroids, and IVIG) in this clinical setting failed to support any improved outcome with IVIG.[36] The catastrophic antiphospholipid syndrome is an often-fatal disorder characterized by multiple, rapidly progressive, arterial and venous thrombotic events. A large registry-based study suggests that plasma exchange or IVIG together with intensive anticoagulation and supportive therapy may be beneficial.[37]

Sjogren Syndrome

IVIG may be indicated in certain highly selected cases where other treatments have not been effective.[38]

Dermatologic Disorders

Autoimmune blistering disorders of the skin include several distinct entities. Immunobullous diseases vary in clinical presentation and have different histopathologic and immunologic features. They are often associated with significant morbidity and mortality if untreated. Pemphigoid is an autoimmune, vesiculobullous, erosive disease that can affect the mucosa. Treatment regimens include prolonged courses of immunosuppressive therapies. An estimated 25% of patients with bullous pemphigoid do not respond to standard treatment.[39] Pemphigus is a group of autoimmune blistering diseases that involve the skin and mucous membranes. The pathognomonic feature of these is acantholysis, which likely results from an autoimmune response to desmoglein. Conventional therapy of pemphigus is immune suppression,[40] although not all patients respond. All the publications related to IVIG are prospective open-label studies or case reports, and controlled studies in these rare conditions are unlikely. Nonrandomized controlled trials and case series studies have shown some benefit of IVIG both as monotherapy and, primarily, as adjuvant therapy for the treatment of pemphigus/pemphigoid blistering diseases. These studies, however, are small and results vary. Indeed, some studies and reports do not show any clear benefit.[41,42] Controlled trials are needed to determine the extent of effect of IVIG, particularly as adjuvant therapy for these disorders. Moreover, controlled trials are needed to determine optimum doses and cycles of therapy for the treatment of these disorders. Guidelines for IVIG treatment in this setting were outlined by the consensus development group of the American Academy of Dermatology.[43]

Toxic Epidermal Necrolysis

Toxic epidermal necrolysis (TEN) is a rare, life-threatening, hypersensitivity reaction to certain medications, such as sulphonamides, antibiotics, nonsteroidal anti-inflammatory drugs, and anticonvulsants. Drug-induced, epidermal apoptosis has been proposed as a possible pathogenesis. The Steven-Johnson syndrome (SJS) is a less extensive manifestation of the same phenomenon. TEN and SJS are characterized by severe bullous reaction with extensive destruction of the epidermis. The term *SJS* is now used to describe patients with blistering and skin detachment involving a total body surface area of <10%. *SJS/TEN* describes patients with 10% to 30% detachment, and *TEN* describes those with >30% skin detachment. A potential immunologic mechanism for IVIG action in these disorders has been proposed that involves the blockade of CD95, promoting cell survival.[44]

Sporadic case reports, as well as prospective and retrospective multicenter studies, have shown that early administration of high-dose IVIG helps to resolve the disease and reduce mortality,[45] but conflicting data exist.[46] One small cohort study (20 patients) without a control group found no significant effect, and that death rate seems to be higher than previously reported.[47] A small randomized study (4 patients) with a control group of two (supportive care only) found that there was some improvement in epithelialization and a significant difference in CD95 receptor between treated patients and controls, although neither IVIG nor its comparison group could completely stop the TEN process.[48] However, given the high risk of mortality, the evidence supports the use of high-dose IVIG as an early therapeutic intervention,[49] and IVIG is recommended in TEN and SJS when other treatments are contraindicated or when the condition is life-threatening (level IIa evidence, grade B recommendation). Although urgent skin biopsy should be performed for confirmation, this should not delay IVIG therapy if indicated.

Bullous Pemphigoid

Bullous pemphigoid (BP) is a rare disease of the elderly characterized by tense blisters and vesicles with a prominent inflammatory component. The cause is unknown. Lesions result from a failure of basal keratinocytes to adhere to the epidermal basement membrane. The course of BP is characterized by exacerbations and remissions. Pruritis is common, and an increase in pruritis may herald an exacerbation. Although in most patients BP is not a life-threatening disease, the side effects of systemic immunosuppressive therapy need to be managed. In most, the disease spontaneously clears within 6 years and all medication can be stopped, but in a small group the disease recurs after cessation of treatment. In open, uncontrolled trials, IVIG as a last resort for the treatment of bullous pemphigoid has shown some benefit.[39,50-52] The Australasian College of Dermatologists recommended IVIG use only in severe cases where improvement with conventional therapy is not readily achieved.[34] The 2003 Harvard consensus statement[53] identified a small study (17 cases) where patients who were on IVIG therapy for at least 3 months benefited from the therapy. Hence, IVIG may be useful 1) in patients who have moderate-to-severe disease, as diagnosed by a dermatologist, and in whom steroids or immunosuppressive agents are contraindicated, 2) if the condition is unresponsive to corticosteroids and immunosuppressive agents, or 3) if the patient has severe side effects of therapy.[1]

Cicatricial Pemphigoid

Cicatricial pemphigoid (CP), or mucous membrane pemphigoid, is a rare, acquired, subepithelial blistering disease characterized by erosive lesions of mucous membranes and skin. Hoarseness, pain, tissue loss, and even upper airway destruction can occur with nasopharyngeal or laryngeal involvement, and oesophageal and urogenital lesions may lead to stenosis or strictures. CP is usually a chronic, progressive disorder. The aim of long-term treatment (steroids and immunosuppressives) is cessation of the self-destructive autoimmune process. Permanent remission is usually possible if the disease is diagnosed early and treated sufficiently for 1 to 5 years. For the 70% of patients who have eye involvement, the disease progresses to conjunctival scarring and shrinkage but may take 10 to 20 years to reach the end stage of bilateral blindness. Two nonrandomized controlled trials[54,55] studied IVIG use as therapy for oral pemphigoid and mucous membrane pemphigoid with ocular involvement, respectively. In the study of Sami et al,[54] IVIG resulted in a faster rate of decline in antibody titers, and sustained clinical and serologic remission as compared to conventional therapy. In the study of Letko et al,[55] IVIG produced a faster control of inflammation, and there were no reoccurences as compared to conventional immunosuppressive therapy. Qualifying criteria for IVIG use are as for BP.[1]

Pemphigus Vulgaris

Pemphigus vulgaris (PV) is a rare but potentially fatal condition accounting for approximately 70% of pemphigus cases. Although the cause is unknown, an immunogenetic predisposition is well established. PV may also be drug induced. The oral cavity is almost always affected, and erosions can be scattered and extensive, with subsequent dysphagia. Pemphigus may occur in patients with other autoimmune diseases, particularly myasthenia gravis and thymoma. The severity and natural history of PV are variable. Before the advent of steroids, most patients with PV died. Treatment with systemic steroids has reduced the mortality rate to 5% to 15%. Most deaths occur during the first few years of disease, and if the patient survives 5 years, the prognosis is good. Early disease is easier to control than widespread disease, and mortality may be higher if therapy is delayed. Morbidity and mortality are related to the extent of disease, the maximum dose of corticosteroid required to induce remission, and the presence of other diseases. In a retrospective cohort, 15 corticosteroid-dependent patients with moderate to severe PV were treated with IVIG and followed over a mean period of 6.2 years.[48] All 15 patients had a satisfactory clinical response to IVIG therapy. IVIG has a demonstrable corticosteroid-sparing effect.[56] Criteria for IVIG use are as for BP above.[1]

Pemphigus Foliaceus

Pemphigus foliaceus (PF) is a rare, autoimmune, blistering skin disease characterized by loss of cohesion of cells (acantholysis) in the superficial layers of the epidermis. The lesions are generally well demarcated and do not coalesce to form large eroded areas (as seen in PV). It is mediated by an autoantibody targeting desmoglein 1, a cell-to-cell protein molecule that binds the desmosomes of neighboring keratinocytes in the epidermis. The disease has a long-term course, with patients maintaining satisfactory health. Spontaneous remissions occasionally occur. Habif[57] and others[58] concluded that IVIG was effective as monotherapy for PF and particularly useful in patients who experienced life-threatening complications from immunosuppression. Sami et al[54,59] observed that autoantibody titers to desmoglein 1 decreased persistently following IVIG therapy. Criteria for IVIG use are as for BP above.[1]

Atopic Dermatitis/Eczema

IVIG treatment has been tried in small, open, uncontrolled trials in patients with atopic dermatitis who failed standard therapeutic regimens.[60-62] A single, small, randomized, evaluator-blinded trial (n = 10) did not support the routine use of IVIG in patients with atopic dermatitis,[63] and small studies using IVIG in eczema failed to show significant effectiveness.[60,63,64] Hence, published data do not support the use of IVIG. Cyclosporin is recommended as first choice for patients with atopic eczema refractory to conventional topical steroid treatment, followed by azathioprine.[65]

Pyoderma Gangrenosum

Most of the six cases of pyoderma gangrenosum reported where other therapies had failed received adjunctive high-dose IVIG and responded over several weeks.[66-71] Improvement in the setting of hypogammaglobulinemia[72,73] has also been described with replacement IVIG.[1] Treatment with IVIG may be considered in select cases of severe pyoderma gangrenosum where patients have failed to respond to all other therapies, particularly where a vital organ or structure is threatened, and in patients for whom immunosuppressants are inappropriate.

Chronic Urticaria

Chronic urticaria is often difficult to treat. One-third of patients with chronic urticaria appear to have an autoimmune disease.[74-76] Ten patients with severe autoimmune chronic urticaria, poorly responsive to conventional treatment, were treated with IVIG, 0.4 g/kg daily for 5 days; clinical benefit was seen in nine patients, with prolonged complete remissions (3 years followup) in three, temporary complete remissions in two, and improved symptoms in four patients.[77] However, similar benefit was not seen in a case report of three patients with severe chronic urticaria.[78] In an open trial of IVIG in patients with delayed-pressure urticaria, one-third of the patients underwent a remission, another third experienced some benefit, and the rest did not respond.[79] In a single case report of an autologous serum test-negative patient treated with low-dose IVIG, the urticaria improved.[80] A single report of five patients with combined variable immunodeficiency and chronic urticaria noted amelioration of the urticaria in response to IVIG therapy.[81] Current data are insufficient to recommend the routine administration of IVIG in patients with urticaria, and additional studies are needed.[1] Patients with pressure urticaria who fail other therapeutic modalities, however, might benefit from high-dose IVIG.

Other Skin Diseases

There is a single case report of benefit from IVIG therapy in psoriasis.[82]

Solid Organ Transplantation

There appears to be a role for the use of IVIG in solid organ transplant recipients who experience acute humoral rejection. Encouraging results have been obtained with plasmapheresis followed by IVIG administration in patients who are presensitized (having reactive antibodies), who are in the midst of an acute antibody-mediated kidney rejection, or both. Economic analysis has suggested that the use of IVIG in these settings might be financially advantageous, and therefore broader application warrants consideration.[83] IVIG might also be useful in solid organ transplant recipients who experience autoimmune cytopenias after transplantation, but currently available evidence is limited to case reports and retrospective analyses.[84]

A recent initiative of Canadian Blood Services and the National Advisory Committee on Blood and Blood Products of Canada was undertaken by Shehata et al[85] to provide guidance for practitioners involved in the care of patients undergoing solid organ transplantation and for transfusion medicine specialists on the use of IVIG. The panel determined key clinical areas of solid organ transplantation that might benefit from treatment with IVIG and generated salient clinical questions: Is there evidence that the use of IVIG reduces morbidity and mortality for patients undergoing solid organ transplantation who are 1) sensitized (HLA or ABO), 2) in the perioperative setting and are sensitized, 3) experiencing acute graft rejection, or 4) experiencing chronic graft rejection? A systematic, expert, and bibliographic literature search up to July 2008 was conducted: 791 citations were retrieved, and 45 reports were used for the guideline.[85] The levels of evidence and grading of recommendations were adapted from the Canadian Task Force on Preventive Health Care and differ from those used otherwise in this chapter.[86] The recommendations identified 1) sensitized patients undergoing solid organ transplantation that would have a better survival and decreased morbidity by receiving IVIG preoperatively, postoperatively, and for the treatment of organ rejection, and 2) patients who may not have any benefit from receiving IVIG. It was noted that reports were limited by inconsistent definitions of sensitization, inconsistent reporting of type and titer of the antibody, assays used to detect anti-HLA, the response criteria, and dosing schedules for IVIG. Because of inadequate evidence, a consensus process was used. Although use of IVIG was associated with decreased sensitization and acceptable morbidity and mortality in living donor kidney transplantation, IVIG was often used with several other therapeutic modalities, and it was difficult to separate outcomes based on an individual modality.

Kidney Transplantation

HLA Sensitization

There were two RCTs[87,88] and 17 cohort/case series[89-104] on the use of IVIG for desensitization of HLA-sensitized renal transplant recipients. The double-blind RCT of Jordan et al[87] reported a trend to improvement in desensitization rates and a statistically significant decrease in time to transplantation for patients treated with IVIG. However, acute rejection was more frequent in those receiving IVIG. Peraldi et al[88] randomized patients having a second deceased donor transplant; it was unclear whether donor-specific antibodies were present because only the panel-reactive antibody test was used. Five-year survival was not different between the groups, but graft survival was superior in IVIG-treated patients. The observational reports were mostly case series. One report compared single-dose IVIG to regimens containing IVIG and plasmapheresis[92]; IVIG as a single agent was associated with inferior desensitization rates and higher rates of rejection. A small observational report[91] using low-dose IVIG (500 mg/kg) was unsuccessful at desensitization, but other reports[92,93,97,99,101,102,105] using lower-dose (100 to 500 mg/kg) IVIG/cytomegalovirus immune globulin (CMVIG) in combination with plasmapheresis and various immunosuppressive regimens (total = 201 patients) had success rates of 63% to 100% for desensitization, with frequency of antibody-mediated rejection ranging from 25% to 43% and graft survival from 79% to 100%. Five reports,[89,92,98,100,104] including 177 adult patients, used higher doses of IVIG (2 g/kg): rates of desensitization ranged from 36% to 100%, and antibody-mediated rejection occurred in 7% to 80% of patients transplanted.

ABO Incompatibility

Seven observational reports described the use of IVIG/CMVIG in patients undergoing ABO-incompatible renal transplantation.[105-111] All used IVIG concurrently with other immune modulating agents. Graft survival ranged from 80% to 100%, and patient survival was over 90%. Two reports compared graft survival and overall survival to patients receiving ABO-compatible transplants and reported comparable outcomes.[106,111]

Transplant Rejection

Rejection of the renal allograft can be categorized as 1) acute antibody-mediated rejection, 2) steroid-resistant acute cellular rejection, 3) "simple" acute cellular rejection, or 4) chronic active antibody-mediated rejection. A mixed picture may also occur. Seven case series included a total of 166 patients who had antibody-mediated rejection.[112-118] These used both IVIG and plasmapheresis and various immunosuppressive agents. Definitions of acute humoral rejection differed. The doses of IVIG administered ranged from 2 to 100 g/kg. Graft survival ranged from 60% to 100% and patient survival from 90% to 100%. This compares with 3-month graft survival of historical controls of 50%.[119] The data are insufficient to draw conclusions regarding treatment of antibody-mediated rejection using IVIG alone, without concomitant plasmapheresis. An RCT,[120] a cohort study,[121] and two case series[122,123] addressed the use of IVIG in patients having steroid-resistant rejection (the cohort may have been a preliminary report of the RCT). RCT patients were treated with IVIG or OKT3. Comparable graft and patient survival were reported.[120] A lower recurrence rate of acute rejection occurred with IVIG (46% vs 75% with OKT3).[120] In one case series,[122] graft survival was similar to that seen in the RCT (71%), in contrast to patients treated with a calcineurin inhibitor-based immunosuppression protocol, where 6-month graft survival was 59%.[124] No studies had a sufficient sample size (ie, more than five patients) to address the use of IVIG for the treatment of simple, acute, cell-mediated rejection or chronic, active, antibody-mediated rejection.

In most published reports, in the setting of transplant rejection, IVIG is used with plasmapheresis. CMVIG has also been administered at some centers with plasmapheresis; however, no data indicate that CMVIG is superior to other IVIG preparations. No trials compare IVIG and plasmapheresis to other rejection therapies or compare IVIG alone to plasmapheresis. Data are limited on the use of IVIG in patients with increased immunologic risk who experience acute, antibody-mediated rejection. However, because immune mechanisms of rejection are similar in such patients, IVIG use may be a treatment option in these patients even though they may be less responsive. IVIG is not presently considered as first-line therapy for the treatment of steroid-resistant rejection as no data indicate that IVIG is superior to alternate therapies. The use of IVIG may be reserved for situations where standard treatments have been ineffective or are contraindicated.

Cardiac Transplantation

There is considerable controversy regarding quantification, evaluation, and management of the sensitized potential cardiac transplant recipient. Highly sensitized patients do have an increased risk of antibody-mediated rejection, cardiac allograft vasculopathy, and early graft loss after transplantation.[125,126] Multiple strategies to desensitize the potential cardiac transplant recipient have included plasmapheresis, mycophenolate mofetil, rituximab, cyclophosphamide, and IVIG, in isolation or in combination, either before transplantation, perioperatively, or immediately following transplantation. Results have been variable, and the interpretation is limited by inconsistent use of classification of outcomes. Six observational studies reported on the use of IVIG in cardiac transplantation[127-132]; three included the same patient cohort treated with IVIG for desensitization to achieve a negative crossmatch.[129,130,132] Four reports did not define response to treatment.[127,128,130,131] The reduction of antibody level with IVIG as a single modality was not measured in any report. A decreased panel-reactive antibody was detected in two reports,[127,131] and four reports did not show a change in panel-reactive antibodies.[128-130,132] Some authors demonstrated a reduced time to transplantation.[129,130] One small study showed a survival benefit in sensitized heart transplant recipients who were treated before transplantation with plasmapheresis and IVIG.[127] In a pediatric population, outcomes were not improved with the use of IVIG.[128] One study reported complications associated with IVIG[130]: the use of IVIG resulted in immune complex disease (fevers, arthralgias, maculopapular rash) in four patients (15%), and four patients also experienced reversible renal insufficiency, which resolved in 3 weeks.

Hence, although one report found a survival benefit,[127] these results have not been reproduced, the numbers are small, and, in the absence of data on donor-specific antibodies, it is difficult to formulate recommendations. Thus, the panel considered that there were insufficient data to formulate a recommendation on the routine use of IVIG for desensitization in cardiac transplantation.

Lung Transplantation

The role of IVIG or any other desensitization therapy in patients undergoing lung transplantation who are sensitized to HLA antigens is unknown. Some studies identified increased morbidity and mortality with sensitization, but others did not.[133-136] Given different diagnostic techniques, interpretation of these reports is difficult. There has been only one report on the use of IVIG in lung transplantation.[137] Twelve patients were treated with IVIG and extracorporeal immunoadsorption for removal of preformed antibodies beginning from the time of transplantation. There were no statistically significant differences in freedom from bronchiolitis obliterans or acute rejection. An additional 8 patients who developed de novo antibodies and declining graft function were treated with 500 mg IVIG weekly as "rescue therapy." There was no statistically significant effect on declining lung function. No other studies have substantiated these results.

Liver Transplantation

Antibody-mediated rejection is rare after liver transplantation. Therefore, desensitizing protocols with IVIG have not been performed. IVIG has, however, been used as specific therapy for posttransplant complications, including hypogammaglobulinemia,[138] thrombocytopenia,[139] and demyelinating polyradiculoneuropathy.[140] In adults receiving ABO-incompatible liver transplants, IVIG has been incorporated into successful protocols but always added to various combinations of immunosuppressive agents such as plasmapheresis, extracorporeal photopheresis, and anti-CD20 antibody therapy.[141] Benefits from the immunomodulatory effects of IVIG have been proposed in the existing literature (eg, CMVIG prophylaxis appeared to offer a survival benefit independent of its anti-viral effect in one report[142]), but no studies have been specifically designed to prospectively assess the role of IVIG/CMVIG in rejection and survival following liver transplantation.

Summary of Recommendations for Transplantation

Key recommendations from the Canadian initiative[85] were as follows:
1. When transplantation will involve use of a kidney from a living donor to whom the patient is sensitized, IVIG is recommended to decrease donor-specific sensitization (level I-II 2-3 evidence, grade B recommendation). For patients who are sensitized as defined by a complement-dependent cytotoxicity crossmatch, IVIG, 2 g/kg/month for up to 4 months, may be given to achieve a negative antihuman globulin complement-dependent cytotoxicity (AHG-CDC) crossmatch before transplantation. Alternate strategies such as plasmapheresis followed by IVIG (100-200 mg/kg) are considered acceptable. Plasmapheresis followed by IVIG (100-200 mg/kg/dose) is generally restricted to the perioperative period. A negative AHG-CDC crossmatch is what should be aimed for, and not a change in the percentage of panel-reactive antibody. Emerging studies suggest that high-titer (ie, AHG-CDC crossmatch higher than 1:16) donor-specific HLA antibodies may limit the effectiveness of desensitization.[88]

For patients who are sensitized and require a deceased donor, desensitization with IVIG is generally not used because of limited availability of deceased donors. Although the evidence from this systematic review supports the use of IVIG for desensitization before transplantation for highly sensitized patients receiving kidneys from deceased donors, the routine use of IVIG would result in unnecessary wastage, as it is not guaranteed that recipients will have access to donors within 2 years. The recommendation against the use of IVIG for recipients of deceased donor transplants is subject to the availability of deceased donors; should deceased donor kidneys become readily available, IVIG would be recommended for desensitization of the sensitized recipient.

2. There is insufficient evidence to make a recommendation for or against the use of IVIG for ABO-incompatible transplantation; however, other factors may influence decision-making (level II-2-III evidence, grade B recommendation).
3. IVIG is recommended perioperatively for patients who have donor-specific antibodies to reduce the incidence of accelerated acute humoral rejection (level III evidence, grade B recommendation).
4. IVIG is not recommended for patients who do not have donor-specific antibodies (level III evidence, grade D recommendation).
5. IVIG may be given with plasmapheresis for patients who have received a living-donor or deceased-donor transplant and who have acute antibody-mediated rejection, to improve graft survival (level II-3 evidence, grade B recommendation). IVIG is typically administered as part of a treatment protocol that includes plasmapheresis. Regimens for administration of IVIG include IVIG after each plasmapheresis treatment (100 mg/treatment day) or as a set dose of 2 g/kg total, usually after the final plasmapheresis treatment. CMVIG has also been administered at a dose of 100 mg/kg after each plasmapheresis treatment.
6. In patients who have received a living- or deceased-donor transplant and who have steroid-resistant rejection, IVIG may be considered, to improve graft survival when other therapies are deemed unacceptable or ineffective (level I, II2, III evidence, grade B recommendation). IVIG can be administered over a period of up to 10 consecutive days, at a total dose of 2 to 3.5 g/kg. Longer administration periods with smaller doses can be used where fluid overload is a potential risk.
7. Evidence is insufficient to make a recommendation for or against the routine use of IVIG for other forms of rejection (level III evidence).
8. Evidence is insufficient to recommend for or against the routine use of IVIG for desensitization for patients undergoing heart, lung, or liver transplantation to improve graft or overall survival or to treat rejection; however, other factors may influence decision-making (level II-2-III evidence).

In summary, there is limited methodologically rigorous evidence for the use of IVIG for solid organ transplantation. Future studies are needed to delineate the effect of IVIG on desensitization using standardized methods for assessing desensitization; the effect of IVIG on acute rejection rates, graft survival, and overall survival; the use of the combined modality IVIG and plasmapheresis compared to plasmapheresis or IVIG alone; and the optimum dosage of IVIG.

Cardiac Disorders

Kawasaki Disease

Kawasaki disease (KD) is a systemic vasculitis occurring primarily in young children; those of Japanese and Korean origin are at highest risk. There is convincing evidence for the use of IVIG in KD from meta-analyses and prospective, multicenter trials. KD is an acute, febrile, childhood vasculitis of medium-sized vessels, commonly affecting the coronary arteries. The cause of illness remains unknown. Several clinical, laboratory, and epidemiologic features strongly support an infectious or postinfectious origin,[143] but there is evidence that characteristic vasculitis results from an immune reaction involving T-cell and macrophage activation to an unknown antigen, secretion of cytokines, polyclonal B-cell hyperactivity, and the formation of autoantibodies to endothelial cells and smooth muscle cells. It is likely that, in genetically susceptible individuals, one or more uncharacterized common infectious agents, possibly with super-antigen activity, may trigger the disease.

IVIG with aspirin is the standard of care for children during the first 10 days of the syndrome to prevent the development of coronary aneurysms.[144] Limited evidence suggests that treatment by the fifth day of illness might be associated with even better outcomes,[145] but these data have been challenged.[146] Reductions in fever, neutrophil counts, and acute-phase reactants typically occur within 24 hours after IVIG at 2 g/kg.[147] Although alternative IVIG regimens have been described, including 4 daily infusions (0.4 g/kg), they are less efficacious, as shown in a prospective multicenter trial.[147] The frequency of coronary artery abnormalities and duration of fever were significantly greater with the multidose regimen. A meta-analysis of RCTs of IVIG in KD also supported the use of a single 2-g/kg dose of IVIG and found that this regimen resulted in a significant decrease in new coronary artery abnormalities 30 days after diagnosis.[148] Another meta-analysis including more than 3400 patients also demonstrated that a single high dose of IVIG was superior to other IVIG regimens in preventing coronary aneurysms[149]; this analysis also found that low-dose aspirin (<80 mg/kg) was comparable with high-dose aspirin (>80 mg/kg) when combined with high-dose IVIG. Hence, IVIG in conjunction with aspirin is the treatment of choice for KD (level Ia evidence, grade A recommendation).[150]

Patients should receive a single 2-g/kg dose as soon as the diagnosis is established (5-10 days after start of fever). Some patients require a second dose if there is no response or a relapse within 48 hours; if a second dose fails to elicit a response, high-dose pulsed steroids are the next line of treatment.[150] Up to 15% of patients do not respond to initial IVIG therapy. Although the exact mechanism of action of IVIG in KD is not clear, it could involve neutralization of bacteria superantigen toxins that lead to vascular endothelial inflammation and damage associated with KD.[151,152] Other proposed mechanisms include anti-idiotype inhibition of antiendothelial antibodies, effects on the cytokine milieu, inhibition of vascular endothelial activation, and inhibition of complement-mediated tissue damage.[153,154]

Acute Myocarditis and Dilated Cardiomyopathy

Inflammation of the myocardium is a condition of serious clinical importance, with inflammatory etiologies ranging from viral myocarditis, Chagas' disease, AIDS, and noninfectious causes, including posttransplant cardiac rejection. Treatment for acute myocarditis and dilated cardiomyopathy is not readily available, but there is some evidence from case reports[155-158] and a Cochrane review[159] that high-dose IVIG improves cardiac function in children with proven or likely viral myocarditis. However, placebo-controlled trials evaluating the benefit of IVIG use in recent-onset cardiomyopathy showed no benefit over placebo.[160] High-dose IVIG might provide help to patients with acute myocarditis but has no therapeutic role in recent-onset dilated cardiomyopathy. The purported mechanism of action of IVIG in myocarditis may be the capacity of IVIG to deviate deleterious complement activation to innocuous targets, with the IgG molecule itself binding C3b.[161]

Miscellaneous Disorders

Neonatal Hemachromatosis

Neonatal hemachromatosis (NH) manifests in the fetus and newborn and is characterized by abnormal accumulation of iron in the liver and extra-hepatic tissues. Affected neonates present with fulminant liver failure, usually in the context of a history of prematurity, intrauterine growth retardation, and oligohydramnios. NH differs from most other causes of neonatal liver disease, other than congenital infections, in that the condition begins in utero, and fulminant liver disease is manifested in the first few days of life. The etiology and pathogenesis remain uncertain and may be the outcome of numerous disease processes. There is also evidence, however, that NH is an alloimmune disorder. First, there is an approximate 80% likelihood of NH once a woman has had an affected baby. Second, mothers can have affected babies with different fathers. Diagnosis is made after other causes of neonatal liver failure have been excluded. NH is rare, but the rate of recurrence after the index case in a sibship is up to 80%, and survival is about 20% with medical treatment. It has therefore been suggested that IVIG may be used in women who are pregnant or attempting to conceive and whose most recent pregnancy ended in delivery of a fetus shown to have had NH.[162-166]

Stiff-Person Syndrome

Patients with stiff-person syndrome present with symptoms related to muscular rigidity and superimposed episodic spasms. The rigidity spreads insidiously, involving axial muscles, primarily abdominal and thoracolumbar, as well as proximal limb muscles. Typically, cocontraction of truncal agonist and antagonistic muscles leads to a board-like appearance with hyperlordosis. Less frequently, respiratory muscle involvement leads to breathing difficulty and facial muscle involvement to a mask-like face. Investigations that may be useful for diagnosis include those for autoantibodies to GAD-65 or GAD-67, electromyogram recordings from stiff muscles, and cerebrospinal fluid oligoclonal bands. There is one randomized, double-blind, placebo-controlled trial with a crossover design of 16 patients with stiff-person syndrome and anti-GAD-65.[167] A significant treatment effect with IVIG was seen, resulting in decreased stiffness and heightened sensitivity scores. According to expert consensus,[168-170] considering the disabling progressive course of stiff-person syndrome, IVIG should be offered as the first-line treatment. Although periodic infusions would be required in most, further studies are needed to determine optimal dosage and duration.

Autoimmune Uveitis

Birdshot retinochoroidopathy is an autoimmune posterior uveitis that may threaten sight and frequently requires immunosuppressive therapy, but it may be resistant to standard immunosuppression. An open trial with IVIG treatment for 6 months (1.6 g/kg every 4 weeks with transition to every 6-8 weeks) has shown promise.[171] Visual acuity improved in 53.8% and decreased in 7.7% of patients during treatment. When present, macular edema improved in half of the eyes during treatment. In another trial with therapy-resistant autoimmune uveitis, clinical benefit was seen in half of the patients treated with IVIG.[172] These data suggest that IVIG therapy might be an effective alternative for patients with immune-mediated, sight-threatening uveitis with persistent activity despite both oral corticosteroid and systemic immunosuppressive therapy.[1] IVIG is not indicated for uveitis of nonimmune origin.

Autoimmune Graves Ophthalmopathy

A randomized trial of patients with active Graves ophthalmopathy compared systemic corticosteroids with 6 courses of IVIG at 1 g/kg for 2 days every 3 weeks. Both treatment modalities were equally successful, but the side effects were more frequent and severe in the steroid-treated group.[173] In a separate case report, IVIG was also noted to be superior to systemic corticosteroids in controlling Graves ophthalmopathy.[174] Hence, IVIG may be indicated where steroids have failed or are contraindicated.

Autoimmune Diabetes Mellitus

Antibodies against islet cell antigens are implicated in the pathogenesis of insulin-dependent (type 1) diabetes mellitus. A case report of a patient with newly diagnosed type 1 diabetes treated with immunoadsorption plasmapheresis showed a decrease in those antibodies correlated directly with a decreased requirement for insulin.[175] A review of IVIG administration to 77 subjects with newly diagnosed diabetes was summarized from 6 different studies and compared with 56 newly diagnosed diabetic case control subjects also reported in those studies.[176] In most patients, no benefits were found, but two of the six studies reported decreased insulin requirement in IVIG-treated patients; all six studies, however, identified subpopulations of patients who responded to IVIG therapy with a preserved C-peptide release, higher rate of remission, and longer duration of remission.[176] In contrast, a single RCT evaluating the effect of IVIG administered every 2 months to children and adults with type 1 diabetes failed to demonstrate any benefits associated with IVIG therapy.[177]

Autoimmune Liver Disease

In one case report of a patient with autoimmune chronic active hepatitis, IVIG treatment was used with a successful outcome.[178] Specifically, liver enzymes normalized, circulating immune complexes were no longer detectable, and periportal mononuclear cell infiltrates improved after treatment.

PANDAS

Pediatric Autoimmune Neuropsychiatric Disorder Associated with Streptococcus (PANDAS) was first described in the early 1990s. PANDAS is characterized by rapid-onset tics associated with obsessive-compulsive disorder in the context of recovery from streptococcal infection. Molecular mimicry between streptococcal antigens and the central nervous system is thought to underlie the cause. Symptomatic therapy is used with variable response. A single, randomized, placebo-controlled trial[179] using IVIG and plasmapheresis for PANDAS showed prolonged and significant improvement in obsessive-compulsive symptoms, anxiety, depression, emotional lability, and overall function compared with placebo.

Paraneoplastic Disorders

There are no randomized trials in paraneoplastic encephalomyelitis, limbic encephalitis, cerebellar degeneration, peripheral neuropathy, or opsoclonus myoclonus. Case reports and small series provide conflicting results in these rare disorders. Such anecdotal reports are impossible to interpret because paraneoplastic disorders may stabilize or improve spontaneously. IVIG has been of little benefit, except possibly in opsoclonus myoclonus.[180]

Potassium Channel Antibody-Associated, Nonneoplastic Limbic Encephalitis

There are no RCTs in potassium channel antibody-associated, nonneoplastic limbic encephalitis, but case series suggest that a variety of immunomodulatory interventions, including IVIG, plasma exchange, and corticosteroids, give encouraging results.[181,182]

Asthma

Asthma is a heterogeneous disease, and some patients are found to have antibody deficiency.[183-188] In some patients with immune abnormalities and infection-associated asthma, replacement doses of IVIG might eliminate the triggering infections, reducing the frequency and severity of pulmonary symptoms.[188,189] Most asthmatic patients, however, do not have a humoral immunodeficiency; in the former, the treatment may be corticosteroids, but severely affected patients often require high doses, with unacceptable side effects.

The potent anti-inflammatory properties of IVIG have led to open trials of its use as an anti-inflammatory or steroid-sparing agent. An open-label trial of 2 g/kg per month IVIG in eight steroid-dependent, asthmatic children showed a significant reduction in steroid dose and improved peak expiratory flow rate and symptoms.[190] Subsequently, another open-label study in 11 children from the same institution found that an IVIG treatment regimen allowed significant reduction in steroid requirements and resulted in decreased hospitalizations, effects attributed to increased responsiveness of patients' lymphocytes to dexamethasone, and increased glucocorticoid receptor-binding affinity.[191] Other in-vitro studies have shown a suppressive effect for IVIG on IgE production[192,193] and neutralization of inflammatory mediators that induce bronchospasm.[194] Other open trials of IVIG[195,196] have shown similar results, and a case series of seven highly refractory adult asthmatics unresponsive to immunosuppressive drugs reported a small but statistically significant reduction in daily prednisone and in the number of hospital admissions, but no significant improvement in lung function.[197] Thus, open-label studies, which include a total of 56 patients, suggest that IVIG might have beneficial steroid-sparing effects in some patients with asthma.

There have been three double-blind, placebo-controlled studies of IVIG in asthma.[198-200] The first included 31 patients randomized to receive a loading dose of 2 g/kg IVIG, followed by 2 monthly doses of 1 g/kg each or the equivalent amount of albumin as a control; there was no difference in number of days of systemic steroid treatment, dose of inhaled steroid, pulmonary function, or symptoms, although there were fewer days with symptoms in the IVIG group.[198] The duration of this study was only 2 months, in contrast to most others, which were 6 months. A second study had 3 arms in which 40 patients were randomized to receive either 2 g/kg IVIG per month, 1 g/kg IVIG per month, or 2 g/kg albumin per month.[199] Effects on asthma were not significantly different among the three groups, and severe adverse effects (severe headaches) resulted in premature termination of the study. The third study evaluated 28 patients who could not be weaned off steroids during an initial treatment-optimization phase, followed by randomization to receive a loading dose of 2 g/kg IVIG, followed by 400 mg/kg every 3 weeks for 9 months vs albumin placebo.[200] Oral steroid doses were reduced in both the IVIG and albumin groups, and the difference between the groups was not significant. There were no differences in pulmonary function test results, inhaled steroid use, symptoms, or days lost from work or school.[200] Hence, despite data suggesting efficacy in uncontrolled studies, two of three RCTs showed no significant effect of IVIG in asthma, and at this time the literature does not support a recommendation for the routine use of IVIG in patients with severe asthma.

Recurrent Spontaneous Abortion

The underlying cause of recurrent miscarriage in some cases might be immune mediated. Prospective studies[201,202] have suggested that the use of IVIG in pregnant women with a history of recurrent abortions gave a protective benefit. Other studies, however, suggested no benefit,[203] and a review of the randomized, placebo-controlled, multicenter studies found that IVIG did not provide benefit.[204] This indication nonetheless remains controversial because of the studies that claim benefits, along with the paucity of effective therapies available to such patients. Given the reviews of randomized trials,[36,204] however, cumulative evidence does not presently support the widespread use of IVIG for the prevention of recurrent spontaneous abortions (with or without antiphospholipid syndrome).

Chronic Fatigue Syndrome

Chronic fatigue syndrome is a clinically defined disorder that has often been associated with mild immune dysfunction. There have been numerous anecdotal reports of IVIG use having subjective benefits; however, as demonstrated in a double-blind, placebo-controlled trial,[205] IVIG is not effective in the treatment of typical chronic fatigue syndrome.

Cystic Fibrosis

Patients with cystic fibrosis and normal immune systems do not benefit from the addition of IVIG therapy. RCTs comparing the benefit of IVIG with that of placebo showed no added benefit for the use of IVIG.[206] Between 2% and 10% of patients with cystic fibrosis have hypogammaglobulinemia.[207] Some studies do not suggest any associated additional morbidity because of this,[207] but some anecdotal reports indicate benefit for IVIG in cystic fibrosis with hypogammaglobulinemia.[208,209] There is no randomized trial in this setting.

Alzheimer Disease

Antibodies in IVIG against amyloid beta peptide (Abeta) that recognize conformation-specific epitopes as well as linear epitopes from different regions of the Abeta peptide may have a neuroprotective effect.[210] Natural Abeta antibodies have the capacity to prevent Abeta oligomer-induced neurotoxicity in neuroblastoma cells, and this neuroprotective effect may reflect a therapeutic potential of the natural Abeta antibodies found in IVIG for the treatment of patients with Alzheimer disease. Relkin et al in 2008 performed an open-label, dose-ranging study in eight mild Alzheimer disease patients in which IVIG was added to approved Alzheimer disease therapies for 6 months, discontinued, and then resumed for another 9 months.[211] Anti-Abeta in the serum from Alzheimer disease patients increased in proportion to IVIG dose. Cerebrospinal fluid Abeta decreased significantly at 6 months, returned to baseline after washout, and decreased again after IVIG was readministered for an additional 9 months. Mini-mental state was improved after 6 months, returned to baseline during washout, and remained stable during subsequent IVIG treatment. These findings confirmed and extended those obtained by Dodel et al[212] from a 6-month trial of IVIG in five Alzheimer disease patients. Although the sample sizes of these studies are too small to draw clear conclusions, they suggest that a more detailed investigation of IVIG use in Alzheimer disease may be warranted.

Conclusions

IVIG has been used for a great many disorders, often as a "last-resort" therapy. Although in a number of disorders there is reasonable evidence of its efficacy, the use of IVIG has often not been accompanied by good evidence but is based on current understanding of the theoretical activity of the mechanisms of action of IVIG in exerting immune modulation. Where safe, effective, and affordable alternative therapies exist, these should be considered preferable to IVIG. When IVIG is used, the lowest dose for the shortest duration required to achieve the desired outcome should be chosen. For ongoing therapy, the achievement of measurable clinical outcomes is a requirement, and IVIG should not be continued in patients with no demonstrable clinical benefit. Properly designed ongoing and future studies will continue to delineate the appropriate uses of this expensive therapeutic modality.

References

1. Orange JS, Hossny EM, Weiler CR, et al. Use of intravenous immunoglobulin in human disease: A review of evidence by members of the Primary Immunodeficiency Committee of the American Academy of Allergy, Asthma and Immunology. J Allergy Clin Immunol 2006; 117:S525-53.
2. Dalakas MC. Immunopathogenesis of inflammatory myopathies. Ann Neurol 1995;37 (Suppl 1):S74-86.
3. Dalakas MC, Illa I, Dambrosia JM, et al. A controlled trial of high-dose intravenous immune globulin infusions as treatment for dermatomyositis. N Engl J Med 1993;329:1993-2000.
4. Cherin P, Piette JC, Wechsler B, et al. Intravenous gamma globulin as first line therapy in polymyositis and dermatomyositis: An open study in 11 adult patients. J Rheumatol 1994; 21:1092-7.
5. Sansome A, Dubowitz V. Intravenous immunoglobulin in juvenile dermatomyositis—four year review of nine cases. Arch Dis Child 1995; 72:25-8.
6. Choy EHS, Hoogendijk JE, Lecky B, Winer JB. Immunosuppressant and immunomodulatory treatment for dermatomyositis and polymyositis. Cochrane Database Syst Rev 2005;(3): CD003643.
7. Lang BA, Laxer RM, Murphy G, et al. Treatment of dermatomyositis with intravenous gammaglobulin. Am J Med 1991;91:169-72.
8. Collet E, Dalac S, Maerens B, et al. Juvenile dermatomyositis: Treatment with intravenous gammaglobulin. Br J Dermatol 1994;130:231-4.
9. Roifman CM. Use of intravenous immune globulin in the therapy of children with rheumatological diseases. J Clin Immunol 1995;15(6 Suppl):42S-51S.
10. Tsai MJ, Lai CC, Lin SC, et al. Intravenous immunoglobulin therapy in juvenile dermatomyositis. Zhonghua Min Guo Xiao Er Ke Yi Xue Hui Za Zhi 1997;38:111-15.
11. Al-Mayouf SM, Laxer RM, Schneider R, et al. Intravenous immunoglobulin therapy for juve-

nile dermatomyositis: Efficacy and safety. J Rheumatol 2000;27:2498-503.
12. Zipitis CS, Baildam EM, Ramanan AV. Treatment approaches to juvenile dermatomyositis. Expert Opin Pharmacother 2004;5:1509-15.
13. Amato AA, Barohn RJ, Jackson CE, et al. Inclusion body myositis: Treatment with intravenous immunoglobulin. Neurology 1994;44:1516-8.
14. Dalakas MC, Koffman B, Fujii M, et al. A controlled study of intravenous immunoglobulin combined with prednisone in the treatment of IBM. Neurology 2001;56:323-7.
15. Cherin P, Pelletier S, Teixeira A, et al. Results and long-term follow up of intravenous immunoglobulin infusions in chronic, refractory polymyositis: An open study with thirty-five adult patients. Arthritis Rheum 2002;46:467-74.
16. Moriya Y, Yamaji K, Kanai Y, Tsuda H. The effectiveness of intravenous human immunoglobulin treatment after plasmapheresis in restoring serum immunoglobulin levels: A preliminary study. Ther Apher 2002;6:154-8.
17. Savery F. Intravenous immunoglobulin treatment of rheumatoid arthritis-associated immunodeficiency. Clin Ther 1988;10:527-9.
18. Ballow M. Mechanisms of action of intravenous immunoglobulin therapy and potential use in autoimmune connective tissue diseases. Cancer 1991;68:1430-6.
19. Kanik KS, Yarboro CH, Naparstek Y, et al. Failure of low-dose intravenous immunoglobulin therapy to suppress disease activity in patients with treatment-refractory rheumatoid arthritis. Arthritis Rheum 1996;39:1027-9.
20. Prieur AM. Intravenous immunoglobulins in Still's disease: Still controversial, still unproven. J Rheumatol 1996;23:797-800.
21. Uziel Y, Laxer RM, Schneider R, Silverman ED. IVIG therapy in systemic onset JRA: A follow-up study. J Rheumatol 1996;23:910-18.
22. Rutter A, Luger TA. Intravenous immunoglobulin: An emerging treatment for immune-mediated skin diseases. Curr Opin Investig Drugs 2002;3:713-9.
23. Arnal C, Piette JC, Leone J, et al. Treatment of severe immune thrombocytopenia associated with systemic lupus erythematosus: 59 cases. J Rheumatol 2002;29:75-83.
24. Meissner M, Sherer Y, Levy Y, et al. Intravenous immunoglobulin therapy in a patient with lupus serositis and nephritis. Rheumatol Int 2000;19:199-201.
25. Silvestris F, D'Amore O, Cafforio P, et al. Intravenous immune globulin therapy of lupus nephritis: Use of pathogenic anti-DNA-reactive IgG. Clin Exp Immunol 1996;104(Suppl 1):91-7.
26. Lesprit P, Mouloud F, Bierling P, et al. Prolonged remission of SLE-associated polyradiculoneuropathy after a single course of intravenous immunoglobulin. Scand J Rheumatol 1996;25:177-9.
27. Levy Y, Sherer Y, George J, et al. Serologic and clinical response to treatment of systemic vasculitis and associated autoimmune disease with intravenous immunoglobulin. Int Arch Allergy Immunol 1999;119:231-8.
28. Aharon A, Levy Y, Bar-Dayan Y, et al. Successful treatment of early secondary myelofibrosis in SLE with IVIG. Lupus 1997;6:408-11.
29. Aharon A, Zandman-Goddard G, Shoenfeld Y. Autoimmune multiorgan involvement in elderly men: Is it SLE? Clin Rheumatol 1994;13:631-4.
30. Pasatiempo AM, Kroser JA, Rudnick M, Hoffman BI. Acute renal failure after intravenous immunoglobulin therapy. J Rheumatol 1994;21:347-9.
31. Jayne DR, Chapel H, Adu D, et al. Intravenous immunoglobulin for ANCA-associated systemic vasculitis with persistent disease activity. QJM 2000;93:433-9.
32. Jayne DR, Esnault VL, Lockwood CM. ANCA anti-idiotype antibodies and the treatment of systemic vasculitis with intravenous immunoglobulin. J Autoimmun 1993;6:207-19.
33. Aries PM, Hellmich B, Gross WL. Intravenous immunoglobulin therapy in vasculitis: Speculation or evidence? Clin Rev Allergy Immunol 2005;29:237-45.
34. National Blood Authority, Australia. Criteria for the clinical use of intravenous immunoglobulin (IVIg) in Australia (effective from 3 March 2008). Canberra, ACT, Australia: NBA, 2010. [Available at www.nba.gov.au/ivig/index.html (accessed February 26, 2010).]
35. Galli M, Cortelazzo S, Barbui T. In vivo efficacy of intravenous gammaglobulins in patients with lupus anticoagulant is not mediated by an anti-idiotypic mechanism. Am J Hematol 1991;38:184-8.
36. Empson M, Lassere M, Craig J, Scott J. Prevention of recurrent miscarriage for women with antiphospholipid antibody or lupus anticoagulant. Cochrane Database Syst Rev 2005;(2):CD002859.

37. Bucciarelli S, Espinosa G, Cervera R, et al. European Forum on Antiphospholipid Antibodies. Mortality in the catastrophic antiphospholipid syndrome: Causes of death and prognostic factors in a series of 250 patients. Arthritis Rheum 2006;54:2568-76.
38. Smith A, Jackson M, Wang F, et al. Neutralisation of muscarinic receptor autoantibodies by intravenous immunoglobulin in Sjogren's syndrome. Hum Immunol 2005;66:411-16.
39. Fontaine J, Joly P, Roujeau JC. Treatment of bullous pemphigoid. J Dermatol 2003;30:83-90.
40. Scully C, Challacombe SJ. Pemphigus vulgaris: Update on etiopathogenesis, oral manifestations, and management. Crit Rev Oral Biol Med 2002;13:397-408.
41. Wetter DA, Davis MD, Yiannias JA, et al. Effectiveness of intravenous immunoglobulin therapy for skin disease other than toxic epidermal necrolysis: A retrospective review of Mayo Clinic experience. Mayo Clinic Proc 2005;80: 41-7.
42. Jolles S, Hughes J, Rustin M. Therapeutic failure of high-dose intravenous immunoglobulin in pemphigus vulgaris. J Am Acad Dermatol 1999;40:499-500.
43. Ahmed AR, Dahl MV. Consensus statement on the use of intravenous immunoglobulin therapy in the treatment of autoimmune mucocutaneous blistering diseases. Arch Dermatol 2003;139:1051-9.
44. Viard I, Wehrli P, Bullani R, et al. Inhibition of toxic epidermal necrolysis by blockade of CD95 with human intravenous immunoglobulin. Science 1998;282:490-3.
45. Prins C, Vittorio C, Padilla RS, et al. Effect of high-dose intravenous immunoglobulin therapy in Stevens-Johnson syndrome: A retrospective, multicenter study. Dermatology 2003; 207:96-9.
46. Bachot N, Revuz J, Roujeau JC. Intravenous immunoglobulin treatment for Stevens-Johnson syndrome and toxic epidermal necrolysis: A prospective noncomparative study showing no benefit on mortality or progression. Arch Dermatol 2003;139:33-6.
47. Trent JT, Kirsner RS, Romanelli P, Kerdel FA. Analysis of intravenous immunoglobulin for the treatment of toxic epidermal necrolysis using SCORTEN: The University of Miami experience. Arch Dermatol 2003;139:39-43.
48. Biotext, commissioned by the National Blood Authority on behalf of all Australian Governments. A systematic literature review and report on the efficacy of intravenous immunoglobulin therapy and its risks. Final report v04. Appendix 2: Summary data on conditions and papers. (September 6, 2004) Canberra, ACT, Australia: NBA, 2004:190-1. [Available at http://www.nba.gov.au/pubs/pdf/ivig-appendix2.pdf (accessed February 26, 2010).]
49. Frommer M, Madronio C. The use of intravenous immunoglobulin in Australia. A report for the National Blood Authority, Part B: Systematic literature review, 2006. Sydney, NSW, Australia: Sydney Health Projects Group, University of Sydney, 2006:55-6.
50. Ahmed AR. Intravenous immunoglobulin therapy for patients with bullous pemphigoid unresponsive to conventional immunosuppressive treatment. J Am Acad Dermatol 2001;45:825-35.
51. Ahmed AR. Intravenous immunoglobulin therapy in the treatment of patients with pemphigus vulgaris unresponsive to conventional immunosuppressive treatment. J Am Acad Dermatol 2001;45:679-90.
52. Sami N, Bhol KC, Ahmed AR. Treatment of oral pemphigoid with intravenous immunoglobulin as monotherapy. Long-term follow-up: Influence of treatment on antibody titres to human alpha6 integrin. Clin Exp Immunol 2002;129:533-40.
53. Ahmed AR, Dahl MV, for the Consensus Development Group. Consensus statement on the use of intravenous immunoglobulin therapy in the treatment of autoimmune mucocutaneous blistering diseases. Arch Dermatol 2003; 139:1051-9.
54. Sami N, Bhol KC, Razzaque A. Influence of IVIG therapy on autoantibody titres to desmoglein 1 in patients with pemphigus foliaceus. Clin Immunol 2002;105:192-8.
55. Letko E, Miserocchi E, Daoud YJ, et al. A nonrandomized comparison of the clinical outcome of ocular involvement in patients with mucous membrane (cicatricial) pemphigoid between conventional immunosuppressive and intravenous immunoglobulin therapies. Clin Immunol 2004;111:303-10.
56. Sami N, Oureshi A, Ruocco E, et al. Corticosteroid-sparing effect of intravenous immunoglobulin therapy in patients with pemphigus vulgaris. Arch Dermatol 2002;138:1158-62.
57. Habif TP. Clinical dermatology. 4th ed. St Louis, MO: Mosby, 2004:547-86.

58. Ahmed AR, Sami N. Intravenous immunoglobulin therapy for patients with pemphigus foliaceus unresponsive to conventional therapy. J Am Acad Dermatol 2002;46:42-9.
59. Sami N, Ali S, Bhol KC, Ahmed AR. Influence of intravenous immunoglobulin therapy on autoantibody titres to BP Ag1 and BP Ag2 in patients with bullous pemphigoid. J Eur Acad Dermatol Venereol 2003;17:641-5.
60. Jolles S, Sewell C, Webster D, et al. Adjunctive high-dose intravenous immunoglobulin treatment for resistant atopic dermatitis: Efficacy and effects on intracellular cytokine levels and CD4 counts. Acta Derm Venereol 2003;83:433-7.
61. Jolles S, Hughes J, Rustin M. The treatment of atopic dermatitis with adjunctive high-dose intravenous immunoglobulin: A report of three patients and review of the literature. Br J Dermatol 2000;142:551-4.
62. Kimata H. High dose gammaglobulin treatment for atopic dermatitis. Arch Dis Child 1994;70:335-6.
63. Paul C, Lahfa M, Bachelez H, et al. A randomized controlled evaluator-blinded trial of intravenous immunoglobulin in adults with severe atopic dermatitis. Br J Dermatol 2002;147:518-22.
64. Wakim M, Alazard M, Yajima A, et al. High dose intravenous immunoglobulin in atopic dermatitis and hyper-IgE syndrome. Ann Allergy Asthma Immunol 1998;81:153-8.
65. Schmitt J, Schakel K, Schmitt N, Meurer M. Systemic treatment of severe atopic eczema: A systematic review. Acta Derm Venereol 2007;87:100-11.
66. Budde M, Gusek-Schneider GC, Mayer U, Seitz B. Annular crystalline keratopathy in association with immunoglobulin therapy for pyoderma gangrenosum. Cornea 2003;22:82-5.
67. Dobson CM, Parslew RA, Evans S. Superficial granulomatous pyoderma treated with intravenous immunoglobulin. J Am Acad Dermatol 2003;48:456-60.
68. Dirschka T, Kastner U, Behrens S, Altmeyer P. Successful treatment of pyoderma gangrenosum with intravenous human immunoglobulin. J Am Acad Dermatol 1998;39:789-90.
69. Hagman JH, Carrozzo AM, Campione E, et al. The use of high-dose immunoglobulin in the treatment of pyoderma gangrenosum. J Dermatolog Treat 2001;12:19-22.
70. Gleichmann US, Otte HG, Korfer R, Stadler R. Post-traumatic pyoderma gangrenosum: Combination therapy with intravenous immunoglobulins and systemic corticosteroids. Hautarzt 1999;50:879-83.
71. Gupta AK, Shear NH, Sauder DN. Efficacy of human intravenous immune globulin in pyoderma gangrenosum. J Am Acad Dermatol 1995;32:140-2.
72. Bloom D, Fisher D, Dannenberg M. Pyoderma gangrenosum associated with hypogammaglobulinemia. Arch Dermatol 1958;77:412-21.
73. Marcussen PV. Hypogammaglobulinemia in pyoderma gangrenosum. J Invest Dermatol 1955;24:275-80.
74. Greaves MW. Pathophysiology of chronic urticaria. Int Arch Allergy Immunol 2002;127:3-9.
75. Fiebiger E, Maurer D, Holub H, et al. Serum IgG autoantibodies directed against the alpha chain of Fc epsilon RI: A selective marker and pathogenetic factor for a distinct subset of chronic urticaria patients? J Clin Invest 1995;96:2606-12.
76. Kikuchi Y, Kaplan AP. Mechanisms of autoimmune activation of basophils in chronic urticaria. J Allergy Clin Immunol 2001;107:1056-62.
77. O'Donnell BF, Barr RM, Black AK, et al. Intravenous immunoglobulin in autoimmune chronic urticaria. Br J Dermatol 1998;138:101-6.
78. Asero R. Are IVIG for chronic unremitting urticaria effective? Allergy 2000;55:1099-101.
79. Dawn G, Urcelay M, Ah-Weng A, et al. Effect of high-dose intravenous immunoglobulin in delayed pressure urticaria. Br J Dermatol 2003;149:836-40.
80. Kroiss M, Vogt T, Landthaler M, Stolz W. The effectiveness of low-dose intravenous immunoglobulin in chronic urticaria. Acta Derm Venereol 2000;80:225.
81. Altschul A, Cunningham-Rundles C. Chronic urticaria and angioedema as the first presentations of common variable immunodeficiency. J Allergy Clin Immunol 2002;110:664-5.
82. Gurmin V, Mediwake R, Fernando M, et al. Psoriasis: Response to high-dose intravenous immunoglobulin in three patients. Br J Dermatol 2002;147:554-7.
83. Jordan S, Cunningham-Rundles C, McEwan R. Utility of intravenous immune globulin in kidney transplantation: Efficacy, safety, and cost implications. Am J Transplant 2003;3:653-64.
84. Riechsteiner G, Speich R, Schanz U, et al. Haemolytic anaemia after lung transplantation:

An immune-mediated phenomenon? Swiss Med Wkly 2003;133:143-7.
85. Shehata N, Palda VA, Meyer RM, et al. Immunoglobulin for patients undergoing solid organ transplantation: An evidence based practice guideline (review). Transfus Med Rev 2010; 24(Suppl 1):S7-27.
86. New grades for recommendations from the Canadian Task Force on Preventive Health Care. CMAJ 2003;169:207-8.
87. Jordan SC, Tyan D, Stablein D, et al. Evaluation of intravenous immunoglobulin as an agent to lower allosensitization and improve transplantation in highly sensitized adult patients with end-stage renal disease: Report of the NIH IG02 trial. J Am Soc Nephrol 2004;15:3256-62.
88. Peraldi MN, Akposso K, Haymann JP, et al. Long-term benefit of intravenous immunoglobulins in cadaveric kidney retransplantation. Transplantation 1996;62:1670-3.
89. Anglicheau D, Loupy A, Suberbielle C, et al. Posttransplant prophylactic intravenous immunoglobulin in kidney transplant patients at high immunological risk: A pilot study. Am J Transplant 2007;7:1185-92.
90. Bielmann D, Honger G, Lutz D, et al. Pretransplant risk assessment in renal allograft recipients using virtual crossmatching. Am J Transplant 2007;7:626-32.
91. Mahmoud KM, Sobh MA, El SF, et al. Management of sensitized patients awaiting renal transplantation: Does sequential therapy of intravenous immunoglobulin and simvastatin offer a solution? Eur J Pharmacol 2007;561:202-5.
92. Stegall MD, Gloor J, Winters JL, et al. A comparison of plasmapheresis versus high-dose IVIG desensitization in renal allograft recipients with high levels of donor specific alloantibody. Am J Transplant 2006;6:346-51.
93. Thielke J, DeChristopher PJ, Sankary H, et al. Highly successful living donor kidney transplantation after conversion to negative of a previously positive flow-cytometry cross-match by pretransplant plasmapheresis. Transplant Proc 2005;37:643-4.
94. Akalin E, Ames S, Sehgal V, et al Intravenous immunoglobulin and thymoglobulin induction treatment in immunologically high-risk kidney transplant recipients. Transplantation 2005; 79:742.
95. Mahmoud K, Sobh M, El-Shenawy F, et al. Effect of high-dose intravenous immunoglobulin on suppression of alloantibodies against HLA in highly sensitized transplant candidates. Transplant Proc 2004;36:1850-2.
96. Akalin E, Ames S, Sehgal V, et al. Intravenous immunglobulin (IVIG) and thymoglobulin facilitate kidney transplantation in complement dependent cytotoxicity (CDC) B cell and flow cytometry (FC) T and/or B cell cross-match positive patients. Transplantation 2003;76:1444.
97. Gloor JM, DeGoey SR, Pineda AA, et al. Overcoming a positive crossmatch in living-donor kidney transplantation. Am J Transplant 2003; 3:1017-23.
98. Jordan SC, Vo A, Bunnapradist S, et al. Intravenous immune globulin treatment inhibits crossmatch positivity and allows for successful transplantation of incompatible organs in living-donor and cadaver recipients. Transplantation 2003;76:631-6.
99. Zachary AA, Montgomery RA, Ratner LE, et al. Specific and durable elimination of antibody to donor HLA antigens in renal-transplant patients. Transplantation 2003;76:1519-25.
100. Glotz D, Antoine C, Julia P, et al. Desensitization and subsequent kidney transplantation of patients using intravenous immunoglobulins (IVIG). Am J Transplant 2002;2:758-60.
101. Sonnenday CJ, Ratner LE, Zachary AA, et al. Preemptive therapy with plasmapheresis/intravenous immunoglobulin allows successful live donor renal transplantation in patients with a positive cross-match. Transplant Proc 2002; 34:1614-16.
102. Schweitzer EJ, Wilson JS, Fernandez-Vina M, et al. A high panel-reactive antibody rescue protocol for cross-match-positive live donor kidney transplants. Transplantation 2000;70:1531-6.
103. Glotz D, Haymann JP, Niaudet P, et al. Successful kidney transplantation of immunized patients after desensitization with normal human polyclonal immunoglobulins. Transplant Proc 1995;27:1038-9.
104. Vo AA, Lukovsky M, Toyoda M, et al. Rituximab and intravenous immune globulin for desensitization during renal transplantation. N Engl J Med 2008;359:242-51.
105. Kayler L, Farber JL, Clombe B, et al. Characterization of rejection episoded in patients following positive crossmatch and ABO-incompatible liver donor renal transplantation. Transplant International 2006;19:128-39.

106. Tyden G, Donauer J, Wadstrom J, et al. Implementation of a protocol for ABO-incompatible kidney transplantation—a three-center experience with 60 consecutive transplantations. Transplantation 2007;83:1153-5.
107. Tyden G, Kumlien G, Genberg H, et al. The Stockholm experience with ABO-incompatible kidney transplantations without splenectomy. Xenotransplantation 2006;13:105-7.
108. Tyden G, Kumlien G, Genberg H, et al. ABO incompatible kidney transplantations without splenectomy, using antigen-specific immunoadsorption and rituximab. Am J Transplant 2005;5:145-8.
109. Winters JL, Gloor JM, Pineda AA, et al. Plasma exchange conditioning for ABO-incompatible renal transplantation. J Clin Apher 2004;19:79-85.
110. Sonnenday CJ, Warren DS, Cooper M, et al. Plasmapheresis, CMV hyperimmune globulin, and anti-CD20 allow ABO-incompatible renal transplantation without splenectomy. Am J Transplant 2004;4:1315-22.
111. Gloor JM, Lager DJ, Moore SB, et al. ABO-incompatible kidney transplantation using both A2 and non-A2 living donors. Transplantation 2003;75:971-7.
112. Vasilescu ER, Ho EK, Colovai AI, et al. Alloantibodies and the outcome of cadaver kidney allografts. Human Immunol 2006;67:597-604.
113. Jordan SC, Vo AA, Toyoda M, et al. Post-transplant therapy with high-dose intravenous gammaglobulin: Applications to treatment of antibody-mediated rejection. Pediatr Transpl 2005;9:155-61.
114. Lehrich RW, Rocha PN, Reinsmoen N, et al. Intravenous immunoglobulin and plasmapheresis in acute humoral rejection: Experience in renal allograft transplantation. Human Immunol 2005;66:350-8.
115. White NB, Greenstein SM, Cantafio AW, et al. Successful rescue therapy with plasmapheresis and intravenous immunoglobulin for acute humoral renal transplant rejection. Transplantation 2004;78:772-4.
116. Rocha PN, Butterly DW, Greenberg A, et al. Beneficial effect of plasmapheresis and intravenous immunoglobulin on renal allograft survival of patients with acute humoral rejection. Transplantation 2003;75:1490-5.
117. Montgomery RA, Zachary AA, Racusen LC, et al. Plasmapheresis and intravenous immune globulin provides effective rescue therapy for refractory humoral rejection and allows kidneys to be successfully transplanted into cross-match-positive recipients. Transplantation 2000;70:887-95.
118. Jordan SC, Quartel AW, Czer LSC, et al. Post-transplant therapy using high-dose human immunoglobulin (intravenous gammaglobulin) to control acute humoral reaction in renal and cardiac allograft recipients and potential mechanism of action. Transplantation 1998;66:800-8.
119. Trpkov K, Campbell P, Pazderka F, et al. Pathologic features of acute renal allograft rejection associated with donor-specific antibody: Analysis using the Banff grading schema. Transplantation 1996;61:1586-92.
120. Casadei DH, del C Rial M, Opelz G, et al. A randomized and prospective study comparing treatment with high-dose intravenous immunoglobulin with monoclonal antibodies for rescue of kidney grafts with steroid-resistant rejection. Transplantation 2001;71:53-8.
121. Casadei D, Rial M, Argento J, et al. Preliminary results from a randomized and prospective study of high-dose immunoglobulin versus monoclonal antibody in the rescue of steroid-resistant rejections. Transplant Proc 1998;30:2164.
122. Luke PP, Scantlebury VP, Jordan ML, et al. Reversal of steroid- and anti-lymphocyte antibody-resistant rejection using intravenous immunoglobulin (IVIG) in renal transplant recipients. Transplantation 2001;72:419-22.
123. Casadei D, Rial M, Raimondi E, et al. Immunoglobulin i.v. high dose (IVIGHD): New therapy as a rescue treatment of grafted kidneys. Transplant Proc 1996;28:3290-1.
124. Petrie JJ, Rigby RJ, Hawley CM, et al. Effect of OKT3 in steroid-resistant renal transplant rejection. Transplantation 1995;59:347-52.
125. Nwakanma LU, Williams JA, Weiss ES, et al. Influence of pre-transplant panel-reactive antibody on outcomes in 8,160 heart transplant recipients in recent era. Ann Thorac Surg 2007;84:1556-62; discussion, 1562-3.
126. Tambur AR, Pamboukian SV, Costanzo MR, et al. The presence of HLA-directed antibodies after heart transplantation is associated with poor allograft outcome. Transplantation 2005;80:1019-25.
127. Leech SH, Lopez-Cepero M, LeFor WM, et al. Management of the sensitized cardiac recipient: The use of plasmapheresis and intrave-

nous immunoglobulin. Clin Transplant 2006; 20:476-84.
128. Jacobs JP, Quintessenza JA, Boucek RJ, et al. Pediatric cardiac transplantation in children with high panel-reactive antibody. Ann Thor Surg 2004;78:1703-9.
129. John R, Lietz K, Schuster M, et al. Immunologic sensitization in recipients of left ventricular assist devices. J Thorac Cardiovasc Surg 2003; 125:578-91.
130. Itescu S, Burke E, Lietz K, et al. Intravenous pulse administration of cyclophosphamide is an effective and safe treatment for sensitized cardiac allograft recipients. Circulation 2002; 105:1214-19.
131. Pisani BA, Mullen GM, Malinowska K, et al. Plasmapheresis with intravenous immunoglobulin G is effective in patients with elevated panel-reactive antibody prior to cardiac transplantation. J Heart Lung Transplant 1999;18: 701-6.
132. John R, Lietz K, Burke E, et al. Intravenous immunoglobulin reduces anti-HLA alloreactivity and shortens waiting time to cardiac transplantation in highly sensitized left ventricular assist device recipients. Circulation 1999;100 (19 Suppl):II229-35.
133. Shah AS, Nwakanma L, Simpkins C, et al. Pretransplant panel-reactive antibodies in human lung transplantation: An analysis of over 10,000 patients. Ann Thorac Surg 2008;85: 1919-24.
134. Hadjiliadis D, Chaparro C, Reinsmoen NL, et al. Pre-transplant panel-reactive antibody in lung transplant recipients is associated with significantly worse post-transplant survival in a multicenter study. J Heart Lung Transplant 2005;24(7 Suppl):S249-54.
135. Lau CL, Palmer SM, Posther KE, et al. Influence of panel-reactive antibodies on posttransplant outcomes in lung transplant recipients. Ann Thorac Surg 2000;69:1520-4.
136. Gammie JS, Pham SM, Colson YL, et al. Influence of panel-reactive antibody on survival and rejection after lung transplantation. J Heart Lung Transplant 1997;16:408-15.
137. Appel JZ 3rd, Hartwig MG, Davis RD, Reinsmoen NL. Utility of peritransplant and rescue intravenous immunoglobulin and extracorporeal immunoadsorption in lung transplant recipients sensitized to HLA antigens. Human Immunol 2005;66:378-86.
138. Ganschow R, Englert C, Grabhorn E, et al. Hypogammaglobulinemia in pediatric liver transplant recipients. Pediatr Transplant 2005; 9:215-19.
139. Nascimbene A, Iannacone M, Brando B, De Gasperi A. Acute thrombocytopenia after liver transplant: Role of platelet activation, thrombopoietin deficiency and response to high dose intravenous IgG treatment. J Hepatol 2007;47: 651-7.
140. Echaniz-Laguna A, Battaglia F, Ellero B, et al. Chronic inflammatory demyelinating polyradiculoneuropathy in patients with liver transplantation. Muscle Nerve 2004;30:501-4.
141. Urbani L, Mazzoni A, De Simone P, et al. Treatment of antibody-mediated rejection with high-dose immunoglobulins in ABO-incompatible liver transplant recipient. Transpl Int 2007; 20:467-70.
142. Falagas ME, Snydman DR, Ruthazer R, et al. Cytomegalovirus immune globulin (CMVIG) prophylaxis is associated with increased survival after orthotopic liver transplantation. The Boston Center for Liver Transplantation CMVIG Study Group. Clin Transplant 1997; 11:432-7.
143. Lloyd AJ, Walker C, Wilkinson M. Kawasaki disease: Is it caused by an infectious agent? Br J Biomed Sci 2001;58:122-8.
144. Sundel RP. Update on the treatment of Kawasaki disease in childhood. Curr Rheumatol Rep 2002;4:474-82.
145. Tse SM, Silverman ED, McCrindle BW, Yeung RS. Early treatment with intravenous immunoglobulin in patients with Kawasaki disease. J Pediatr 2002;140:450-5.
146. Muta H, Ishii M, Egami K, et al. Early intravenous gamma-globulin treatment for Kawasaki disease: The nationwide surveys in Japan. J Pediatr 2004;144:496-9.
147. Newburger JW, Takahashi M, Beiser AS, et al. A single intravenous infusion of gamma globulin as compared with four infusions in the treatment of acute Kawasaki syndrome. N Engl J Med 1991;324:1633-9.
148. Oates-Whitehead R, Baumer J, Haines L, et al. Intravenous immunoglobulin for the treatment of Kawasaki disease in children. Cochrane Database Syst Rev 2003;(4):CD004000.
149. Durongpisitkul K, Gururaj VJ, Park JM, Martin CF. The prevention of coronary artery aneurysm in Kawasaki disease: A meta-analysis on the efficacy of aspirin and immunoglobulin treatment. Pediatrics 1995;96:1057-61.
150. UK Department of Health. Clinical guidelines for immunoglobulin use. 2nd ed. (June 4,

2008). London: DH, 2008. [Available at http://www.dh.gov.uk/en/Publicationsandstatistics/Publications/PublicationsPolicyAndGuidance/DH_085235 (accessed February 26, 2010).]
151. Leung DY. Kawasaki syndrome: Immunomodulatory benefit and potential toxin neutralization by intravenous immune globulin. Clin Exp Immunol 1996;104(Suppl 1):49-54.
152. Leung DY. Superantigens related to Kawasaki syndrome. Springer Semin Immunopathol 1996;17:385-96.
153. Wolf HM, Eibl MM. Immunomodulatory effect of immunoglobulins. Clin Exp Rheumatol 1996;14(Suppl 15):S17-25.
154. Xu C, Poirier B, Van Huyen JP, et al. Modulation of endothelial cell function by normal polyspecific human intravenous immunoglobulins: A possible mechanism of action in vascular diseases. Am J Pathol 1998;153:1257-66.
155. Drucker NA, Colan SD, Lewis AB, et al. Gamma-globulin treatment of acute myocarditis in the pediatric population. Circulation 1994;89:252-7.
156. Briassoulis G, Papadopoulos G, Zavras N, et al. Cardiac troponin I in fulminant adenovirus myocarditis treated with a 24-hour infusion of high-dose intravenous immunoglobulin. Pediatr Cardiol 2000;21:391-4.
157. Takeda Y, Yasuda S, Miyazaki S, et al. High-dose immunoglobulin G therapy for fulminant myocarditis. Jpn Circ J 1998;62:871-2.
158. Tedeschi A, Airaghi L, Giannini S, et al. High-dose intravenous immunoglobulin in the treatment of acute myocarditis. A case report and review of the literature. J Intern Med 2002;251:169-73.
159. Robinson J, Hartling L, Vandermeer B, et al. Intravenous immunoglobulin for presumed viral myocarditis in children and adults. Cochrane Database Syst Rev 2005;(1):CD004370.
160. McNamara DM, Holubkov R, Starling RC, et al. Controlled trial of intravenous immune globulin in recent-onset dilated cardiomyopathy. Circulation 2001;103:2254-9.
161. Nydegger UE. Immunoglobulins. In: Simon TL, Snyder EL, Solheim BG, et al, eds. Rossi's principles of transfusion medicine. 4th ed. Bethesda, MD: AABB Press, 2009:260-72.
162. Flynn DM, Mohan N, McKiernan P, et al. Progress in treatment and outcome for children with neonatal haemochromatosis. Arch Dis Child Foetal Neonatal Ed 2003;88:F124-7.
163. Knisely AS, Mieli-Vergani G, Whitington PF. Neonatal haemochromatosis. Gastroenterol Clin North Am 2003;32:877-89.
164. Rodriguez F, Kallas M, Nash R, et al. Neonatal haemochromatosis—medical treatment vs. transplantation: The King's experience. Liver Transpl 2005;11:1417-24.
165. Whitington PF, Hibbard, JU. High-dose immunoglobulin during pregnancy for recurrent neonatal haemochromatosis. Lancet 2004;364:1690-8.
166. Whittington PF, Kelly S, Ekong UD. Neonatal haemochromatosis: Foetal liver disease leading to liver failure in the foetus and newborn. Paediatr Transplant 2005;9:640-5.
167. Dalakas MC, Fujii M, Li M, et al. High-dose intravenous immune globulin for stiff-person syndrome (see comment). N Engl J Med 2001;345:1870-6.
168. Kornberg AJ, for the Asia-Pacific IVIG Advisory Board. Bringing consensus to the use of IVIG in neurology. Expert consensus statements on the use of IVIG in neurology. 1st ed. Melbourne, Australia: Asia-Pacific IVIG Advisory Board, 2004:70-2.
169. Dalakas MC. The role of IVIG in the treatment of patients with stiff person syndrome and other neurological diseases associated with anti-GAD antibodies. J Neurol 2005;252 (Suppl 1):119-25.
170. Rowland LP, Layzer RB. Stiff man syndrome (Moersch-Woltman syndrome). In: Rowland LP, ed. Merritt's Neurology. 11th ed. Philadelphia: Lippincott Williams and Wilkins, 2005:927.
171. LeHoang P, Cassoux N, George F, et al. Intravenous immunoglobulin (IVIG) for the treatment of birdshot retinochoroidopathy. Ocul Immunol Inflamm 2000;8:49-57.
172. Rosenbaum JT, George RK, Gordon C. The treatment of refractory uveitis with intravenous immunoglobulin. Am J Ophthalmol 1999;127:545-9.
173. Kahaly G, Pitz S, Muller-Forell W, Hommel G. Randomized trial of intravenous immunoglobulins versus prednisolone in Graves' ophthalmopathy. Clin Exp Immunol 1996;106:197-202.
174. Philipsen EK, Larsen S, Helin P. A preliminary trial of high-dose intravenous immunoglobulin to a patient with euthyroid ophthalmopathy. Thyroidology 1989;1:93-5.

175. Richter WO, Donner MG, Schwandt P. Elimination of islet cell antibodies and glutamic acid decarboxylase antibodies II in a patient with newly diagnosed insulin-dependent diabetes mellitus. J Clin Apher 1997;12:196-9.
176. Heinze E. Immunoglobulins in children with autoimmune diabetes mellitus. Clin Exp Rheumatol 1996;14(Suppl):S99-102.
177. Colagiuri S, Leong GM, Thayer Z, et al. Intravenous immunoglobulin therapy for autoimmune diabetes mellitus. Clin Exp Rheumatol 1996;14(Suppl 15):S93-7.
178. Carmassi F, Morale M, Puccetti R, et al. Efficacy of intravenous immunoglobulin therapy in a case of autoimmune-mediated chronic active hepatitis. Clin Exp Rheumatol 1992;10:13-7.
179. Perlmutter SJ, Leitman SF, Garvey MA, et al. Therapeutic plasma exchange and intravenous immunoglobulin for obsessive-compulsive disorder and tic disorders in childhood. Lancet 1999;354:1153-8.
180. Hadden RDM, Nobile-Orazio E, Sommer C, et al. European Federation of Neurological Societies/Peripheral Nerve Society guideline on management of paraproteinaemic demyelinating neuropathies: Report of a joint task force of the European Federation of Neurological Societies and the Peripheral Nerve Society. Eur J Neurol 2006;13:809-18.
181. Vincent A, Buckley C, Schott JM, et al. Potassium channel antibody-associated encephalopathy: A potentially immunotherapy responsive form of limbic encephalitis. Brain 2004;127:701-12.
182. Jacob S, Irani SR, Rajabally YA, et al. Hypothermia in VGKC antibody-associated limbic encephalitis. J Neurol Neurosurg Psychiatry 2008;79:202-4.
183. Hamilos DL, Young RM, Peter JB, et al. Hypogammaglobulinemia in asthmatic patients. Ann Allergy 1992;68:472-81.
184. Moss RB, Carmack MA, Esrig S. Deficiency of IgG4 in children: Association of isolated IgG4 deficiency with recurrent respiratory tract infection. J Pediatr 1992;120:16-21.
185. Klaustermeyer WB, Wong SC, Schoettler JJ, et al. Quantitative immunoglobulins and IgG subclasses in patients with corticosteroid-dependent reversible airway obstruction. Ann Allergy 1989;63:327-30.
186. Loftus BG, Price JF, Lobo-Yeo A, Vergani D. IgG subclass deficiency in asthma. Arch Dis Child 1988;63:1434-7.
187. Oxelius VA, Hanson LA, Bjorkander J, et al. IgG3 deficiency: Common in obstructive lung disease. Hereditary in families with immunodeficiency and autoimmune disease. Monogr Allergy 1986;20:106-15.
188. Page R, Friday G, Stillwagon P, et al. Asthma and selective immunoglobulin subclass deficiency: Improvement of asthma after immunoglobulin replacement therapy. J Pediatr 1988;112:127-31.
189. Schwartz HJ, Berger M. Intravenous gammaglobulin therapy in bronchial asthma. Allergy Asthma Proc 2002;23:15-8.
190. Mazer BD, Gelfand EW. An open-label study of high-dose intravenous immunoglobulin in severe childhood asthma. J Allergy Clin Immunol 1991;87:976-83.
191. Spahn JD, Leung DY, Chan MT, et al. Mechanisms of glucocorticoid reduction in asthmatic subjects treated with intravenous immunoglobulin. J Allergy Clin Immunol 1999;103:421-6.
192. Sigman K, Ghibu F, Sommerville W, et al. Intravenous immunoglobulin inhibits IgE production in human B lymphocytes. J Allergy Clin Immunol 1998;102:421-7.
193. Zhuang Q, Mazer B. Inhibition of IgE production in vitro by intact and fragmented intravenous immunoglobulin. J Allergy Clin Immunol 2001;108:229-34.
194. Basta M, Van Goor F, Luccioli S, et al. F(ab)92-mediated neutralization of C3a and C5a anaphylatoxins: A novel effector function of immunoglobulins. Nat Med 2003;9:431-8.
195. Jakobsson T, Croner S, Kjellman NI, et al. Slight steroid-sparing effect of intravenous immunoglobulin in children and adolescents with moderately severe bronchial asthma. Allergy 1994;49:413-20.
196. Landwehr LP, Jeppson JD, Katlan MG, et al. Benefits of high-dose i.v. immunoglobulin in patients with severe steroid-dependent asthma. Chest 1998;114:1349-56.
197. Haque S, Boyce N, Thien FC, et al. Role of intravenous immunoglobulin in severe steroid-dependent asthma. Intern Med J 2003;33:341-4.
198. Niggemann B, Leupold W, Schuster A, et al. Prospective, double-blind, placebo-controlled, multicentre study on the effect of high-dose, intravenous immunoglobulin in children and adolescents with severe bronchial asthma. Clin Exp Allergy 1998;28:205-10.
199. Kishiyama JL, Valacer D, Cunningham-Rundles C, et al. A multicenter, randomized, double-

blind, placebo-controlled trial of high-dose intravenous immunoglobulin for oral corticosteroid-dependent asthma. Clin Immunol 1999; 91:126-33.
200. Salmun LM, Barlan I, Wolf HM, et al. Effect of intravenous immunoglobulin on steroid consumption in patients with severe asthma: A double-blind, placebo-controlled, randomized trial. J Allergy Clin Immunol 1999;103:810-15.
201. Bulletti C, Flamigni C, Giacomucci E. Reproductive failure due to spontaneous abortion and recurrent miscarriage. Hum Reprod Update 1996;2:118-36.
202. Carp HJ, Ahiron R, Mashiach S, et al. Intravenous immunoglobulin in women with five or more abortions. Am J Reprod Immunol 1996; 35:360-2.
203. Daya S, Gunby J, Porter F, et al. Critical analysis of intravenous immunoglobulin therapy for recurrent miscarriage. Hum Reprod Update 1999;5:475-82.
204. Scott JR. Immunotherapy for recurrent miscarriage. Cochrane Database Syst Rev 2003;(1): CD000112; update in 2006;(2):CD000112.
205. Vollmer-Conna U, Hickie I, Hadzi-Pavlovic D, et al. Intravenous immunoglobulin is ineffective in the treatment of patients with chronic fatigue syndrome. Am J Med 1997;103:38-43.
206. Winnie GB, Cowan RG, Wade NA, Cairo MS. Intravenous immune globulin treatment of pulmonary exacerbations in cystic fibrosis. J Pediatr 1989;114:309-14.
207. Garside JP, Kerrin DP, Brownlee KG, et al. Immunoglobulin and IgG subclass levels in a regional pediatric cystic fibrosis clinic. Pediatr Pulmonol 2005;39:135-40.
208. Bentur L, McKlusky I, Levison H, Roifman CM. Advanced lung disease in a patient with cystic fibrosis and hypogammaglobulinemia: Response to intravenous immune globulin therapy. J Pediatr 1990;117:741-3.
209. Matthews WJ Jr, Williams M, Oliphint B, et al. Hypogammaglobulinemia in patients with cystic fibrosis. N Engl J Med 1980;302:245-9.
210. Szabo P, Relkin N, Weksler ME. Natural human antibodies to amyloid beta peptide. Autoimmun Rev 2008;7:415-20.
211. Relkin NR, Szabo P, Adamiak B, Burgut T, et al. 18-Month study of intravenous immunoglobulin for treatment of mild Alzheimer disease. Neurobiol Aging 2009;30:1728-36.
212. Dodel RC, Du Y, Depboylu C, Hampel H, et al. Intravenous immunoglobulins containing antibodies against beta-amyloid for the treatment of Alzheimer's disease. J Neurol Neurosurg Psychiatry 2004;75:1472-4.

8

Anti-D: Basic Concepts and Mechanisms of Action in Hemolytic Disease of the Fetus and Newborn

Davor Brinc, PhD, and Alan H. Lazarus, PhD

ANTI-D IMMUNE GLOBULIN IS used for the prevention of the antibody response to D-positive red cells in pregnant women at risk for hemolytic disease of the fetus and newborn (HDFN). Despite its effectiveness in nonimmune individuals, anti-D fails to protect from HDFN in cases of preexisting immunity to the D antigen. Furthermore, the current anti-D product is prepared from pooled human plasma, and as such, the supply is limited and the potential to transmit infectious agents is always a concern. Several monoclonal and recombinant anti-Ds have recently been developed and tested; the variable and unpredictable effects of these products have precluded their clinical application.

Human studies of polyclonal anti-D have established an effective dose and treatment schedule. With respect to the mechanism of anti-D, human studies indicate a correlation between the anti-D effect and D-positive red cell clearance, which has been taken to suggest that red cell clearance is the major mechanism of the IgG effect. However, monoclonal/recombinant anti-D studies have failed to establish such a correlation for all antibodies. The ability of IgG to prevent the antigen-specific antibody response has also been observed in animal models using a variety of different antigens;

Davor Brinc, PhD, Postdoctoral Fellow in Clinical Chemistry, University of Toronto, and Alan H. Lazarus, PhD, Scientist, Canadian Blood Services, St Michael's Hospital, and Associate Professor of Medicine and Associate Professor, Laboratory Medicine and Pathobiology, University of Toronto, Toronto, Ontario, Canada

This work was supported by grants from the Canadian Blood Services (Lazarus) and a Graduate Student Fellowship Award from the Canadian Blood Services (Brinc).

The authors have disclosed no conflicts of interest.

this phenomenon has been referred to as antibody-mediated immune suppression (AMIS), and this use of IgG predates the use of anti-D by over half a century. Animal studies of AMIS have provided evidence that IgG may impair early B-cell responses to the antigen independently of antigen clearance. However, AMIS suppresses only primary antibody responses, the suppression is only partial in many cases, and these models are not associated with HDFN. The applicability of AMIS studies for understanding the true mechanism of anti-D is therefore uncertain, but the studies nevertheless provide insight into potential mechanisms of action of red cell antibodies.

Historical Overview

HDFN was first recorded in 1609 and has historically been described as hydrops fetalis, icterus gravis neonatorum, congenital anemia, or hemolytic anemia based on its varying clinical presentation.[1] Erythroblastosis fetalis, the term used to describe the hematologic findings in the presence of generalized neonatal edema,[2] was often present along with severe anemia. In 1932, Diamond et al reported that the various syndromes were manifestations of the same disease.[3] The understanding of HDFN progressed after the identification of the Rh blood group system and the finding that HDFN is usually presented by Rh-negative mothers pregnant with Rh-positive children.[1,4] Subsequently, maternal antibody transfer across the placenta was correlated with fetal red cell destruction.[1,4]

It is now known that HDFN is caused by the destruction of fetal or newborn red cells by maternal antibodies directed against their surface antigens, most commonly against the D polypeptide. The individuals who do not express the D polypeptide (15%-17% of people of European ethnicity; 5%-7%, African ethnicity; and 0-1%, Asian ethnicity) can develop antibodies to this antigen following exposure to D-positive red cells from transfusion or pregnancy.[1,4,5]

The original work that used anti-D to suppress the humoral immune response in the setting of HDFN was based on two independent lines of reasoning[6,7]: 1) the reduced incidence of HDFN in cases of ABO incompatibility between mother and child and reduced incidence of primary D immunization following transfusion of D-positive red cells in male volunteers,[8,9] and 2) the inhibitory effect of antiserum in different animal models, originally described by von Dungern[10] and later termed *AMIS*.

It was first shown in 1961 that red cells coated in vitro with anti-D serum could prevent the anti-D response in male recipients.[9] This was followed by landmark reports of the successful use of anti-D in human male volunteers using plasma[11] or IgG-enriched plasma fractions[12,13] from immunized donors. These early studies established that only IgG anti-D, and not IgM, could prevent the antibody response to the D antigen.[11] Comprehensive clinical trials were subsequently conducted in Canada, England, and the United States,[7,14-19] leading to the introduction of standard anti-D prophylaxis programs.

In the initial protocol, anti-D was administered to D-negative mothers within 72 hours of delivery of D-positive pregnancy.[5,20] This postnatal anti-D administration reduced the incidence of primary D immunization from 17% to 1.5% in ABO-compatible pregnancies.[5,20] It was believed that most of the remaining cases of D immunization occurred during pregnancy, before administration of anti-D. As a result, studies were initiated in which anti-D was administered at the 28th and 34th week of pregnancy, and then again within 72 hours of delivery. Antenatal administration of anti-D resulted in the transfer of some of the injected anti-D to the fetus; however, the dose was insufficient to cause any significant clinical condition in the fetus or newborn.[5,20] The successful outcome of clinical trials of antenatal anti-D treatment led to the introduction of routine combined antenatal and postnatal anti-D prophylaxis.[20-27]

The current clinical anti-D product is the IgG fraction of plasma prepared from D-positive-red-cell-immunized individuals and likely rich in polyclonal anti-D specificities. To further minimize the risk of infectious disease transmission as well as to increase the supply of anti-D, there have been attempts to develop monoclonal and recombinant anti-D as replacements for the current product.[28-30] Monoclonal anti-D has been prepared from an Epstein-Barr virus (EBV)-transformed B-lymphoblastoid cell line (B-LCL) or from heterohybridomas (hybridomas prepared by fusion of anti-D-secreting B cells and murine myelomas).[29] Recombinant anti-D has been prepared using cDNA for D-specific Fab and the human Fc region of IgG, which have been cloned in an expression vector in rat YB2/0 myelomas or Chinese hamster ovary (CHO) cell lines.[28,29]

Immune Response to the D Antigen and Immune Response Suppression

The D antigen can induce a potent antibody response against D-positive red cells in D-negative individuals. Several studies have shown that T cells are necessary for the antibody response to red cells in animal models.[31-33] Based on this evidence, T cells specific to the D polypeptide, which have recently been identified in humans, are also likely necessary for the anti-D response.[34,35]

The immune response to the D antigen has been predominantly studied in human male volunteers immunized with D-positive red cells.[1,5] On the basis of these early studies, more than 80% of D-negative male volunteers make anti-D within 6 months after transfusion of 200 mL of group O D-positive red cells[5,36] or 500 mL of whole blood.[5,37] Following transfusion of lower blood volumes—for example, 0.5 to 1 mL of D-positive red cells—around 50% of subjects respond.[5] A cumulative dose of 0.03 mL red cells has been suggested to be capable of stimulating an anti-D response.[5] The incidence of D alloimmunization in D-negative oncology/hematology patients receiving D-positive red cells is much lower, reported at 9% to 30.4%.[38-40] The anti-D response can usually be detected several weeks after primary D immunization.[5] The secondary antibody response is restricted primarily to the IgG1 and IgG3 isotypes.[41] Interestingly, it has been observed in some individuals that immunization may occur without serologically detectable anti-D.[5,42] The second injection of D-positive red cells in these individuals can result in rapid clearance of transfused D-positive red cells and rapid appearance of anti-D, suggesting a secondary antibody response.[5] As a result, lack of detection of anti-D following primary immunization need not necessarily indicate a suppressed immune response against the D antigen. Anti-D has been reported as being one of the most persistent red cell alloantibodies.[43] However, in a subset of D-negative recipients, termed nonresponders, repeated injection of small amounts of D-positive red cells can fail to induce an antibody response or lead to accelerated clearance of red cells.[5]

The antibody response to the D antigen in D-negative mothers is thought to be induced after fetal D-positive red cells have gained access to the maternal circulation during pregnancy and/or delivery. Fetomaternal hemorrhage (FMH), or the leakage of fetal red cells across the placenta into the maternal circulation, can lead to an immune response to the D antigen.[1] The frequency of FMH and the amount of fetal red cells present in the maternal circulation increase with gestational age and then significantly increase during delivery.[20] ABO incompatibility reduces the observed incidence and the quantity of fetal red cells detected in the maternal circulation, and this is thought to underlie the observed reduction in the incidence of D immunization and HDFN in ABO-incompatible pregnancies.[20] The extent of FMH is linked to the probability of an anti-D immune response in the mother, as there is a correlation between the level of fetal red cells in the maternal circulation after delivery and the anti-D response.[6]

Following D-positive pregnancy, only a subset of D-negative women becomes alloimmunized.[1,5,44] The incidence of D immunization in D-negative women 6 months after the delivery of a D-positive ABO-compatible child is 4% to 9%.[20] The incidence increases to 17% by the end of the second D-positive pregnancy.[20] In the case of ABO incompatibility, the incidence following delivery is 2%,[1] which is thought to reflect increased destruction of ABO-incompatible red cells by A or B antibodies, as appropriate. Combined antenatal and postnatal administration of anti-D has reduced the incidence of D alloimmunization and subsequent HDFN by as much as 99%[22-25,45,46] and the HDFN-related infant mortality rate by 97%.[47,48] Nevertheless, red cell alloimmunization can still occur in D-negative mothers. A recent study in the central-west region of Sweden reported a total red cell alloimmunization rate for all pregnancies excluding ABO immunizations at 0.4%[49]; 60% of these alloimmunized subjects made anti-D, followed by anti-Fy^a at 10%, anti-c at 7%, and anti-K at 4%.[49]

Anti-D Studies in Humans

Chapter 10 describes clinical use of anti-D in detail. In brief, human studies of anti-D have been designed in two formats. Autologous red cells opsonized in vitro with anti-D were injected into D-positive individuals and the clearance rate of the injected red cells determined.[29,50] Alternatively, anti-D was given before or after (24-72 hours) red cells were injected into D-negative subjects.[29] In some cases, subjects were rechallenged with D-positive red cells after 6 and 9 months to determine if primary or secondary responses were initiated after rechallenge.[29,51] The latter studies measured red cell clearance as well as the anti-D response. Anti-D-mediated suppression was judged effective if the anti-D response was not detected within 6 months of the first challenge with D-positive red cells.[29,51] To additionally confirm that the anti-D response has not developed, after 6 months, subjects were sometimes rechallenged with D-positive red cells but without anti-D coadministration.[29,51] The concept of these studies was that a secondary anti-D response would be induced if immune memory developed against the D antigen following the primary challenge, even though the antibody response was not initially detected. The (secondary) response detected after this red cell rechallenge was interpreted to indicate that anti-D failed to prevent the immune response to the D antigen.[29,51]

The studies of the anti-D effect in humans allowed development of clinical protocols for the administration of anti-D, including the dose and timing of the anti-D administration. A dose of anti-D given intramuscularly that is sufficient for prevention of primary D immunization is 20 µg of anti-D per mL of D-positive red cells.[5,37,52] Intravenous administration of anti-D appears to be effective at a slightly lower dose.[5] The standard dose of anti-D for postnatal prophylaxis has been, for example, 100 µg in the United Kingdom or 300 µg in the United States. For antenatal prophylaxis, in addition to postnatal administration of anti-D, two modalities have been in use: 100 µg administered at 28 and 34 weeks or 300 µg administered at 28 weeks.[26,27]

In addition, human studies of anti-D have shown that the anti-D effect is restricted to the primary antibody response against D-positive red cells; anti-D cannot prevent the antibody response once the antibody response to D antigen has been initiated.[53,54] Furthermore, a delayed administration of anti-D reduces its effectiveness.[55] Anti-D, therefore, cannot be used to prevent HDFN in previously D-immunized individuals.

Anti-D in Animal Models

Animal models have been used to measure anti-D-mediated red cell clearance. The clearance rate mediated by monoclonal anti-D was tested in chimpanzees[56,57] and nonobese/diabetic severe combined immunodeficient (NOD-SCID) mice[58,59] infused with D-positive red cells.

The major obstacle to the development of a murine model of D immunization is the inability of mice to respond to the human D antigen. Two strategies have been used to address this issue. In one approach, SCID mice were reconstituted with peripheral blood lymphocytes from a D-immunized human donor. Following challenge with D-positive red cells, these human-blood-reconstituted mice showed a secondary response to D-positive red cells.[60] In a different and more recent approach, mice expressing a major histocompatibility complex (MHC) Class II molecule capable of D antigen presentation (HLA-DR15) were generated. These mice presented D peptides to T cells, and T-cell responses were detected following challenge with purified D protein or peptides.[61] However, the effect of anti-D has not yet been studied in these models.

An animal model that shows some of the features of HDFN has also recently been developed. This model was based on the blood group system in rabbits containing red cell antigen allotypes expressed from the Hg locus (Hg^A, Hg^D, Hg^F). In this model, female rabbits are first immunized against allogeneic red cells and then mated with male rabbits homozygous for the incompatible allotype.[62,63] The maternal red cell antibody response and fetal red cell lysis were observed. The ability of antibodies against different allotypes to prevent the maternal response has not yet been tested.

Monoclonal/Recombinant Anti-D

As part of the efforts to replace polyclonal anti-D, several monoclonal/recombinant D antibodies have been developed.[28-30,64] The criteria suggested for selection of clinically useful anti-D include red cell clearance, prevention of D alloimmunization, and long plasma half-life.[29] It has further been suggested that monoclonal anti-D-mediated red cell clearance should resemble the clearance characteristics mediated by polyclonal anti-D; ie, red cell clearance should be achieved at a low dose of anti-D below D antigen saturation.[28] The success of these products in clinical trials has been variable, and none have yet been licensed for use in HDFN prevention.

To test the newly developed monoclonal/recombinant anti-D, both in-vitro and in-vivo assays have been developed based on the ability of IgG to interact with the Fcγ receptors (FcγRs) on effector cells and induce red cell clearance by phagocytosis (eg, monocyte chemiluminescence assay) or extracellular lysis (eg, monocyte/macrophage/natural-killer-mediated, antibody-dependent, cytotoxicity assays).[65] In-vivo assays similarly measure the ability of anti-D to clear red cells from the circulation.[51,56-59,66-68]

FcγRs come in two different functional varieties, either activating (human FcγRI, FcγRIIA, and FcγRIII; murine FcγRI, FcγRIII, and FcγRIV) or inhibitory (human or murine FcγRIIB). The relative ratio of activating vs inhibitory FcγRs on effector cells can affect the outcome of the IgG-FcγR interaction in mice,[69-71] and thus macrophage-mediated phagocytosis of anti-D-opsonized red cells may or may not occur.

Different IgG isotypes bind FcγRs with varying affinity and, as a result, vary in the ability to induce FcγR-mediated effector functions. For example, in mice, IgG3 does not bind FcγRs and fails to induce FcγR-mediated effector functions. As different IgG isotypes in mice bind the inhibitory FcγRIIB with varying affinities, they can exhibit differential sensitivity to FcγRIIB-mediated inhibition. For example, mouse IgG1 has 10-fold higher affinity for the inhibitory FcγRIIB than for the activating FcγRIII, whereas mouse IgG2a has 70-fold higher affinity for the activating FcγRIV than for the inhibitory FcγRIIB. As a result, effector functions induced by mouse monoclonal IgG1 can be more sensitive to negative regulation by the inhibitory FcγRIIB than the effects induced by IgG2a.[72,73]

IgG contains a single N-linked oligosaccharide chain at the Asn^{297} amino-acid position; different IgG glycoforms have different affinities for the FcγR and, as a result, vary in the ability to induce effector functions.[73,74] For example, a change in the IgG glycosylation pattern can promote or inhibit inflammatory reactions mediated by the same IgG.[74,75] Thus, the glycosylation pattern of particular monoclonal IgG antibodies may be an important factor to consider in predicting the anti-D effect.[29]

Several monoclonal/recombinant D antibodies have been selected largely based on their ability to mediate red cell clearance for clinical trials, albeit with limited success.[29,30] The ability of anti-D to mediate phagocytosis in vitro or clearance in vivo has not always predicted the successful inhibition of the anti-D response in vivo.[28] Monoclonal/recombinant anti-D preparations vary in their ability to prevent the antibody response and can cause an enhanced antibody response to the D antigen under certain conditions, despite efficient antigen clearance.[28,29] As discussed above, IgG gylosylation may be one of the reasons for discrepant findings.[29] Monoclonal anti-Ds prepared in different cell lines or by recombinant technology will exist in different glycoforms. Different affinities of IgG glycoforms for activating vs inhibitory FcγRs may also explain variable clearance rates of fully opsonized incompatible red cells. In addition, sialylated IgG species can bind the C-type lectin SIGN-R1 [specific intercellular adhesion molecule (ICAM)-3-grabbing, nonintegrin-related 1] receptor on splenic murine macrophages and elicit the ability of effector macrophages to upregulate the inhibitory FcγRs and downregulate phagocytosis.[74] SIGN-R1 is a mouse homolog of human DC-SIGN, expressed on human dendritic cells.[76,77] Carbohydrates attached to the IgG molecule may also stimulate antigen-presenting cells, which may account for the observed enhancing anti-D effect.[29]

Antibody-Mediated Immune Suppression

The ability of antigen-specific IgG, such as anti-D, to prevent or downregulate the antibody response had been observed well before the introduction of anti-D prophylaxis. The antibody response against a variety of different antigens has been inhibited using antigen-specific antiserum or the IgG fraction in a large number of animal studies.[68,78-81] This IgG effect has often been described as AMIS.[80,82-92]

The earliest reference to AMIS dates to 1900: antiserum against xenogeneic (cattle) red cells prevented the antibody response to these red cells in rabbits.[10,44] In 1909, it was discovered that an excess of antitoxin downregulated the immune response against diphtheria toxin in guinea pigs[93]; this finding was reported in several other studies.[94-98] The same effect of antiserum has been observed following immunization with other bacteria products, such as tetanus toxoid[99-102] and bacterial flagellum,[103] as well as with viruses, such as poliomyelitis virus[104,105] and bacteriophages.[106-108]

The ability of antibodies to downregulate the antibody response to an antigen has also been detected following immunization with protein antigens in adjuvants, such as bovine gamma globulin,[109,110] keyhole limpet hemocyanin,[111] bovine serum albumin,[109] ovalbumin,[109] and several haptens, such as dinitrophenyl conjugated to bovine gamma globulin[112] or rabbit gamma globulin.[113] Finally, the inhibitory IgG effect has been observed upon challenge with blood cells: red cells [such as sheep red cells (SRBCs)[114-117] and rabbit red cells[85,118]], platelets,[119-121] and leukocytes.[122,123]

Early studies of this inhibitory IgG effect used only crude serum prepared from animals immunized with toxins or heterologous red cells as an antibody source, but more purified IgM or IgG serum fractions were applied in the later studies.[93,112,115] The availability of distinct antibody fractions allowed later studies to show that only IgG effectively prevented the antibody response to particulate antigens, including bacteriophage ΦX174,[108] SRBCs,[117] and trinitrophenyl-horse red cells,[124] and also to soluble antigens administered in adjuvants.[93]

The inhibitory IgG effect on the host antibody response was studied in several other models developed in the late 1980s and 1990s. Antigen-specific IgG was used to prevent the antibody response following human platelet transfusion into SCID mice reconstituted with human peripheral blood lymphocytes.[119-121,125] In this model, peripheral blood lymphocytes from female blood donors previously immunized against Class I HLA were adoptively transferred into SCID mice, followed by challenge with allogeneic platelets. The HLA antibody response could be prevented if the platelets were presensitized with

IgG specific to the HLA or to the associated β₂ microglobulin. IgG specific for other platelet antigens in this model (eg, CD42a and FcγRII) were ineffective in preventing the antibody response.[120,121]

The maternal IgG transferred across the placenta during pregnancy can also downregulate the antibody response following vaccination in infants.[126-128] This IgG effect has been observed using several different vaccines, such as measles,[129] polio,[130] influenza,[131] rotavirus,[132] pertussis,[133,134] tetanus and diphtheria toxoid,[96,135-137] Haemophilus influenzae,[138,139] and hepatitis A[140-142] vaccines.

Whether AMIS is relevant for understanding the mechanism of action of anti-D is controversial.[80] Animal models study the IgG effect on the immune response rather than in preventing HDFN: it is not known if the type of suppression observed in animal models of AMIS is sufficient for prevention of HDFN. Human studies of anti-D in male volunteers may have a similar limitation. Furthermore, the immune response against model antigens in AMIS is designed to occur early after immunization in up to 100% of recipients. In contrast, the anti-D response is slower with fewer respondents.[80] However, the conditions that lead to an immune response following transfusion of D-positive red cells are not completely known, preventing a more specific comparison between the anti-D effect and AMIS.

Mechanisms of Anti-D

An Overview of the Hypotheses

Several hypotheses concerning the mechanism of AMIS, which have also been applied to the anti-D effect, have been suggested (see Table 8-1). The "antigen clearance" hypothesis proposes that IgG removes the antigen before it can be recognized by the immune system.[51,68,78,80,144] The "steric-hindrance" or "epitope-masking" hypothesis suggests that IgG binds the antigen and sterically blocks the site recognized by antigen-specific B cells.[78,79,81] The "FcγRIIB-mediated B-cell inhibition" hypothesis proposes that the IgG-antigen complex co-ligates the B-cell receptor (BCR) and the inhibitory IgG receptor FcγRIIB on the B-cell surface and delivers a negative signal to inactivate antigen-specific B cells.[90,145,146]

Studies of anti-D effects in human male volunteers have suggested other possible mechanisms, such as a long-term suppressive effect of anti-D on the host immune system,[80,147] transforming growth factor beta (TGFβ)-mediated B-cell inhibition, or Fc-independent antigen clearance of IgG-opsonized red cells.[80] There is limited support for the role of cytokines and other soluble factors in anti-D-mediated prevention of D immunization and HDFN. It has been shown that anti-D increases TGF-β1 and prostaglandin E2 levels in some women, which probably correlated with the amount of D-positive red cells in the circulation.[148] The level of

Table 8-1. Potential Mechanisms of Action of Anti-D

Accelerated red cell clearance
Immunosuppression
Inhibitory Fc receptor (FcγRIIB)
Steric hindrance
Altered cytokines
Inhibition of synapse formation between the B cell and the red cell[143]
Altered B-cell antigen processing and presentation[143]

interleukin-1 receptor antagonist is also slightly decreased in some women.[148]

Antigen Clearance

The antigen clearance hypothesis remains at the forefront of the proposed mechanisms for anti-D.[68] According to this hypothesis, IgG prevents the antibody response by accelerating the phagocytosis and removal of antigens, such as red cells, from the circulation by the mononuclear phagocytic system (particularly by macrophages) before their recognition by the immune system.[80] The antigen opsonized with the IgG may be cleared by sequestration and phagocytosis in the liver, spleen, and/or other secondary lymphoid tissue or by direct complement-mediated lysis. Specifically, macrophage FcγRs can interact with IgG-opsonized antigen, resulting in antigen removal. The IgG on the red cell surface can also trigger complement activation resulting in direct lysis of cellular antigens and/or deposition of complement fragments onto the antigen surface, leading to interaction with complement receptors on macrophages and dendritic cells and subsequent phagocytosis. Anti-D itself does not activate complement[149] but can interact with FcγRs and mediate adhesion and phagocytosis of red cells.[65]

Anti-D

In support of the antigen clearance hypothesis of anti-D, ABO incompatibility reduced the incidence of anti-D responders in male volunteers.[8,9] It was assumed that A or B IgM antibodies destroy the incompatible fetal red cells and that this prevented their recognition by the immune system. Furthermore, the clearance of IgG-opsonized red cells has been repeatedly observed and appears to be related to the ability of the IgG to prevent the antibody response in humans.[6,28,29,44,51,67,150-155] Also, the ability of IgG to prevent the response against antigens on human red cells was not found to be antigen specific. In a single study, IgG specific to the Kell antigen was demonstrated to prevent the response to both Kell and D antigens following challenge of D/Kell-negative male volunteers with D/Kell-positive red cells.[144] Finally, anti-D failed to accelerate red cell clearance and prevent an anti-D response in a splenectomized D-negative subject.[44]

Antibody-Mediated Immune Suppression

In the SRBC model of AMIS, virtually all detectable red cells can be cleared within 10 minutes of intravenous injection,[87] and no difference has been observed between SRBC clearance and IgG-opsonized-SRBC clearance.[87,156] In this model of AMIS, therefore, the correlation between clearance and the IgG effect could not be established.

The antigen clearance hypothesis requires the Fc portion of the IgG for inhibition of the humoral immune response because this IgG region is necessary for the interaction with FcγRs as well as for complement activation. Several studies in the SRBC model have shown that the whole IgG, but not the $F(ab')_2$ fragments, can reduce the antibody response,[90,157-160] although other studies have come to the opposite conclusion.[121,161-163]

A multitude of other studies in mice has suggested that the inhibitory IgG effect on the antibody response may not be dependent on antigen clearance. In particular, the AMIS effect correlates with the number of IgG molecules attached to the SRBC, rather than the ability of the IgG to fix complement or bind FcγRs.[164] The inhibitory IgG effect was also found to be independent of complement.[165] Last, it has been shown that the FcR γ chain, which associates with FcγRs and is absolutely required for FcγR-mediated phagocytosis, is not at all necessary for the AMIS effect in a murine model using SRBCs as foreign red cells.[163]

The antigen clearance hypothesis assumes that antigen removal by macrophages is sufficient to prevent the antibody response. However, antibody-sensitized red cells should also interact with dendritic cells, which would logically be expected to promote an immune response by presenting red cell antigens to B and T cells.[166-171] To test the likelihood of these seemingly opposite potential mechanisms, the authors recently examined whether the transfusion of IgG-opsonized SRBCs preinternalized or prebound by adherent mononuclear cells (rich in phagocytic cells and dendritic cells) inhibited the immune response. Rather than inhibiting the response as would be expected based on the antigen clearance model, transfusion of the mononuclear cells incubated with IgG-opsonized red cells instead elicited a potent antibody response upon infusion into naive recipient mice.[156]

The Role of T Cells

T cells are necessary for the B-cell response to red cells.[31-33,172] The inhibition of the T-cell response would therefore be sufficient for protection from D alloimmunization and HDFN.

Anti-D

T cells responding to D-derived peptides have recently been cloned,[34] although the effect of anti-D on T-cell responses has not yet been tested. HDFN is usually caused by a secondary antibody response in pregnancies subsequent to the D alloimmunization initiating event.[1] It is likely that this secondary antibody response is dependent on T-cell memory. The effect of anti-D on T-cell memory, as with T-cell responses, has not been tested. However, under these assumptions, the demonstrated protection from HDFN suggests that anti-D can prevent or inhibit the T-cell response and T-cell memory. Anti-D may inhibit T-cell responses by causing nonimmunogenic red cell clearance by dendritic cells or macrophages[68] or by inhibiting B-cell antigen-presenting cell function. A recent study in an animal model has shown that dendritic cells mediate T-cell responses to incompatible red cells[173] and B cells were also shown to be able to induce T-cell activation against SRBCs.[174,175]

Antibody-Mediated Immune Suppression

T cells are necessary for the B cell response to SRBCs.[176,177] However, anti-SRBC has not been found to prevent the antigen-induced expansion and priming of SRBC-specific T cells in mice under AMIS conditions.[156,163,178] IgG can enhance, rather than inhibit, T-cell proliferation in vitro in the presence of an antigen and antigen-presenting cells.[179] Maternal IgG antibodies, while inhibiting the antibody responses in infants following vaccination, do not affect T-cell priming nor change the type of cytokines produced by these T cells in humans[180,181] or mice.[182,183] Finally, IgG does not prevent immunologic memory in animal models of AMIS.[88,163,184]

In contrast, IgG prevents the proliferation of lymphocytes from human donors in response to allogeneic platelets in vitro.[120] Also, the proliferation of antigen-specific T-cell clones can be prevented by IgG targeting MHC-bound peptides in vitro.[185] It has also been shown that repeated injection of allogeneic leukocytes or platelets,[122,123] following the primary challenge under AMIS conditions, fails to induce the antibody response. This response can be absent even after subsequent multiple transfusions of uncoated platelets or leukocytes, suggesting that the IgG may have a dominant inhibitory effect on the immune system in the recipient.[123] The dominant inhibitory effect may be mediated by T cells.[186] However, in other studies it has been observed that multiple transfusions of uncoated cells could eventually overcome the inhibitory effect mediated by IgG.[187]

In addition, it has been suggested that IgG may prevent the antibody response by preventing B/T-cell cooperation.[188] The AMIS effect on the antibody response could be reversed in vitro by the provision of T-cell help using "tumor necrosis serum," obtained from mice treated with bacillus Calmette-Guérin and lipopolysaccharide.[188] However, it has been difficult to determine specific cytokines in tumor necrosis serum that can reverse the AMIS effect, and this approach has not been further pursued.

B-Cell Inhibition via the Inhibitory FcγR (FcγRIIB)

According to the B-cell inhibition hypothesis, upon antibody production and subsequent class-switching to IgG, the concentration of IgG increases. When antigen-specific IgG is present at sufficient quantities, immune complexes form between the IgG and the antigen. These immune complexes then act in a feedback pathway by cross-linking the inhibitory FcγR (FcγRIIB) on B cells with the BCR. FcγRIIB possesses an amino-acid sequence in the intracellular portion of the molecule, termed the immune receptor tyrosine-based inhibitory motif (ITIM). This sequence expressed by FcγRIIB is necessary and sufficient for FcγRIIB-mediated inhibition of B-cell activation upon co-ligation with the BCR.[189] When a B cell encounters an antigen, the simultaneous engagement of the BCR and FcγRIIB initiates inhibitory signaling in B cells.[189-195] This physiologic effect thus downregulates the production of new antibodies.[192,195-201] Under conditions where the antigen and IgG are administered concurrently, feedback is then artificially induced and B-cell responses are decreased.[79,145]

Anti-D

The role of the inhibitory receptor on B cells, FcγRIIB, has not been directly addressed in anti-D studies. In addition to a potential contribution by FcγRIIB, several novel FcR-like molecules (FCRL,[202] previously referred to as FcR homologs, or FcRH) have been identified in mice and humans.[203-206] FCRLs are predominantly expressed by B-cell lineages,[207] and some of these FCRLs, theoretically, can mediate B-cell inhibition instead of the classical FcγRIIB. For example, FCRL4, upon co-ligation with the BCR, can inhibit the activation of human memory B cells.[208] Also, the engagement of FCRL5 by monoclonal antibodies can inhibit marginal-zone B-cell activation in mice.[209] However, it has not yet been shown that these FCRLs can bind monovalent or aggregated IgG.[203,204,206,209]

Antibody-Mediated Immune Suppression

The FcγRIIB-mediated B-cell inhibition hypothesis was originally supported by findings that FcγRIIB can downregulate B-cell activation in vitro.[190,191] However, a major and compelling argument against FcγRIIB-mediated B-cell inhibition has been provided in the SRBC model using mice genetically deficient in FcγRIIB (FcγRIIB−/− mice), which showed that FcγRIIB is not necessary for the AMIS effect.[163,210,211] The authors speculate that some of the FCRLs may also mediate B-cell inhibition instead of the classical FcγRIIB, and this should be tested in the future.

Epitope Masking

The epitope-masking hypothesis suggests that IgG binds the antigen and prevents the BCR from recognizing the corresponding epitopes.[78,81,114]

Anti-D

Epitope-masking is not expected to contribute to the anti-D effect. Several studies argue against the epitope-masking hypothesis of the anti-D effect. The amount of IgG that prevents the antibody response does not saturate all the epitopes on D-positive red cells.[51,80,153,212] It is known that as little as 0.06 mL of whole blood (corresponding approximately to 3×10^8 red cells, expressing roughly 3×10^{12} D antigens[5,80]) is sufficient to induce an alloimmune response to the D antigen. A dose of 20 µg of anti-D can effectively prevent the antibody response to 1 mL of D-positive red cells,[5] which contains 10^{10} red cells and 10^{14} D antigens. It was estimated using the law of mass action that only 5% of D antigen sites are bound under these conditions[44]; this leaves 95% of the D antigens free (9.5×10^{13} D antigens) in the 1 mL of D-positive red cells. Thus, given that only 3×10^{12} D antigens are required for immunization and 9.5×10^{13} D antigens are free after an optimal dose of anti-D, it is difficult to understand how simple steric hindrance is possible. Even if anti-D bound to 97% of the D sites, an immunogenic dose of D antigens would still be available. Thus, if simple steric hindrance was the major mechanism by which anti-D mediated its effects, theoretically, the currently used dose of anti-D would not be able to suppress the response.

Antibody-Mediated Immune Suppression

Several studies can be interpreted as good support for the steric-hindrance hypothesis of AMIS. The ability of IgG to prevent the antibody response correlates with the IgG affinity for the antigen and the amount of IgG bound to the antigen.[117,163,164,213,214] Furthermore, it has been shown in vitro that SRBC-specific IgG can prevent the B-cell response to SRBC only if the IgG and BCR share immunoglobulin-variable regions.[215] The adverse effect of the maternal IgG on infant vaccination (an AMIS-like scenario) is also dose dependent and epitope specific.[127]

Notwithstanding the above work, it has been observed that it is not necessary to block all epitopes on the antigen to prevent the antibody response, similar to the conclusions from the anti-D studies.[109] For example, the amount of IgG that prevents the antibody response does not saturate all the epitopes on SRBCs[216] and platelets.[121] This indicates that free antigens are available under AMIS conditions. Furthermore, the authors have recently shown that if a fully immunogenic dose of nonsensitized SRBCs is given concurrently with a desensitizing dose of washed SRBCs pre-opsonized with IgG, the resulting anti-SRBC response is proportionally reduced.[184] According to the steric-hindrance hypothesis, the normal antibody response against the unopsonized SRBCs, with freely available antigens, should have fully occurred.

Future Considerations

Current data in animal models of AMIS show that T cells and antigen-presenting cells need not be inhibited for AMIS to occur. This suggests that AMIS may in fact be an entirely B-cell-restricted phenomenon. The authors propose a new potential mechanism to explain the AMIS effect: B-cell antigen-presenting function is altered under AMIS conditions. Red cell antigens bound to IgG are not acquired, processed, or presented by red-cell-specific B cells; red-cell-specific T cells are not recruited; and full B-cell activation and differentiation into antibody-secreting cells does not occur. In the case of anti-D, because this immune response is much less robust than the SRBC model, this lack of interaction between the B cell and the T cell may lead to decreased T-cell stimulation and inhibition/prevention of appropriate T-cell memory. The ability of IgG to suppress antigen processing was previously observed, although the effect of this suppressed antigen processing on the antibody response was not studied.[217]

It should be pointed out that there are major differences between the SRBC model of AMIS and anti-D-mediated prevention of HDFN.[80,218] In particular, frequency of responders, rapid IgG-independent red-cell clearance (~10 minutes), and rapid induction of an antibody response (~3 days) in the mice are some of the important differences between the anti-SRBC response and the anti-D response in humans.[80] Furthermore, a high IgG:red-cell ratio and dose-dependent IgG effects differentiate anti-SRBC from the anti-D-mediated protective effect.[80] However, in both cases, the immune response is directed against antigens on the red cell. The specific conditions leading to the response against red cells in either setting are currently unknown but may be common to both the SRBC model and anti-D responses in humans. A better knowledge of the normal physiologic response against "foreign" red cells in both settings may allow more meaningful comparison between the AMIS effect in animal models and anti-D effects in humans. For example, it has recently been shown that an inflammatory stimulus can promote an immune response against foreign red cells in mice.[173] SRBCs may provide such stimulus directly, whereas the response against D-positive red cells may depend on additional signals that are not present at the time of transfusion.

Caution is necessary when the various models of AMIS reviewed here are used to explain the prevention of HDFN. The B-cell-restricted AMIS effect may in fact not be sufficient to prevent HDFN. Although B-cell-restricted AMIS prevents the primary B-cell response, it does not prevent the T-cell response[156,163,178] or immunologic memory in the mouse model.[88,163,184,219] Because HDFN is caused by secondary antibody responses, the question arises whether anti-D needs to prevent T-cell responses and memory to prevent HDFN. It may be necessary to differentiate between the AMIS effect restricted to the primary B-cell response and the more general IgG effect involving T cells, B cells, and memory. These effects may occur by different mechanisms. Alternatively, the putative suppressive IgG effect on T cells and memory may simply be a consequence of a central role of B-cell antigen-presenting cell function in anti-D responses. Therefore, the role of B cells in T-cell responses and immunologic memory in the animal models of AMIS vs D immunization should be determined and then the appropriate animal model of anti-D effect designed. Finally, the knowledge of potentially different mechanisms of the IgG effect can help in the evaluation of monoclonal/recombinant anti-Ds.

Conclusion

Anti-D has been successfully used for the prevention of HDFN. The ability of IgG to inhibit the antibody response to a coadministered antigen has also been observed in a variety of different animal models using vastly different antigens, including red cell antigens. Despite a century of efforts, the mechanisms of anti-D and inhibitory IgG effects in animal models have not yet been clearly established, likely owing to the technical limitations of all current models. Whereas the anti-D effect tends to correlate with antigen clearance, simple antigen clearance fails to explain the inhibitory IgG effect in animal models. Instead, the latter IgG effect may be restricted to B-cell activation. Whether IgG must also inhibit other components of the immune response to red cells—particularly T cells and immunologic memory—to prevent HDFN, and whether the current polyclonal anti-D is effective against HDFN because of the putative effect on T cells and memory remain critical questions.

References

1. Urbaniak SJ, Greiss MA. RhD haemolytic disease of the fetus and the newborn. Blood Rev 2000;14:44-61.
2. Rautmann H. Uber Blutbildungbei fotaler allgemeiner Wassersucht. Beitr Path Anat Allg Path 1912;54:332-9.
3. Diamond LK, Blackfan KD, Bathy JM. Erythroblastosis fetalis and its association with universal edema of the fetus, icterus gravis neonatorum, and anemia of the newborn. J Pediatr 1932;1:269-309.
4. Bowman JM. The prevention of Rh immunization. Transfus Med Rev 1988;2:129-50.
5. The Rh blood group system (and LW). In: Klein HG, Anstee DJ. Mollison's blood transfusion in clinical medicine. 11th ed. Malden, MA: Blackwell Publishing, 2005:163-208.
6. Finn R, Clarke CA, Donohoe WT, et al. Experimental studies on the prevention of Rh haemolytic disease. Br Med J 1961;5238:1486-90.
7. Freda VJ, Gorman JG, Pollack W. Rh Factor: Prevention of isoimmunization and clinical trial on mothers. Science 1966;151:828-30.
8. Davidsohn I, Masaitis L, Stern K. Experimental studies on Rh immunization. Am J Clin Pathol 1956;26:833-43.
9. Stern K, Goodman HS, Berger M. Experimental isoimmunization to hemoantigens in man. J Immunol 1961;87:189-98.
10. von Dungern E. Beitrage zur Immunitatslehre. Munch Med Wochenschr 1900;47:677-80.
11. Clarke CA, Donohoe WT, McConnell CR, et al. Further experimental studies on the prevention of Rh haemolytic disease. Br Med J 1963;5336:979-84.
12. Freda VJ, Gorman JG, Pollack W. Successful prevention of experimental Rh sensitization in man with an anti-Rh gamma2-globulin antibody preparation: A preliminary report. Transfusion 1964;77:26-32.
13. Zipursky A, Israels LG. The pathogenesis and prevention of Rh immunization. Can Med Assoc J 1967;97:1245-57.
14. Gorman JG, Freda VJ, Pollack WJ, Robertson JG. Protection from immunization in Rh-incompatible pregnancies: A progress report. Bull N Y Acad Med 1966;42:458-73.
15. Combined study. Prevention of Rh-haemolytic disease: Results of the clinical trial. A com-

bined study from centres in England and Baltimore. Br Med J 1966;2:907-14.
16. Freda VJ, Gorman JG, Pollack W, et al. Prevention of Rh isoimmunization. Progress report of the clinical trial in mothers. JAMA 1967; 199:390-4.
17. Pollack W, Gorman JG, Freda VJ, et al. Results of clinical trials of RhoGAM in women. Transfusion 1968;8:151-3.
18. Combined study. Prevention of primary Rh immunization: First report of the Western Canadian trial, 1966-1968. Can Med Assoc J 1969;100:1021-4.
19. Combined study. Controlled trial of various anti-D dosages in suppression of Rh sensitization following pregnancy. Report to the Medical Research Council by the Working Party on the Use of Anti-D-Immunoglobulin for the Prevention of Isoimmunization of Rh-Negative Women During Pregnancy. Br Med J 1974;2: 75-80.
20. Haemolytic disease of the fetus and the newborn. In: Klein HG, Anstee DJ. Mollison's blood transfusion in clinical medicine. 11th ed. Malden, MA: Blackwell Publishing, 2005:496-545.
21. Bowman JM, Chown B, Lewis M, Pollock JM. Rh isoimmunization during pregnancy: Antenatal prophylaxis. Can Med Assoc J 1978;118: 623-7.
22. Bowman JM, Pollock JM. Antenatal prophylaxis of Rh isoimmunization: 28-weeks'-gestation service program. Can Med Assoc J 1978;118: 627-30.
23. Tovey LA, Townley A, Stevenson BJ, Taverner J. The Yorkshire antenatal anti-D immunoglobulin trial in primigravidae. Lancet 1983;2: 244-6.
24. Huchet J, Dallemagne S, Huchet C, et al. [Antepartum administration of preventive treatment of Rh-D immunization in rhesus-negative women. Parallel evaluation of transplacental passage of fetal blood cells. Results of a multicenter study carried out in the Paris region]. J Gynecol Obstet Biol Reprod (Paris) 1987;16: 101-11.
25. Thornton JG, Page C, Foote G, et al. Efficacy and long term effects of antenatal prophylaxis with anti-D immunoglobulin. BMJ 1989;298: 1671-3.
26. Contreras M. The prevention of Rh haemolytic disease of the fetus and newborn—general background. Br J Obstet Gynaecol 1998;105 (Suppl 18):7-10.
27. Lee D, Contreras M, Robson SC, et al. Recommendations for the use of anti-D immunoglobulin for Rh prophylaxis. British Blood Transfusion Society and the Royal College of Obstetricians and Gynaecologists. Transfus Med 1999;9:93-7.
28. Beliard R. Monoclonal anti-D antibodies to prevent alloimmunization: Lessons from clinical trials. Transfus Clin Biol 2006;13:58-64.
29. Kumpel BM. Efficacy of RhD monoclonal antibodies in clinical trials as replacement therapy for prophylactic anti-D immunoglobulin: More questions than answers. Vox Sang 2007;93: 99-111.
30. Kumpel BM. Lessons learnt from many years of experience using anti-D in humans for prevention of RhD immunization and haemolytic disease of the fetus and newborn. Clin Exp Immunol 2008;154:1-5.
31. Naysmith JD, Ortega-Pierres MG, Elson CJ. Rat erythrocyte-induced anti-erythrocyte autoantibody production and control in normal mice. Immunol Rev 1981;55:55-87.
32. Coutelier JP, Johnston SJ, El Idrissi Me-A, Pfau CJ. Involvement of CD4+ cells in lymphocytic choriomeningitis virus-induced autoimmune anaemia and hypergammaglobulinaemia. J Autoimmun 1994;7:589-99.
33. Oliveira GG, Hutchings PR, Roitt IM, Lydyard PM. Production of erythrocyte autoantibodies in NZB mice is inhibited by CD4 antibodies. Clin Exp Immunol 1994;96:297-302.
34. Stott LM, Barker RN, Urbaniak SJ. Identification of alloreactive T-cell epitopes on the Rhesus D protein. Blood 2000;96:4011-19.
35. Hall AM, Ward FJ, Vickers MA, et al. Interleukin-10-mediated regulatory T-cell responses to epitopes on a human red blood cell autoantigen. Blood 2002;100:4529-36.
36. Urbaniak SJ, Robertson AE. A successful program of immunizing Rh-negative male volunteers for anti-D production using frozen/thawed blood. Transfusion 1981;21:64-9.
37. Pollack W, Ascari WQ, Crispen JF, et al. Studies on Rh prophylaxis. II. Rh immune prophylaxis after transfusion with Rh-positive blood. Transfusion 1971;11:340-4.
38. Schonewille H, Haak HL, van Zijl AM. Alloimmunization after blood transfusion in patients with hematologic and oncologic diseases. Transfusion 1999;39:763-71.
39. Frohn C, Dumbgen L, Brand JM, et al. Probability of anti-D development in D− patients receiving D+ RBCs. Transfusion 2003;43:893-8.

40. Gonzalez-Porras JR, Graciani IF, Perez-Simon JA, et al. Prospective evaluation of a transfusion policy of D+ red blood cells into D− patients. Transfusion 2008;48:1318-24.
41. Mattila PS, Seppala IJ, Eklund J, Makela O. Quantitation of immunoglobulin classes and subclasses in anti-Rh (D) antibodies. Vox Sang 1985;48:350-6.
42. Nevanlinna HR. Factors affecting maternal Rh immunisation. Ann Med Exp Biol Fenn 1953; 31:1-80.
43. Reverberi R. The persistence of red cell alloantibodies. Blood Transfus 2008;6:225-34.
44. Immunology of red cells. In: Klein HG, Anstee DJ. Mollison's blood transfusion in clinical medicine. 11th ed. Malden, MA: Blackwell Publishing, 2005:48-113.
45. Chavez GF, Mulinare J, Edmonds LD. Epidemiology of Rh hemolytic disease of the newborn in the United States. JAMA 1991;265:3270-4.
46. Urbaniak SJ. The scientific basis of antenatal prophylaxis. Br J Obstet Gynaecol 1998;105 (Suppl 18):11-18.
47. McSweeney E, Kirkham J, Vinall P, Flanagan P. An audit of anti-D sensitisation in Yorkshire. Br J Obstet Gynaecol 1998;105:1091-4.
48. Robson SC, Lee D, Urbaniak S. Anti-D immunoglobulin in RhD prophylaxis. Br J Obstet Gynaecol 1998;105:129-34.
49. Gottvall T, Filbey D. Alloimmunization in pregnancy during the years 1992-2005 in the central west region of Sweden. Acta Obstet Gynecol Scand 2008;87:843-8.
50. Chapman GE, Ballinger JR, Norton MJ, et al. The clearance kinetics of autologous RhD-positive erythrocytes coated ex vivo with novel recombinant and monoclonal anti-D antibodies. Clin Exp Immunol 2007;150:30-41.
51. Kumpel BM, Goodrick MJ, Pamphilon DH, et al. Human Rh D monoclonal antibodies (BRAD-3 and BRAD-5) cause accelerated clearance of Rh D+ red blood cells and suppression of Rh D immunization in Rh D− volunteers. Blood 1995;86:1701-9.
52. Pollack W, Ascari WQ, Kochesky RJ, et al. Studies on Rh prophylaxis. 1. Relationship between doses of anti-Rh and size of antigenic stimulus. Transfusion 1971;11:333-9.
53. Bowman JM, Pollock JM. Reversal of Rh alloimmunization. Fact or fancy? Vox Sang 1984;47:209-15.
54. de Silva M, Contreras M, Mollison PL. Failure of passively administered anti-Rh to prevent secondary Rh responses. Vox Sang 1985;48: 178-80.
55. Samson D, Mollison PL. Effect on primary Rh immunization of delayed administration of anti-Rh. Immunology 1975;28:349-57.
56. Blancher A, Socha WW, Roubinet F, et al. Human monoclonal anti-D-induced clearance of human D-positive red cells in a chimpanzee model. Vox Sang 1993;65:47-54.
57. Eder G, Fritsch S, Dauber E, et al. Pharmacokinetics of human rhesus immunoglobulin. 26th Congress of the International Society of Blood Transfusion, Vienna. Vox Sang 2000;78(Suppl 1):197-201.
58. Bazin R, Aubin E, Boyer L, et al. Functional in vivo characterization of human monoclonal anti-D in NOD-SCID mice. Blood 2002;99: 1267-72.
59. Siberil S, de Romeuf C, Bihoreau N, et al. Selection of a human anti-RhD monoclonal antibody for therapeutic use: Impact of IgG glycosylation on activating and inhibitory Fc gamma R functions. Clin Immunol 2006;118: 170-9.
60. Leader KA, Macht LM, Steers F, et al. Antibody responses to the blood group antigen D in SCID mice reconstituted with human blood mononuclear cells. Immunology 1992;76: 229-34.
61. Hall AM, Cairns LS, Altmann DM, et al. Immune responses and tolerance to the RhD blood group protein in HLA-transgenic mice. Blood 2005;105:2175-9.
62. Moise KJ Jr, Rodkey LS, Saade G, et al. An animal model for hemolytic disease of the fetus and newborn. I. Alloimmunization techniques. Am J Obstet Gynecol 1995;173:51-5.
63. Moise KJ Jr, Rodkey LS, Saade GR, et al. An animal model for hemolytic disease of the fetus and newborn. II. Fetal effects in New Zealand rabbits. Am J Obstet Gynecol 1995;173:747-53.
64. Kumpel BM. Monoclonal anti-D development programme. Transpl Immunol 2002;10:199-204.
65. Kumpel BM, Beliard R, Brossard Y, et al. Section 1C: Assessment of the functional activity and IgG Fc receptor utilisation of 64 IgG Rh monoclonal antibodies. Coordinator's report. Transfus Clin Biol 2002;9:45-53.
66. Thomson A, Contreras M, Gorick B, et al. Clearance of Rh D-positive red cells with monoclonal anti-D. Lancet 1990;336:1147-50.

67. Kumpel BM. In vivo studies of monoclonal anti-D and the mechanism of immune suppression. Transfus Clin Biol 2002;9:9-14.
68. Kumpel BM. On the immunologic basis of Rh immune globulin (anti-D) prophylaxis. Transfusion 2006;46:1652-6.
69. Clynes R, Maizes JS, Guinamard R, et al. Modulation of immune complex-induced inflammation in vivo by the coordinate expression of activation and inhibitory Fc receptors. J Exp Med 1999;189:179-85.
70. Boruchov AM, Heller G, Veri MC, et al. Activating and inhibitory IgG Fc receptors on human DCs mediate opposing functions. J Clin Invest 2005;115:2914-23.
71. Nimmerjahn F, Ravetch JV. Fcgamma receptors as regulators of immune responses. Nat Rev Immunol 2008;8:34-47.
72. Nimmerjahn F, Bruhns P, Horiuchi K, Ravetch JV. FcgammaRIV: A novel FcR with distinct IgG subclass specificity. Immunity 2005;23:41-51.
73. Nimmerjahn F, Ravetch JV. Divergent immunoglobulin G subclass activity through selective Fc receptor binding. Science 2005;310:1510-12.
74. Kaneko Y, Nimmerjahn F, Ravetch JV. Anti-inflammatory activity of immunoglobulin G resulting from Fc sialylation. Science 2006;313:670-3.
75. Anthony RM, Nimmerjahn F, Ashline DJ, et al. Recapitulation of IVIG anti-inflammatory activity with a recombinant IgG Fc. Science 2008;320:373-6.
76. Geijtenbeek TB, Torensma R, van Vliet SJ, et al. Identification of DC-SIGN, a novel dendritic cell-specific ICAM-3 receptor that supports primary immune responses. Cell 2000;100:575-85.
77. Park CG, Takahara K, Umemoto E, et al. Five mouse homologues of the human dendritic cell C-type lectin, DC-SIGN. Int Immunol 2001;13:1283-90.
78. Uhr JW, Moller G. Regulatory effect of antibody on the immune response. Adv Immunol 1968;8:81-127.
79. Heyman B. Regulation of antibody responses via antibodies, complement, and Fc receptors. Annu Rev Immunol 2000;18:709-37.
80. Kumpel BM, Elson CJ. Mechanism of anti-D-mediated immune suppression—a paradox awaiting resolution? Trends Immunol 2001;22:26-31.
81. Hjelm F, Carlsson F, Getahun A, Heyman B. Antibody-mediated regulation of the immune response. Scand J Immunol 2006;64:177-84.
82. Wigzell H. Antibody synthesis at the cellular level. Antibody-induced suppression of 7S antibody synthesis. J Exp Med 1966;124:953-69.
83. Freda VJ, Gorman JG, Pollack W. Suppression of the primary Rh immune response with passive Rh IgG immunoglobulin. N Engl J Med 1967;277:1022-3.
84. Greenbury CL, Moore DH. Non-specific antibody-induced suppression of the immune response. Nature 1968;219:526-7.
85. Pollack W, Gorman JG, Hager HJ, et al. Antibody-mediated immune suppression to the Rh factor: Animal models suggesting mechanism of action. Transfusion 1968;8:134-45.
86. Siskind GW. The role of circulating antibody in the control of antibody synthesis: Mechanism for the suppressive effect of passive antibody on active antibody synthesis. Transfusion 1968;8:127-33.
87. Dennert G. The mechanism of antibody-induced stimulation and inhibition of the immune response. J Immunol 1971;106:951-5.
88. Safford JW Jr, Tokuda S. Antibody-mediated suppression of the immune response: Effect on the development of immunologic memory. J Immunol 1971;107:1213-25.
89. Sinclair NR, Chan PL. Relationship between antibody-mediated immunosuppression and tolerance induction. Nature 1971;234:104-5.
90. Chan PL, Sinclair NR. Regulation of the immune response. VI. Inability of F(ab') 2 antibody to terminate established immune responses and its ability to interfere with IgG antibody-mediated immunosuppression. Immunology 1973;24:289-301.
91. Hoffmann MK, Kappler JW. Two distinct mechanisms of immune suppression by antibody. Nature 1978;272:64-5.
92. Hutchinson IV, Zola H. Antigen-reactive cell opsonization: A mechanism of antibody-mediated immune suppression. Cell Immunol 1978;36:161-9.
93. Smith T. Active immunity produced by so-called balanced or neutral mixtures of diphteria toxin and antitoxin. J Exp Med 1909;11:241-56.
94. Glenny AT, Sudmersen HJ. Notes on the production of immunity to diphtheria toxin. J Hyg (Lond) 1921;20:176.

95. Di Sant Agnese PA. Combined immunization against diphtheria, tetanus and pertussis in newborn infants, duration of antibody levels; antibody titers after booster dose; effect of passive immunity to diphtheria on active immunization with diphtheria toxoid. Pediatrics 1949; 3:181-94.
96. Barr M, Glenny AT, Randall KJ. Diphtheria immunization in young babies; a study of some factors involved. Lancet 1950;1:6-10.
97. Osborn JJ, Dancis J, Julia JF. Studies of the immunology of the newborn infant. II. Interference with active immunization by passive transplacental circulating antibody. Pediatrics 1952;10:328-34.
98. Mason JH, Robinson M, Christensen PA. The active immunization of guinea-pigs passively immunized with homologous antitoxic serum. J Hyg (Lond) 1955;53:172-9.
99. Buxton JB, Glenny AT. The active immunization of horses against tetanus. Lancet 1921; 2:1109.
100. Ramon G, Zoeller C. Sur la valeur et la duree de l'immunite conferee par l'anatoxin tetanique dans la vaccination de l'homme contre le tetanus. C R Seances Soc Biol Fil 1933;112:347.
101. Otto L, Hennemann IP. Combined (simultaneous) immunization against tetanus. J Pathol Bacteriol 1939;49:213.
102. Regamey RH, Aegerter W. Experimental sero-anatoxin therapy of tetanus. Schweiz Z Pathol Bakteriol 1951;14:554-9.
103. Horibata K, Uhr JW. Antibody content of single antibody-forming cells. J Immunol 1967;98:972-8.
104. Rhoads CP. Immunity following the injection of monkeys with mixtures of poliomyelitis virus and convalescent human serum. J Exp Med 1931;53:115.
105. Brodie M. Active immunization against poliomylitis. J Exp Med 1932;56:493-505.
106. Kalmanson GM, Bronfenbrenner J. Restoration of activity of neutralized biologic agents by removal of the antibody with papain. J Immunol 1943;47:387-407.
107. Magano Y, Takenti S. Etudes serologiques sur le bacteriophage. Jpn J Exp Med 1951;21:427.
108. Finkelstein MS, Uhr JW. Specific inhibition of antibody formation by passively administered 19s and 7s antibody. Science 1964;146:67-9.
109. Uhr JW, Baumann JB. Antibody formation. I. The suppression of antibody formation by passively administered antibody. J Exp Med 1961; 113:935-57.
110. Sahiar K, Schwartz RS. Inhibition of 19s antibody synthesis by 7s antibody. Science 1964; 145:395-7.
111. Dixon FJ, Jacot-Guillarmod H, McConahey PJ. The effect of passively administered antibody on antibody synthesis. J Exp Med 1967;125:1119-35.
112. Walker JG, Siskind GW. Studies on the control of antibody synthesis. Effect of antibody affinity upon its ability to suppress antibody formation. Immunology 1968;14:21-8.
113. Brody NI, Walker JG, Siskind GW. Studies on the control of antibody synthesis. Interaction of antigenic competition and suppression of antibody formation by passive antibody on the immune response. J Exp Med 1967;126:81-91.
114. Freter GG, Talmage DW, Thomson A. The effect of whole body x radiation on the specific anamnestic response in the rabbit. J Infect Dis 1956;99:246-52.
115. Rowley DA, Fitch FW. Homeostasis of antibody formation in the adult rat. J Exp Med 1964;120:987-1005.
116. Moeller G, Wigzell H. Antibody synthesis at the cellular level. Antibody-induced suppression of 19S and 7S antibody response. J Exp Med 1965;121:969-89.
117. Henry C, Jerne NK. Competition of 19S and 7S antigen receptors in the regulation of the primary immune response. J Exp Med 1968;128:133-52.
118. Smith GN, Mollison PL. Suppression of primary immunization to the rabbit red cell alloantigen HgA by passively administered anti-HgA. Immunology 1974;26:885-92.
119. Lazarus AH, Crow AR, Semple JW, et al. Induction of a secondary human anti-HLA alloimmune response in severe combined immunodeficient mice engrafted with human lymphocytes. Transfusion 1997;37:1192-9.
120. Crow AR, Freedman J, Hannach B, et al. Antibody-mediated inhibition of the human alloimmune response to platelet transfusion in Hu-PBL-SCID mice. Br J Haematol 1999;104:919-24.
121. Crow AR, Freedman J, Hannach B, Lazarus AH. Monoclonal antibody-mediated inhibition of the human HLA alloimmune response to platelet transfusion is antigen specific and independent of Fcgamma receptor-mediated immune suppression. Br J Haematol 2000; 110:481-7.

122. Terness P, Susal C, Opelz G. IgG-anti-immunoglobulin induced by immunization with antibody-coated blood cells: Mechanism for B-cell suppression? Transplant Proc 1989;21:153-5.
123. Susal C, Terness P, Opelz G. An experimental model for preventing alloimmunization against platelet transfusions by pretreatment with antibody-coated cells. Vox Sang 1990;59:209-15.
124. Enriquez-Rincon F, Klaus GG. Differing effects of monoclonal anti-hapten antibodies on humoral responses to soluble or particulate antigens. Immunology 1984;52:129-36.
125. Lazarus AH, Crow AR, Freedman J, et al. Inhibition of a secondary human alloimmune response via the soluble active component of CD154 (CD40L) in severe combined immunedeficient mice engrafted with human lymphocytes. Transfusion 1999;39:818-23.
126. Osborn JJ, Dancis J, Julia JF. Studies of the immunology of the newborn infant. II. Interference with active immunization by passive transplacental circulating antibody. Pediatrics 1952;10:328.
127. Siegrist CA. Mechanisms by which maternal antibodies influence infant vaccine responses: Review of hypotheses and definition of main determinants. Vaccine 2003;21:3406-12.
128. Lambert PH, Liu M, Siegrist CA. Can successful vaccines teach us how to induce efficient protective immune responses? Nat Med 2005;11:S54-62.
129. Albrecht P, Ennis FA, Saltzman EJ, Krugman S. Persistence of maternal antibody in infants beyond 12 months: Mechanism of measles vaccine failure. J Pediatr 1977;91:715-18.
130. Perkins FT, Yetts R, Gaisford W. A comparison of the responses of 100 infants to primary poliomyelitis immunization with two and with three doses of vaccine. Br Med J 1959;1:1083-6.
131. Karron RA, Steinhoff MC, Subbarao EK, et al. Safety and immunogenicity of a cold-adapted influenza A (H1N1) reassortant virus vaccine administered to infants less than six months of age. Pediatr Infect Dis J 1995;14:10-16.
132. Ruiz-Palacios GM, Guerrero ML, Bautista-Marquez A, et al. Dose response and efficacy of a live, attenuated human rotavirus vaccine in Mexican infants. Pediatrics 2007;120:e253-61.
133. Burstyn DG, Baraff LJ, Peppler MS, et al. Serological response to filamentous hemagglutinin and lymphocytosis-promoting toxin of Bordetella pertussis. Infect Immun 1983;41:1150-6.
134. Englund JA, Anderson EL, Reed GF, et al. The effect of maternal antibody on the serologic response and the incidence of adverse reactions after primary immunization with acellular and whole-cell pertussis vaccines combined with diphtheria and tetanus toxoids. Pediatrics 1995;96:580-4.
135. Booy R, Aitken SJ, Taylor S, et al. Immunogenicity of combined diphtheria, tetanus, and pertussis vaccine given at 2, 3, and 4 months versus 3, 5, and 9 months of age. Lancet 1992;339:507-10.
136. Sarvas H, Kurikka S, Seppala IJ, et al. Maternal antibodies partly inhibit an active antibody response to routine tetanus toxoid immunization in infants. J Infect Dis 1992;165:977-9.
137. Bjorkholm B, Granstrom M, Taranger J, et al. Influence of high titers of maternal antibody on the serologic response of infants to diphtheria vaccination at three, five and twelve months of age. Pediatr Infect Dis J 1995;14:846-50.
138. Claesson BA, Schneerson R, Robbins JB, et al. Protective levels of serum antibodies stimulated in infants by two injections of Haemophilus influenzae type b capsular polysaccharide-tetanus toxoid conjugate. J Pediatr 1989;114:97-100.
139. Daum RS, Siber GR, Ballanco GA, Sood SK. Serum anticapsular antibody response in the first week after immunization of adults and infants with the Haemophilus influenzae type b-Neisseria meningitidis outer membrane protein complex conjugate vaccine. J Infect Dis 1991;164:1154-9.
140. Troisi CL, Hollinger FB, Krause DS, Pickering LK. Immunization of seronegative infants with hepatitis A vaccine (HAVRIX; SKB): A comparative study of two dosing schedules. Vaccine 1997;15:1613-17.
141. Dagan R, Amir J, Mijalovsky A, et al. Immunization against hepatitis A in the first year of life: Priming despite the presence of maternal antibody. Pediatr Infect Dis J 2000;19:1045-52.
142. Kanra G, Yalcin SS, Ceyhan M, Yurdakok K. Clinical trial to evaluate immunogenicity and safety of inactivated hepatitis A vaccination starting at 2-month-old children. Turk J Pediatr 2000;42:105-8.
143. Brinc D, Lazarus AH. Mechanisms of anti-D action in the prevention of hemolytic disease of the fetus and newborn. Hematology Am Soc Hematol Educ Program 2009:185-191.

144. Woodrow JC, Clarke CA, Donohow WT, et al. Mechanism of Rh prophylaxis: An experimental study on specificity of immunosuppression. Br Med J 1975;2:57-9.
145. Sinclair N, Chan P. Regulation of the immune response. IV. The role of the Fc-fragment in feedback inhibition by antibody. Adv Exp Med Biol 1971;12:609-15.
146. Sinclair NR. Fc-signalling in the modulation of immune responses by passive antibody. Scand J Immunol 2001;53:322-30.
147. Derrick Tovey LA, Robinson AE. Reduced severity of Rh-haemolytic disease after anti-D immunoglobulin. Br Med J 1975;4:320-2.
148. Branch DR, Shabani F, Lund N, Denomme GA. Antenatal administration of Rh-immune globulin causes significant increases in the immunomodulatory cytokines transforming growth factor-beta and prostaglandin E2. Transfusion 2006;46:1316-22.
149. Freedman J, Massey A, Chaplin H, Monroe MC. Assessment of complement binding by anti-D and anti-M antibodies employing labelled antiglobulin antibodies. Br J Haematol 1980;45:309-18.
150. Jones NC, Mollison PL, Veall N. Removal of incompatible red cells by the spleen. Br J Haematol 1957;3:125-33.
151. Mollison PL, Crome P, Hughes-Jones NC, Rochna E. Rate of removal from the circulation of red cells sensitized with different amounts of antibody. Br J Haematol 1965;11:461-70.
152. Mollison PL, Hughes-Jones NC. Clearance of Rh-positive red cells by low concentrations of Rh antibody. Immunology 1967;12:63-73.
153. Kumpel BM, Judson PA. Quantification of IgG anti-D bound to D-positive red cells infused into D-negative subjects after intramuscular injection of monoclonal anti-D. Transfus Med 1995;5:105-12.
154. Stucki M, Schnorf J, Hustinx H, et al. Anti-D immunoglobulin in Rh(D) negative volunteers: Clearance of Rh(D) positive red cells and kinetics of serum anti-D levels. Transfus Clin Biol 1998;5:180-8.
155. Miescher S, Spycher MO, Amstutz H, et al. A single recombinant anti-RhD IgG prevents RhD immunization: Association of RhD-positive red blood cell clearance rate with polymorphisms in the FcgammaRIIA and FcgammaIIIA genes. Blood 2004;103:4028-35.
156. Brinc D, Le-Tien H, Crow AR, et al. IgG-mediated immunosuppression is not dependent on erythrocyte clearance or immunological evasion: Implications for the mechanism of action of anti-D in the prevention of haemolytic disease of the newborn? Br J Haematol 2007; 139:275-9.
157. Sinclair NR, Lees RK, Elliott EV. Role of the Fc fragment in the regulation of the primary immune response. Nature 1968;220:1048-9.
158. Nicholas R, Sinclair SC. Regulation of the immune response. I. Reduction in ability of specific antibody to inhibit long-lasting IgG immunological priming after removal of the Fc fragment. J Exp Med 1969;129:1183-201.
159. Sinclair NR, Lees RK, Chan PL, Khan RH. Regulation of the immune response. II. Further studies on differences in ability of F(ab')2 and 7S antibodies to inhibit an antibody response. Immunology 1970;19:105-16.
160. Chan PL, Sinclair NR. Regulation of the immune response. V. An analysis of the function of the Fc portion of antibody in suppression of an immune response with respect to interaction with components of the lymphoid system. Immunology 1971;21:967-81.
161. Tao TW, Uhr JW. Capacity of pepsin-digested antibody to inhibit antibody formation. Nature 1966;212:208-9.
162. Cerottini JC, McConahey PJ, Dixon FJ. The immunosuppressive effect of passively administered antibody IgG fragments. J Immunol 1969;102:1008-15.
163. Karlsson MC, Wernersson S, Diaz de Stahl T, et al. Efficient IgG-mediated suppression of primary antibody responses in Fcgamma receptor-deficient mice. Proc Natl Acad Sci U S A 1999;96:2244-9.
164. Heyman B, Wigzell H. Immunoregulation by monoclonal sheep erythrocyte-specific IgG antibodies: Suppression is correlated to level of antigen binding and not to isotype. J Immunol 1984;132:1136-43.
165. Heyman B, Wiersma E, Nose M. Complement activation is not required for IgG-mediated suppression of the antibody response. Eur J Immunol 1988;18:1739-43.
166. Wykes M, Pombo A, Jenkins C, MacPherson GG. Dendritic cells interact directly with naive B lymphocytes to transfer antigen and initiate class switching in a primary T-dependent response. J Immunol 1998;161:1313-19.
167. Batista FD, Neuberger MS. B cells extract and present immobilized antigen: Implications for affinity discrimination. EMBO J 2000;19:513-20.

168. Batista FD, Iber D, Neuberger MS. B cells acquire antigen from target cells after synapse formation. Nature 2001;411:489-94.
169. Bergtold A, Desai DD, Gavhane A, Clynes R. Cell surface recycling of internalized antigen permits dendritic cell priming of B cells. Immunity 2005;23:503-14.
170. Huang NN, Han SB, Hwang IY, Kehrl JH. B cells productively engage soluble antigen-pulsed dendritic cells: Visualization of live-cell dynamics of B cell-dendritic cell interactions. J Immunol 2005;175:7125-34.
171. Fleire SJ, Goldman JP, Carrasco YR, et al. B cell ligand discrimination through a spreading and contraction response. Science 2006;312:738-41.
172. Goodnow CC, Crosbie J, Adelstein S, et al. Altered immunoglobulin expression and functional silencing of self-reactive B lymphocytes in transgenic mice. Nature 1988;334:676-82.
173. Hendrickson JE, Chadwick TE, Roback JD, et al. Inflammation enhances consumption and presentation of transfused RBC antigens by dendritic cells. Blood 2007;110:2736-43.
174. Malynn BA, Wortis HH. Role of antigen-specific B cells in the induction of SRBC-specific T cell proliferation. J Immunol 1984;132:2253-8.
175. Malynn BA, Romeo DT, Wortis HH. Antigen-specific B cells efficiently present low doses of antigen for induction of T cell proliferation. J Immunol 1985;135:980-8.
176. Miller JF, De Burgh PM, Grant GA. Thymus and the production of antibody-plaque-forming cells. Nature 1965;208:1332-4.
177. Claman HN, Chaperon EA, Triplett RF. Thymus-marrow cell combinations. Synergism in antibody production. Proc Soc Exp Biol Med 1966;122:1167-71.
178. Kappler JW, Hoffmann M, Dutton RW. Regulation of the immune response. I. Differential effect of passively administered antibody on the thymus-derived and bone marrow-derived lymphocytes. J Exp Med 1971;134:577-87.
179. Zubler RH. Antibody feedback regulation in vitro: T helper cell activation and T-B cell cooperation are not impaired by anti-carrier antibody. Eur J Immunol 1981;11:572-9.
180. Gans HA, Maldonado Y, Yasukawa LL, et al. IL-12, IFN-gamma, and T cell proliferation to measles in immunized infants. J Immunol 1999;162:5569-75.
181. Pabst HF, Spady DW, Carson MM, et al. Cell-mediated and antibody immune responses to AIK-C and Connaught monovalent measles vaccine given to 6 month old infants. Vaccine 1999;17:1910-18.
182. Siegrist CA, Barrios C, Martinez X, et al. Influence of maternal antibodies on vaccine responses: Inhibition of antibody but not T cell responses allows successful early prime-boost strategies in mice. Eur J Immunol 1998;28:4138-48.
183. Siegrist CA, Cordova M, Brandt C, et al. Determinants of infant responses to vaccines in presence of maternal antibodies. Vaccine 1998;16:1409-14.
184. Brinc D, Le-Tien H, Crow AR, et al. Immunoglobulin G-mediated regulation of the murine immune response to transfused red blood cells occurs in the absence of active immune suppression: Implications for the mechanism of action of anti-D in the prevention of haemolytic disease of the fetus and newborn? Immunology 2008;124:141-6.
185. Lamb JR, Zanders ED, Lake P, et al. Inhibition of T cell proliferation by antibodies to synthetic peptides. Eur J Immunol 1984;14:153-7.
186. Waldmann H, Cobbold S. How do monoclonal antibodies induce tolerance? A role for infectious tolerance? Annu Rev Immunol 1998;16:619-44.
187. Oh JH, Whelchel JD. Reversal of blood-induced sensitization by antibody-coated platelets. Transplant Proc 1991;23:316-18.
188. Hoffmann MK. Antibody regulates the cooperation of B cells with helper cells. Immunol Rev 1980;49:79-91.
189. Muta T, Kurosaki T, Misulovin Z, et al. A 13-amino-acid motif in the cytoplasmic domain of Fc gamma RIIB modulates B-cell receptor signalling. Nature 1994;368:70-3.
190. Phillips NE, Parker DC. Cross-linking of B lymphocyte Fc gamma receptors and membrane immunoglobulin inhibits anti-immunoglobulin-induced blastogenesis. J Immunol 1984;132:627-32.
191. Bijsterbosch MK, Klaus GG. Crosslinking of surface immunoglobulin and Fc receptors on B lymphocytes inhibits stimulation of inositol phospholipid breakdown via the antigen receptors. J Exp Med 1985;162:1825-36.
192. Takai T, Ono M, Hikida M, et al. Augmented humoral and anaphylactic responses in Fc gamma RII-deficient mice. Nature 1996;379:346-9.
193. Ono M, Okada H, Bolland S, et al. Deletion of SHIP or SHP-1 reveals two distinct pathways

for inhibitory signaling. Cell 1997;90:293-301.
194. Pearse RN, Kawabe T, Bolland S, et al. SHIP recruitment attenuates Fc gamma RIIB-induced B cell apoptosis. Immunity 1999;10:753-60.
195. Yuasa T, Kubo S, Yoshino T, et al. Deletion of fcgamma receptor IIB renders H-2(b) mice susceptible to collagen-induced arthritis. J Exp Med 1999;189:187-94.
196. Bolland S, Ravetch JV. Spontaneous autoimmune disease in Fc(gamma)RIIB-deficient mice results from strain-specific epistasis. Immunity 2000;13:277-85.
197. Nakamura A, Yuasa T, Ujike A, et al. Fcgamma receptor IIB-deficient mice develop Goodpasture's syndrome upon immunization with type IV collagen: A novel murine model for autoimmune glomerular basement membrane disease. J Exp Med 2000;191:899-906.
198. Qin D, Wu J, Vora KA, et al. Fc gamma receptor IIB on follicular dendritic cells regulates the B cell recall response. J Immunol 2000;164:6268-75.
199. Bolland S, Yim YS, Tus K, et al. Genetic modifiers of systemic lupus erythematosus in FcgammaRIIB(−/−) mice. J Exp Med 2002;195:1167-74.
200. Fukuyama H, Nimmerjahn F, Ravetch JV. The inhibitory Fcgamma receptor modulates autoimmunity by limiting the accumulation of immunoglobulin G+ anti-DNA plasma cells. Nat Immunol 2005;6:99-106.
201. McGaha TL, Sorrentino B, Ravetch JV. Restoration of tolerance in lupus by targeted inhibitory receptor expression. Science 2005;307:590-3.
202. Maltais LJ, Lovering RC, Taranin AV, et al. New nomenclature for Fc receptor-like molecules. Nat Immunol 2006;7:431-2.
203. Davis RS, Wang YH, Kubagawa H, Cooper MD. Identification of a family of Fc receptor homologs with preferential B cell expression. Proc Natl Acad Sci U S A 2001;98:9772-7.
204. Davis RS, Dennis G Jr, Odom MR, et al. Fc receptor homologs: Newest members of a remarkably diverse Fc receptor gene family. Immunol Rev 2002;190:123-36.
205. Guselnikov SV, Ershova SA, Mechetina LV, et al. A family of highly diverse human and mouse genes structurally links leukocyte FcR, gp42 and PECAM-1. Immunogenetics 2002;54:87-95.
206. Davis RS, Stephan RP, Chen CC, et al. Differential B cell expression of mouse Fc receptor homologs. Int Immunol 2004;16:1343-53.
207. Davis RS. Fc receptor-like molecules. Annu Rev Immunol 2007;25:525-60.
208. Ehrhardt GR, Davis RS, Hsu JT, et al. The inhibitory potential of Fc receptor homolog 4 on memory B cells. Proc Natl Acad Sci U S A 2003;100:13489-94.
209. Won WJ, Foote JB, Odom MR, et al. Fc receptor homolog 3 is a novel immunoregulatory marker of marginal zone and B1 B cells. J Immunol 2006;177:6815-23.
210. Karlsson MC, Getahun A, Heyman B. FcgammaRIIB in IgG-mediated suppression of antibody responses: Different impact in vivo and in vitro. J Immunol 2001;167:5558-64.
211. Brinc D, Le-Tien H, Crow AR, et al. Transfusion of IgG-opsonized foreign red blood cells mediates reduction of antigen-specific B cell priming in a murine model. J Immunol 2008;181:948-53.
212. Lubenko A, Williams M, Johnson A, et al. Monitoring the clearance of fetal RhD-positive red cells in FMH following RhD immunoglobulin administration. Transfus Med 1999;9:331-5.
213. Bruggemann M, Rajewsky K. Regulation of the antibody response against hapten-coupled erythrocytes by monoclonal antihapten antibodies of various isotypes. Cell Immunol 1982;71:365-73.
214. Dresser DW. Feedback by early and late primary antisera on the primary and secondary adoptive immune responses of mice to burro erythrocytes. Cell Immunol 1990;127:405-19.
215. Zubler RH. Epitope-specific antibody feedback regulation of the humoral immune response against sheep erythrocytes in vitro: Specific effects of anti-antigen antibody vs nonspecific T cell activities. J Immunol 1981;126:557-62.
216. Haughton G, Nash DR. Specific immunosuppression by minute doses of passive antibody. Transplant Proc 1969;1:616-18.
217. Watts C, Lanzavecchia A. Suppressive effect of antibody on processing of T cell epitopes. J Exp Med 1993;178:1459-63.
218. Pollack W, Gorman JG, Freda VJ. Prevention of Rh hemolytic disease. Prog Hematol 1969;6:121-47.
219. Heyman B, Wigzell H. Specific IgM enhances and IgG inhibits the induction of immunological memory in mice. Scand J Immunol 1985;21:255-66.

9

Anti-D: Basic Concepts and Mechanisms of Action in Autoimmunity

John W. Semple, PhD

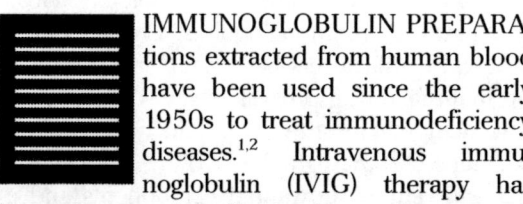IMMUNOGLOBULIN PREPARAtions extracted from human blood have been used since the early 1950s to treat immunodeficiency diseases.[1,2] Intravenous immunoglobulin (IVIG) therapy has been shown to be effective in treating immune deficiency states,[2,3] bacterial/viral infections,[4] and immune regulatory disorders, particularly immunohematologic disorders such as autoimmune neutropenia, autoimmune hemolytic anemia, and immune thrombocytopenia (ITP).[5-10] Although the mechanisms of action of IVIG in immune regulation are complex and not yet fully elucidated, several theories have been postulated in patients with ITP. For example, at least five experimentally supported hypotheses of IVIG's mechanism of action are reticuloendothelial Fc-receptor blockade,[11,12] Fc inhibitory receptor (FcR)-mediated inhibition of phagocytosis,[13] anti-idiotypic regulation,[14-17] cytokine alterations,[18-22] and a new theory, recently proposed by Siragam et al,[23] related to IVIG-mediated dendritic-cell suppression of macrophage function.

In addition, Rh Immune Globulin (anti-D; eg, WinRho SDF, Baxter, Deerfield, IL) has been shown to be effective in raising the platelet counts of patients with ITP,[24-39] but although the above theories may apply, little is known about the mechanisms of action of anti-D. Gammaglobulins (including anti-D) have both

---

John W. Semple, PhD, Head, Transfusion Medicine Research, Keenan Research Centre, Li Ka Shing Knowledge Institute of St Michael's Hospital; Professor, Departments of Pharmacology, Medicine, and Laboratory Medicine and Pathobiology, University of Toronto; and Adjunct Scientist, Canadian Blood Services, Toronto, Ontario, Canada

The author has disclosed no conflicts of interest.

short-term effects, probably related to FcR-mediated events, and long-term effects (ie, immunomodulation beyond the half-life of the infused gammaglobulin[21]), and it is unknown whether the short-term effects have an impact on long-term immunomodulation. This review will focus on the short-term mechanisms of action of anti-D products, particularly related to their efficacy in the autoimmune bleeding disorder, ITP.

Immune Thrombocytopenia

ITP is an autoimmune bleeding disorder characterized by the production of autoreactive antibodies against one's own platelets, resulting in increased platelet destruction by reticuloendothelial system (RES) phagocytes. It is recognized that, in ITP, platelet autoantibodies are primarily of the IgG3 and IgG1 isotypes, although less prevalent IgM and IgA autoantibodies targeted against glycoprotein (GP) IIb/IIIa and GPIb/IX also exist.[40-48] Recently, it has been proposed that the thrombocytopenia in those patients with ITP that do not display platelet autoantibodies is mediated by CD8+ T-cell cytolysis.[49,50] The age-adjusted prevalence of ITP has been estimated to be 9.5 per 100,000 persons in the United States, and its annual incidence is estimated to be 2.68 per 100,000 in Northern Europe (at a cut-off platelet count of $<100 \times 10^9/L$).[51]

ITP used to be understood as having two forms termed *acute* and *chronic,* but an international working group of recognized experts convened a consensus conference in October 2007 and have significantly revised the definitions and recommendations of the clinical diagnosis of ITP.[52] Primary ITP is now defined as an autoimmune disorder characterized by isolated thrombocytopenia (peripheral blood platelet count $<100 \times 10^9/L$) in the absence of other causes or disorders that may be associated with thrombocytopenia.[52] The phases of ITP are divided based on the time since diagnosis: newly diagnosed ITP is the phase within 3 months after diagnosis, persistent ITP falls between 3 and 12 months from diagnosis, and chronic ITP is now defined as thrombocytopenia lasting for more than 12 months.[52] The term *severe ITP* is reserved for those patients with bleeding symptoms at presentation or later that require therapeutic intervention.[52] It was recommended that the term *acute*, which was used to describe a self-limited form of the disease (eg, secondary to viral illness in children), should be avoided because of both its vagueness and its post hoc or retrospective definition.[52] Treatment of chronic ITP has included many first-line therapies, including steroids, IVIG, and anti-D; if these treatments fail, others have been shown to be efficacious, such as azathioprine, rituximab, thrombopoietin, and, ultimately, splenectomy.[40,41]

Overview of Anti-D

The polyclonal gammaglobulin product anti-D is prepared from the pooled plasma of hundreds of previously pregnant, postmenopausal, D-negative females and also from immunized D-negative males. Most anti-D products were originally manufactured by a form of the Cohn cold ethanol fractionation method developed in the 1950s, which did not completely clear aggregates of immunoglobulins. Consequently, various manufacturers have significantly refined the manufacturing process of anti-D, and most now include at least two steps, including an ion-exchange chromatography step to isolate anti-D IgG and remove unwanted components and a solvent/detergent (S/D) treatment to inactivate enveloped viruses (eg, hepatitis B and C viruses and human immunodeficiency virus). Some manufacturers additionally finish the anti-D product with a nanofiltration step to remove enveloped and nonenveloped viruses (eg, hepatitis A virus, parvovirus B19) that the S/D step does not remove.[53-55] Several anti-D preparations are approved for use in ITP in North America and Europe.

In addition to its clear benefit in preventing Rh isoimmunization, anti-D has been shown to be very effective in raising the platelet counts of patients with ITP.[24-39] Although the theories for IVIG may apply, little is known as yet about the mechanism of action of anti-D therapy in ITP. Currently, this appears to relate to several different immune system mechanisms that include RES blockade/inhibition, cytokine alterations, idiotype/anti-idiotype interactions, and alterations in intracellular signaling mechanisms.[24-39]

Reticuloendothelial System Blockade

Most of the platelet clearance in ITP is thought to be mediated by FcR-mediated phagocytosis by the RES, particularly within the spleen. There are several FcRs, which are classed based on the type of antibody they recognize. The FcRs that bind IgG antibodies, for example, are called Fc-gamma receptors (FcγRs), which belong to the immunoglobulin superfamily and are the most important receptors for mediating phagocytosis of opsonized particles such as bacteria, platelets, and/or red cells.[56-59] The FcγR family includes several members: FcγRI (CD64), FcγRIIC, FcγRIIA (CD32), FcγRIIB (CD32), FcγRIIIA (CD16a), and FcγRIIIB (CD16b). These differ in their antibody affinities because of their different molecular structures.[57,60] For example, FcγRI is considered a high-affinity receptor and binds monomeric IgG with relatively strong affinity compared with FcγRII or FcγRIII, which bind only to IgG within an immune complex (Table 9-1).

The first report of successful treatment of ITP with anti-D was by Salama et al,[25] who, at the time, suggested that the efficacy of anti-D in ITP may be the result of competitive inhibition of the RES by sensitized erythrocytes.[25] This theory of RES blockade, subsequently confirmed by other reports,[24-39] has always been thought to be one of the primary mechanisms of action of anti-D in ITP: the relatively small dose of anti-D (μg vs grams for IVIG) opsonizes the patient's D-positive red cells, and these competitively block phagocytosis of platelets within the spleen.[25] This theory was further supported by studies demonstrating anti-D treatment of ITP is ineffective in patients who are RhD antigen negative[62,63] or in patients with chronic ITP who have had a splenectomy.[64] With respect to the latter observation, however, a recent study found that two splenectomized ITP patients did respond to anti-D, suggesting that more research is warranted to determine if anti-D may in fact function in the absence of a spleen.[63]

Several animal models of ITP have been developed over the years, and one of the most successful approaches to study the mechanism of action of gammaglobulin products has been to passively transfer platelet antibodies into mice with concurrent administration of the gammaglonbulins.[65-69] Because mice do not express the D antigen, surrogate antibodies, such as the glycophorin antibody TER-119 or others, have been used in an attempt to mimic anti-D products. Using this approach, Song et al[70] showed that when red-cell-specific antibodies were administered to mice with passively induced thrombocytopenia, platelet counts were significantly increased, and this appeared to be associated with downregulation of the expression of the activating FcγRIIIA on splenic macrophages.[70]

Nevertheless, few, if any, reports have suggested that anti-D or red cell antibodies can modulate the inhibitory FcγRIIB on phagocytic macrophages within the spleen. However, in the passive ITP mouse model, Song et al[71] demonstrated that monoclonal red-cell-reactive antibodies functioned independently of FcγRIIB expression, unlike IVIG. They speculated that these antibodies did not act by regulating FcγRIIB expression, and proposed anti-D and IVIG may function through different mechanisms.[71] Although it is clear that anti-D-opsonized red cells inevitably interact with cells of the RES, the exact mechanisms (eg, passive FcR blockade or active inhibition of phagocytosis) are still unknown.

Cytokines and Anti-D

The earliest study, perhaps, to address whether anti-D-coated red cells could affect cytokine levels was performed by Davenport et al,[72] who

Table 9-1. Summary of the Human FcR Family*

Receptor	Ligand	Affinity	Distribution	IgG-Binding Effect	Alleles
Fcγ RI (CD64)	IgG1 and IgG3	High (Kd ~10^{-9} M)	Macrophages Neutrophils Eosinophils Dendritic cells	Phagocytosis Cell activation Activation of respiratory burst Induction of microbe killing	
Fcγ RIIA (CD32)	IgG	Low (Kd >10^{-7} M)	Macrophages Neutrophils Eosinophils Platelets Langerhans cells	Phagocytosis Degranulation (eosinophils)	Fcγ RIIA^{131H} Fcγ RIIA^{131R}
Fcγ RIIB (CD32)	IgG	Low (Kd >10^{-7} M)	Macrophages Neutrophils Eosinophils B cells Mast cells	No phagocytosis Inhibition of cell activity	Fcγ RIIB^{232I} Fcγ RIIB^{232T}
Fcγ RIIC	IgG	Low (Kd >10^{-7} M)	Macrophages	Inhibition of cell activity	
Fcγ RIIIA (CD16a)	IgG	Low (Kd >10^{-6} M)	Natural killer cells Macrophages (certain tissues)	Induction of antibody-dependent, cell-mediated cytotoxicity Induction of cytokine release by macrophages	Fcγ RIIIA^{158V} Fcγ RIIIA^{158F}
Fcγ RIIIB (CD16b)	IgG	Low (Kd >10^{-6} M)	Eosinophils Macrophages Neutrophils Mast cells Dendritic cells	Induction of microbe killing	NA1 NA2

*Adapted from Nimmerjahn and Ravetch.[61]

showed that anti-D-coated red cells could stimulate peripheral blood mononuclear cells (PBMCs) in vitro to secrete interleukin-1 receptor antagonist (IL-1Ra) within 4 hours. The authors suggested that anti-D-induced cytokine alterations might account for some of the pathophysiologic events seen in IgG-mediated immune hemolysis. However, they did not show whether the secreted IL-1Ra was responsible for any of anti-D's potential effects (eg, inhibition of phagocytosis). IL-1Ra is structurally related to IL-1 and binds to the IL-1 receptor with equal affinity to IL-1.[73] IL-1Ra binding to the IL-1 receptor, however, does not transmit an intracellular signal as IL-1 does, and thus it acts as a potent anti-inflammatory cytokine counteracting IL-1's inflammatory effects (eg, inhibition of phagocytosis).[74,75]

Originally, to examine the mechanism of action of anti-D, Semple et al designed a prospective anti-D dose crossover study in children with chronic ITP.[76] The authors found that early after administration (3 hours), anti-D significantly increased serum levels of several proinflammatory and anti-inflammatory cytokines/chemokines, particularly IL-1Ra, which rose to approximately 60-fold higher (6000 pg/mL) than baseline levels within 3 hours after anti-D administration. By day 8 after treatment, however, all the cytokine/chemokine levels were similar to baseline. These findings were confirmed by two other groups, and they further suggested that, at the cytokine level at least, the mechanism of action of anti-D is different than that of IVIG.[77,78] For example, Cooper et al[78] found that by 2 hours after treatment, anti-D induced the production of IL-6, IL-10, tumor necrosis factor alpha, and monocyte chemoattractant protein-1, whereas 2 hours after IVIG treatment, only IL-10 was increased. This was probably the first study to suggest that IVIG and anti-D treatment ameliorate thrombocytopenia in ITP patients by different mechanisms.

The enhanced early production of IL-1Ra after anti-D administration was also correlated with a significant reduction of platelet phagocytosis by the patients' PBMCs (Fig 9-1).[76] Based

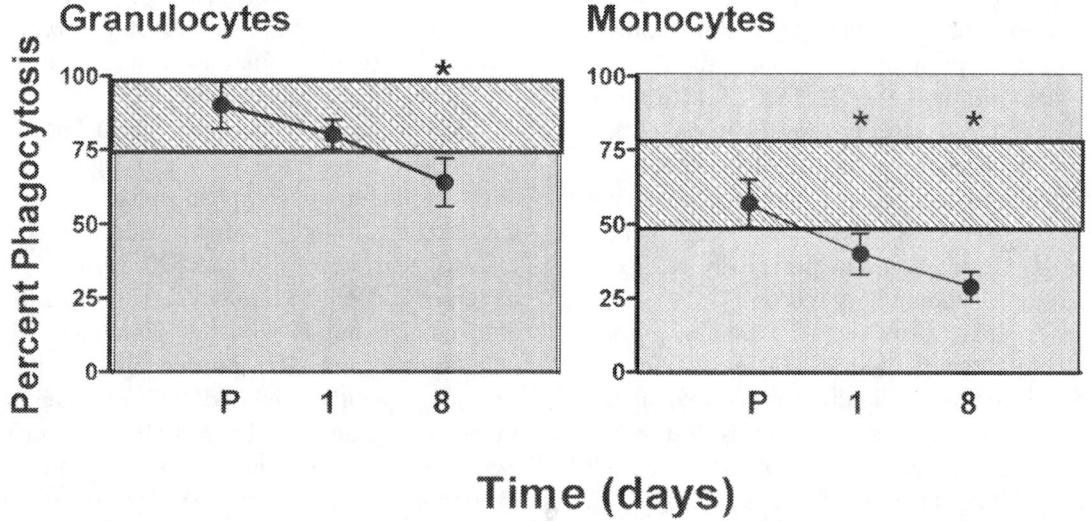

phagocytosis after administration of 50 µg/kg of anti-D. The values were calculated from seven children with chronic ITP.[76] The data are expressed as the mean [± standard deviation (±SD)] percent of opsonized-platelet phagocytosis at preadministration (P) and at 1 day and 8 days after administration. The shaded areas in each panel represent the mean ranges (±SD) for healthy children (n = 8). The stars represent the values that are significantly different from the normal ranges (p <0.05 by Student's t test).

on these results, the author and colleagues hypothesised that anti-D mediated an early but transient stimulation of macrophages and neutrophils within the RES, and the subsequent production of anti-inflammatory cytokines paralyzed their ability to mediate phagocytosis. To test this, a flow-cytometric phagocytosis assay was designed using anti-D-opsonized red cells and peripheral blood leukocytes.[79] It was found that the opsonized red cells significantly stimulated the production of IL-1Ra within 4 hours, supporting Davenport's original observations.[72] Significantly, what the results additionally demonstrated was that when recombinant IL-1Ra was added to the in-vitro assay, it could directly inhibit anti-D-opsonized red cell phagocytosis by both monocytes and granulocytes.[79] This represented one of the first reports linking anti-D-opsonized red cells and FcR-mediated cytokine release with inhibition of phagocytosis of opsonized cells. Overall, the majority of human studies suggest that anti-D-opsonized red cells may actively down-regulate phagocytosis by inducing early events such as the secretion of anti-inflammatory cytokines. The in-vitro phagocytosis assay confirmed these clinical results in that the anti-D-opsonized red cells induced IL-1Ra in both monocytes and granulocytes and demonstrated that IL-1Ra could directly inhibit red cell phagocytosis by cells of the RES. The detection of intracellular IL-1Ra in the phagocytosis assay may indicate that opsonized red cells induce phagocytes to produce IL-1Ra in order to potentially reduce a subsequent inflammatory reaction.[79]

In contrast, Crow et al[80] used a murine model of passively-induced ITP and found that although anti-red cell administration could significantly increase the serum levels of different cytokines, including IL-1Ra, the IL-1Ra itself was not sufficient to mediate the effects of red cell antibodies in raising the platelet counts. Mice deficient in the IL-1 receptor, which are surrogates to those lacking IL-1Ra, still responded to anti-red cell therapy. The apparent differences in results between the murine models and human studies may be for several reasons, including methodologic and/or species differences (eg, mice lack a D antigen). Nonetheless, it appears that anti-D therapy in humans and anti-red cell therapy in mice is associated with significant elevations in IL-1Ra, and it remains to be confirmed whether this cytokine plays a direct role in the mechanism of action of anti-D.

Nevertheless, Coopamah et al found that the in-vitro anti-D-induced cytokine changes were also related to an early but transient burst (within 10 to 30 minutes) of reactive oxygen species (ROS).[79] This was also observed by Shabani et al,[81] who demonstrated that the ROS generation in vitro by human macrophages induced with anti-D-opsonized red cells was either up-regulated or down-regulated depending on the cytokines present (eg, granulocyte-macrophage colony-stimulating factor or transforming growth factor beta, respectively). The production of ROS induced by anti-D-opsonized red cells suggests that anti-D may initially activate the RES, perhaps by inducing danger signals. Phagocytosis is known to be associated with a respiratory burst producing reactive oxygen and nitrogen species, and several studies have demonstrated that erythrocytes and their membranes can inhibit the respiratory burst during erythrophagocytosis.[82-84] In addition, there is literature suggesting that iron derived from red cells can significantly affect mononuclear cell phagocytosis.[85-87] This has also been found in patients with hemochromatosis and iron overload.[88-95] Perhaps the increased red cell accumulation within the RES induced by anti-D initially stimulates RES phagocytosis and ROS production, but these are subsequently inhibited by, for example, excess iron overload. These potential mechanisms will have to be confirmed by further experimentation. Alternatively, the initial activation (eg, ROS production) may subsequently lead to the generation of anti-inflammatory measures such as cytokines that actively down-regulate the RES. Figure 9-2 outlines the major effects of anti-D-opsonized red cells on phagocyte responses.

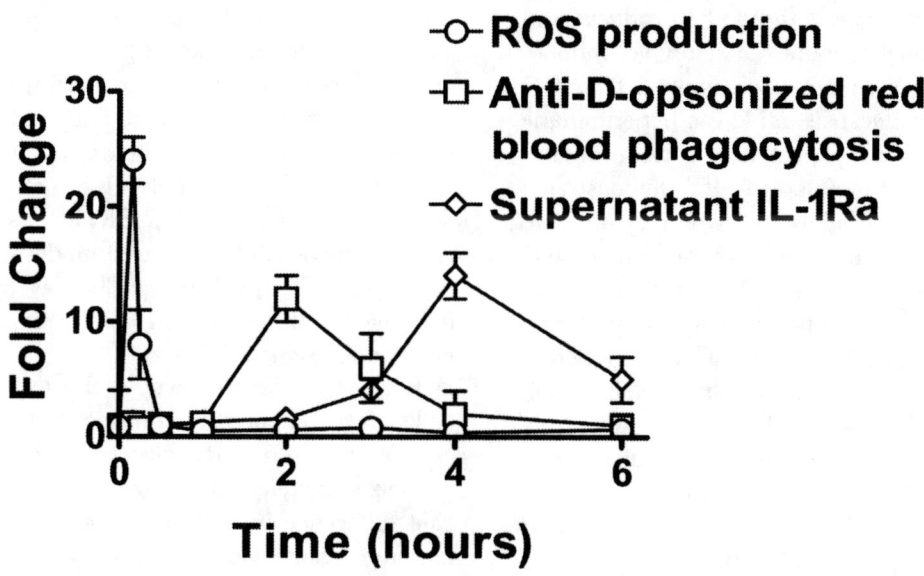

Figure 9-2. Summary of the effects of anti-D-opsonized red cells on phagocyte responses in vitro. Human peripheral blood monocytes were incubated with anti-D-opsonized red cells for various lengths of time, and various responses were measured by flow cytometry [reactive oxygen species (ROS) and phagocytosis] or by cytokine-specific enzyme-linked immunosorbent assay [interleukin-1 receptor antagonist (IL-1Ra)]. Within 10 minutes of incubation, a significant burst of ROS occurred, which was finished by 30 minutes and followed by the phagocytosis of the anti-D-opsonized red cells in 2 hours. Within 6 hours, a significant increase of secreted IL-1Ra was detected in the culture supernatant, which was correlated with a down-regulation of the opsonized-red-cell phagocytosis.

Idiotype Antibodies

An idiotype is defined as the collection of antigenic determinants (termed idiotopes) contained within the variable (V) regions of an antibody molecule.[96] The diversity of variable regions generated during VDJ heavy-chain and VJ light-chain immunoglobulin gene rearrangements and antigen-driven somatic mutation permits the expression of large numbers of potential idiotypes. It has been estimated that there are 15 to 20 idiotopes on the V region of a single immunoglobulin molecule.[97] Some of these idiotopes are topographically distant from the antigen-binding site (paratope) of the immunoglobulin; they are called framework idiotopes.[96,98,99] Other idiotopes overlap partially or fully with the paratope of the immunoglobulin; these are referred to as near-paratopic or paratopic idiotopes.[98,99] Jerne's Nobel-Prize-winning immune network theory originally proposed that the immune system was regulated internally via idiotype regulation; each immunoglobulin variable region contains not only a paratope but also idiotopes, which could be recognized by other antibodies.[100] These latter antibodies are referred to as idiotypic antibodies. Jerne's overall idea was that the immune system is in equilibrium, in that anti-idiotypes hold Ab1 production in check. Anti-idiotypes appear to be a major factor in the development and control of a normal immune response to antigens, and considerable evidence has accumulated to support anti-idiotype-directed regulation of alloantibodies.[101,102]

Although there is a significant amount of research that suggests that IVIG products contain substantial amounts of idiotypic antibodies,[14-17] little work has been applied to anti-D preparations. Because anti-D is a hyperimmune IVIG, one would expect that it also contains anti-idiotypes. Boughton et al[103] demonstrated that patients with active ITP who responded to anti-D treatment had a concomitant decrease in platelet-associated autoantibodies to glycoprotein IIb/IIIa.[104] This finding suggests that anti-D may possess neutralizing idiotype antibodies that down-regulate pathogenic platelet autoantibodies in the disorder. However, results from animal models of ITP have shown that monoclonal red cell antibodies that mimic anti-D and contain no idiotype antibodies are also efficacious in raising platelet counts.[71] Although anti-idiotypic mechanisms in anti-D's therapeutic efficacy cannot be ruled out, further research is clearly needed in order to confirm whether these types of mechanisms are responsible for anti-D ability to raise platelet counts in ITP.

Anti-D and Signaling Mechanisms within the RES

When anti-D is administered to an Rh-positive individual, circulating red cells become quickly opsonized, and as these antibody-bound red cells travel through the spleen, interactions with FcRs of the RES inevitably occur. It is generally assumed that these interactions are at the center of how anti-D is therapeutically efficacious in raising the platelet counts in patients with ITP. FcRs contribute to the internalization of both large and small immune complexes through phagocytosis and endocytosis, respectively.[56-60] The molecular processes underlying these internalization mechanisms differ dramatically and have distinct outcomes in immune clearance and modulation of cell function.[56-60] For example, Huang et al[105] recently demonstrated that there is a differential requirement of intracellular kinases depending on the size of the opsonized particle engulfed. It appears that kinases are not required for FcR-mediated endocytosis of small particles (eg, heat-aggregated IgG) but are crucial for the phagocytosis of larger particles (eg, sheep erythrocytes).[105] Their results suggested that FcR endocytosis and phagocytosis differ in their requirement for intracellular signaling molecules such as Syk, Src-related tyrosine kinases (SRTKs), and PI3K. A competitive inhibition-based model was proposed, in which PI3K and c-Cbl play contrasting roles in the induction of phagocytosis or endocytosis signaling cascades.

Related to these concepts, the author and colleagues compared the phagocytic kinetics of anti-D-opsonized red cells vs autoantibody-opsonized platelets and demonstrated a significant difference in engulfment rates. For example, the phagocytosis of opsonized platelets occurred at significantly higher rates compared to opsonized red cells.[106] Furthermore, the sluggish phagocytic rates of anti-D-opsonized red cells correlated with their ability to induce mononuclear cells to undergo a transient (24- to 48-hour) state of phagocytic refractoriness against further platelet phagocytosis.[106] The early phagocytic refractoriness induced by anti-D is of interest because it may prevent other mononuclear cell functions (eg, antigen presentation) that could affect immunity in the long term. Additionally, similar to the experiments of Huang et al,[105] the author and colleagues found that the slower phagocytic rate of the larger, opsonized red cells and their induction of mononuclear phagocytic refractoriness was related to their ability to differentially modulate intracellular activation of various tyrosine phosphatases compared to the smaller, opsonized platelets.[106] From these data, it appears that opsonized red cells and platelets have different effects on mononuclear phagocytes related to intracellular signaling, suggesting, at least, that anti-D-opsonized red cells may actively inhibit phagocytosis of opsonized platelets by these perhaps competitive intracellular events. If this is true, it may be possible to develop anti-D replacements that target intracellular signaling mechanisms within mononuclear phagocytes.

Monoclonal Anti-D Preparations

Hundreds of human monoclonal D antibodies (eg, BRAD-3, BRAD-5, UCHD4, etc) have been produced with the hope of improving therapy for diseases such as hemolytic disease of the fetus and newborn (HDFN) and reducing usage of polyclonal anti-D, thus reducing patient exposure to blood products.[104,107] It appears that some of these monoclonal D antibodies may be efficacious in HDFN.[108-110] With respect to treatment of ITP patients with monoclonal anti-D, however, only one report has been published[111]; in this study, 6 of 7 patients failed to respond (no increase in platelet count) to the particular IgG1 monoclonal anti-D used. The reasons for this lack of response are unclear, but Kumpel et al[112] suggested that antigen topography of IgG2 red cell antibodies is critical for the interaction with FcRs, and it has been demonstrated recently that IgG1 monoclonal D antibodies are inferior to IgG3 isotypes in modulating opsonized platelet phagocytosis. In addition, reports have documented the efficacy of monoclonal antibodies specific for murine red cell determinants in an animal model of ITP,[70,113] and another recent study has suggested that monoclonal anti-D preparations should be screened before use in humans to ensure the most efficacious activity.[114] Considering these data, it appears that monoclonal anti-D therapy could be made efficacious if there were assays to select the appropriate monoclonal anti-D.

To address this possibility, Kjaersgaard et al studied six human monoclonal D antibodies that were paired according to their isotype or epitope specificity and compared them with polyclonal anti-D for their ability to opsonize red cells and inhibit platelet phagocytosis.[115] It was found that opsonization of erythrocytes with polyclonal anti-D significantly reduced phagocytosis of opsonized platelets in an Fc-dependent manner.[115] Of the monoclonal D antibodies that shared specificity but differed in isotype, only IgG3 antibodies could significantly inhibit platelet phagocytosis.[115] In contrast, with two monoclonal D antibodies that shared isotype but differed in specificity, only one could inhibit platelet phagocytosis.[115] The results suggest that monoclonal anti-D epitope specificity and isotype are important requirements to optimally inhibit platelet phagocytosis, and carefully selecting these different monoclonal D antibodies will be the key to producing efficacious cocktails of monoclonal antibodies for treating ITP.

Recombinant Polyclonal Anti-D

The use of polyclonal IVIG and anti-D preparations derived from plasma has clear advantages in that they reflect the diversity of the natural immune response, but they still carry the risk of inducing recipient adverse reactions such as infectious disease transmission. In an attempt to eliminate these negative attributes, to date, at least 30 monoclonal antibodies of various specificities have been successfully introduced into the drug market to treat a wide spectrum of diseases, and still more are being developed. This second-generation monoclonal antibody approach provides the advantage of specificity and lack of adverse events but still lacks efficacy in the treatment of diseases caused by complex antigens where a polyclonal product would be more advantageous.[117]

A third generation of antibodies is termed *recombinant polyclonal antibodies*. These fully human antibodies can be produced in large scale by a recently developed discovery platform, Symplex (Symphogen, Lyngby, Denmark), which allows for the cloning, screening, and identification of antigen-specific human antibodies.[116] For example, antibody-producing plasma cells can be isolated from human peripheral blood by cell sorting; the antibody heavy- and light-chain mRNA are then reverse-transcribed, amplified, and linked by the Symplex polymerase chain reaction test, which has the advantage of preserving the original pairing of the antibody heavy and light chains (cognate pairing).[116] These types of preparations will have the advantage of eliminating adverse reactions and maintaining the polyclonal nature of the immunoglobulin preparations. With respect to anti-D, one such preparation [rozrolimupab

(Sym001, Symphogen, Lyngby, Denmark)], is a recombinant polyclonal antibody consisting of 25 different IgG1 D antibodies and has been designed to replace existing anti-D hyperimmune immunoglobulins for the treatment of ITP and the prevention of HDFN.[117] In March 2007, Sym001 entered Phase 1 clinical trials, making it the first-ever recombinant polyclonal antibody to enter clinical evaluation. The results from the dose-escalation, placebo-controlled studies showed that Sym001 was safe and well tolerated.[118] Phase 2 trials are currently underway and, if successful, this product may show promise in replacing plasma-derived anti-D preparations. The advantage of these defined monoclonal and recombinant polyclonal anti-D preparations is that they not only may reduce the unwanted adverse effects of anti-D therapy but may be able to effectively elucidate the exact mechanisms of action of anti-D in autoimmune disorders such as ITP.

Summary

Anti-D's efficacy in treating patients with ITP is thought to be related to the product's ability to sensitize red cells that effectively block or inhibit the RES; however, the ability of anti-D to modulate FcR expression and regulate the production of various cytokines suggests that it may exert its efficacious effects via more complex mechanisms. Although IVIG and anti-D may share some pathways in their therapeutic effect, anti-D therapy appears to exhibit distinct mechanisms of action. Future research will not only improve our understanding of these unique mechanisms but potentially allow for the design of replacement therapies for anti-D preparations derived from plasma.

References

1. Bruton OC. Agammaglobulinemia. Pediatrics 1952;9:722-8.
2. Ballow M. Intravenous immunoglobulins: Clinical experience and viral safety. J Am Pharm Assoc 2002;42:449-59.
3. Saulsbury FT, Winkelstein JA, Yolken RH. Chronic rotavirus infection in immunodeficiency. J Pediatrics 1980;97:61-5.
4. Molica S, Musto P, Chiurazzi F, et al. Prophylaxis against infections with low-dose intravenous immunoglobulins (IVIG) in chronic lymphocytic leukemia. Results of a crossover study. Haematologica 1996;81:121-6.
5. Imbach P, Barandum S, d'Appuzo V, et al. High-dose intravenous gammaglobulin for idiopathic thrombocytopenic purpura in childhood. Lancet 1981;1:1228-31.
6. Bussel J, Lalezari P, Hilgartner M, et al. Reversal of neutropenia with intravenous gammaglobulin in autoimmune neutropenia of infancy. Blood 1983;62:398-400.
7. Newland AC, Treleaven JG, Minchinton RM, Waters AH. High-dose intravenous IgG in adults with autoimmune thrombocytopenia. Lancet 1983;1:84-7.
8. Mueller-Eckhardt C, Salama A, Mahn I, et al. Lack of efficacy of high-dose intravenous immunoglobulin in autoimmune haemolytic anaemia: A clue to its mechanism. Scand J Haematol 1985;34:394-400.
9. Bussel JB, Pham LC, Aledort L, Nachman R. Maintenance treatment of adults with chronic refractory immune thrombocytopenic purpura using repeated intravenous infusions of gammaglobulin. Blood 1988;72:121-7.
10. Blanchette VS, Kirby MA, Turner C. Role of intravenous immunoglobulin G in autoimmune hematologic disorders. Semin Hematol 1992;29(Suppl 2):72-82.
11. Fehr J, Hofmann V, Kappeler U. Transient reversal of thrombocytopenia in idiopathic thrombocytopenic purpura by high-dose intravenous gamma globulin. N Engl J Med 1982;306:1254-8.
12. Sacher RA. Intravenous gammaglobulin therapy: Current role in bone marrow transplant, malignancy, and immune hematologic disorders. Semin Hematol 1992;29(Suppl 2):1-5.
13. Samuelsson A, Towers TL, Ravetch JV. Anti-inflammatory activity of IVIG mediated through the inhibitory Fc receptor. Science 2001;291:484-6.
14. Hahn BH, Ebling FM. Suppression of murine lupus nephritis by administration of an anti-idiotypic antibody to anti-DNA. J Immunol 1984;132:187-90.
15. Sultan Y, Kazatchkine MD, Maisonneuve P et al. Anti-idiotypic suppression of autoantibodies to factor VIII (antihaemophilic factor) by

high-dose intravenous gammaglobulin. Lancet 1984;2:765-8.
16. Rossi F, Dietrich G, Kazatchkine MD. Antiidiotypes against autoantibodies in pooled normal human polyspecific Ig. J Immunol 1989;143:4104-9.
17. Rodey GE. Anti-idiotypic antibodies and regulation of immune responses. Transfusion. 1992;32:361-76.
18. Semple JW, Allen D, Hogarth M, et al. In vivo actions of anti-D (WinRho SD) in children with chronic autoimmune thrombocytopenic purpura (ITP) (abstract). Blood 1998;92(Suppl):178a.
19. Bussel J, Heddle N, Richards C, Woloski M. MCP-1, IL10, IL-6 and TNF- levels in patients with ITP before and after IV anti-D and IVIG treatments. Blood 1999;94:15.
20. Aukrust P, Muller F, Svenson M, et al. Administration of intravenous immunoglobulin (IVIG) in vivo—down-regulatory effects on the IL-1 system. Clin Exp Immunol 1999;115:136-43.
21. Blanchette VS, Semple JW, Freedman J. Intravenous immunoglobulin and Rh immunoglobulin as immunomodulators of autoimmunity to blood elements. In: Silberstein LE, ed. Autoimmune disorders of blood. Bethesda, MD: AABB, 1996:35-77.
22. Semple JW, Crow AR, Lazarus AH, et al. Intravenous immunoglobulin products: An update on their mechanisms of action. Vox Sang 2008;3:152-8.
23. Siragam V, Crow AR, Brinc D, et al. Intravenous immunoglobulin ameliorates ITP via activating Fc gamma receptors on dendritic cells. Nat Med 2004;12:688-92.
24. Salama A, Mueller-Eckhardt C, Kiefel V. Effect of intravenous immunoglobulin in immune thrombocytopenia. Lancet 1983;2:193-5.
25. Salama A, Kiefel V, Amberg R, Mueller-Eckhardt C. Treatment of autoimmune thrombocytopenic purpura with rhesus antibodies [anti-RhO(D)]. Blut 1984;49:29-35.
26. Andrew M, Blanchette VS, Adams M, et al. A multicenter study of the treatment of childhood chronic idiopathic thrombocytopenic purpura with anti-D. J Pediatrics 1992;120:522-7.
27. Cooper N, Woloski BM, Fodero EM, et al. Does treatment with intermittent infusions of intravenous anti-D allow a proportion of adults with recently diagnosed immune thrombocytopenic purpura to avoid splenectomy? Blood 2002;99:1922-7.
28. Bussel JB, Graziano JN, Kimberly RP, et al. Intravenous anti-D treatment of immune thrombocytopenic purpura: Analysis of efficacy, toxicity, and mechanism of effect. Blood 1991;77:1884-93.
29. Panzer S, Grfimayer ER, Haas OA, et al. Efficacy of rhesus antibodies [Anti-RhO (D)] in autoimmune thrombocytopenia: Correlation with response to high dose IgG and the degree of haemolysis. Blut 1986;52:117-21.
30. Ambriz-Fernandez R, Martinez-Murillo C, Quintana-Gonzalez S, et al. Fc receptor blockade in patients with refractory chronic immune thrombocytopenic purpura with anti-D IgG. Arch Med Res 2002;33:536-40.
31. Blanchette VS, Luke B, Andrew M, et al. A prospective, randomized trial of high-dose intravenous immune globulin G therapy, oral prednisone therapy, and no therapy in childhood acute immune thrombocytopenic purpura. J Pediatrics 1993;123:989-95.
32. Scaradavou A, Woo B, Woloski BM, et al. Intravenous anti-D treatment of immune thrombocytopenic purpura: Experience in 272 patients. Blood 1997;89:2689-700.
33. Rodeghiero F. First-line therapies for immune thrombocytopenic purpura: Re-evaluating the need to treat. Eur J Haematol 2008;69 (Suppl):19-26.
34. Godeau B, Provan D, Bussel J. Immune thrombocytopenic purpura in adults. Curr Opinion Hematol 2007;14:535-56.
35. Tarantino MD, Bolton-Maggs PH. Update on the management of immune thrombocytopenic purpura in children. Curr Opinion Hematol 2007;14:526-34.
36. Aledort LM, Salama A, Kovaleva L, et al. International Anti-D Study Group. Efficacy and safety of intravenous anti-D immunoglobulin (Rhophylac) in chronic immune thrombocytopenic purpura. Hematol 2007;12:289-95.
37. El Alfy MS, Mokhtar GM, El-Laboudy MA, Khalifa AS. Randomized trial of anti-D immunoglobulin versus low-dose intravenous immunoglobulin in the treatment of childhood chronic idiopathic thrombocytopenic purpura. Acta Haematol 2006;115:46-52.
38. Meyer O, Kiesewetter H, Hermsen M, Salama A. Efficacy and safety of anti-D given by subcutaneous injection to patients with autoimmune thrombocytopenia. Eur J Haematol 2004;73:71-2.

39. Lowe EJ, Buchanan GR. Idiopathic thrombocytopenic purpura diagnosed during the second decade of life. J Pediatrics 2002;141:253-8.
40. Stasi R, Evangelista ML, Stipa E, et al. Idiopathic thrombocytopenic purpura: Current concepts in pathophysiology and management. Thromb Haemost 2008;99:4-13.
41. Cines DB, Blanchette VS. Immune thrombocytopenic purpura. N Eng J Med 2002;346:995-1008.
42. Hou M, Stockelberg D, Kutti J, Wadenvik H. Antibodies against GPIb/IX, GPIIb/IIIa, and other platelet antigens in chronic idiopathic thrombocytopenic purpura. Eur J Haematol 1995;55:307-14.
43. Mehta YS, Pathare AV, Badakere SS, et al. Influence of auto-antibody specificities on the clinical course in patients with chronic and acute ITP. Platelets 2000;11:94-8.
44. Fabris F, Scandellari R, Ruzzon E, et al. Platelet-associated autoantibodies as detected by a solid-phase modified antigen capture ELISA test (MACE) are a useful prognostic factor in idiopathic thrombocytopenic purpura. Blood 2004;103:4562-4.
45. Zhou B, Zhao H, Yang RC, Han ZC. Multi-dysfunctional pathophysiology in ITP. Crit Rev Oncol Hematol 2005;54:107-16.
46. Semple JW, Freedman J. Abnormal cellular immune mechanisms associated with autoimmune thrombocytopenia. Transfus Med Rev 1995;9:327-38.
47. Semple JW. Immunobiology of T helper cells and antigen-presenting cells in autoimmune thrombocytopenic purpura (ITP). Acta Paediatr 1998;424(Suppl):41-5.
48. Coopamah M, Garvey MB, Freedman J, Semple JW. Cellular immune mechanisms in autoimmune thrombocytopenic purpura: An update. Transfus Med Rev 2003;17:69-80.
49. Olsson B, Andersson PO, Jacobsson JM, et al. T-cell-mediated cytotoxicity toward platelets in chronic idiopathic thrombocytopenic purpura. Nat Med 2003;9:1123-4.
50. Zhang F, Chu K, Wang L, et al. Cell-mediated lysis of autologous platelets in chronic idiopathic thrombocytopenic purpura. Eur J Haematol 2006;76:427-31.
51. Michel M. Immune thrombocytopenic purpura: Epidemiology and implications for patients. Eur J Haematol 2009;82(Suppl 71):3-7.
52. Rodeghiero F, Stasi R, Gernsheimer T, et al. Standardization of terminology, definitions and outcome criteria in immune thrombocytopenic purpura of adults and children: Report from an international working group. Blood 2009;113:2386-93.
53. Horowitz B, Chin S, Prince AM, et al. Preparation and characterization of S/D-FFP, a virus sterilized "fresh frozen plasma." J Thromb Haemost 1991;65:1163-8.
54. Horowitz B, Bonomo R, Prince AM, et al. Solvent/detergent-treated plasma: A virus-inactivated substitute for fresh frozen plasma. Blood 1992;79:826-31.
55. MacKenzie IZ, Bichler J, Mason GC, et al. Efficacy and safety of a new, chromatographically purified rhesus (D) immunoglobulin. Eur J Obstetr Gynecol Reprod Biol 2004;117:154-61.
56. Ravetch JV, Bolland S. IgG Fc receptors. Annu Rev Immunol 2001;19:275-90.
57. Cox D, Greenberg S. Phagocytic signaling strategies: Fc(gamma)receptor-mediated phagocytosis as a model system. Semin Immunol 2001;13:339-45.
58. McKenzie SE, Schreiber AD. Fc gamma receptors in phagocytes. Curr Opin Hematol 1998;5:16-21.
59. Garcia-Garcia,E, Rosales C. Signal transduction during Fc receptor-mediated phagocytosis. J Leuk Biol 2002;72:1092-1108.
60. Nimmerjahn F, Bruhns P, Horiuchi K, Ravetch JV. FcgammaRIV: A novel FcR with distinct IgG subclass specificity. Immunity 2005;23:41-51.
61. Nimmerjahn F, Ravetch JV. Fc receptors as regulators of immune responses. Nat Rev Immunol 2008;8;34-47.
62. Bussel JB, Graziano JN, Kimberly RP. Anti-D Ig for treatment of immune thrombocytopenic purpura (letter). Blood 1991:2157-8.
63. Oksenhendler E, Bierling P, Brossard Y, et al. Anti-RH immunoglobulin therapy for human immunodeficiency virus-related immune thrombocytopenic purpura. Blood 1988;71:1499-502.
64. Bussel JB, Graziano JN, Kimberly RP, et al. Intravenous anti-D treatment of immune thrombocytopenic purpura: Analysis of efficacy, toxicity, and mechanism of effect. Blood 1991;77:1884-93.
65. Nieswandt B, Bergmeier W, Rackebrandt K, et al. Identification of critical antigen-specific mechanisms in the development of immune thrombocytopenic purpura in mice. Blood 2000;96:2520-7.

66. Alves-Rosa F, Stanganelli C, Cabrera J, et al. Treatment with liposome-encapsulated clodronate as a new strategic approach in the management of immune thrombocytopenic purpura in a mouse model. Blood 2000;96:2834-40.
67. Samuelsson A, Towers TL, and Ravetch JV. Anti-inflammatory activity of IVIG mediated through the inhibitory Fc receptor. Science 2001;291:484-6.
68. Teeling JL, Jansen-Hendriks T, Kuijpers TW, et al. Therapeutic efficacy of intravenous immunoglobulin preparations depends on the immunoglobulin G dimers: Studies in experimental immune thrombocytopenia. Blood 2001;98: 1095-9.
69. Crow AR, Song S, Semple JW, et al. IVIG inhibits reticuloendothelial system function and ameliorates murine passive-immune thrombocytopenia independent of anti-idiotype reactivity. Br J Haematol 2001;115:679-86.
70. Song S, Crow AR, Siragam V, et al. Monoclonal antibodies that mimic the action of anti-D in the amelioration of murine ITP act by a mechanism distinct from that of IVIG. Blood 2005;105:1546-8.
71. Song S, Crow AR, Freedman J, et al. Monoclonal IgG can ameliorate immune thrombocytopenia in a murine model of ITP: An alternative to IVIG. Blood 2003;101:3708-13.
72. Davenport RD, Burdick MD, Strieter RM, Kunkel SL. In vitro production of interleukin-1 receptor antagonist in IgG-mediated red cell incompatibility. Transfusion 1994;34:297-303.
73. Dripps DJ, Brandhuber BJ, Thompson RC, Eisenberg SP. Interleukin-1 (IL-1) receptor antagonist binds to the 80-kDa IL-1 receptor but does not initiate IL-1 signal transduction. J Biol Chem 1991;266:10331-6.
74. Evans RJ, Bray J, Childs JD, et al. Mapping receptor binding sites in interleukin (IL)-1 receptor antagonist and IL-1 beta by site-directed mutagenesis. Identification of a single site in IL-1ra and two sites in IL-1 beta. J Biol Chem 1995;270:11477-83.
75. Aderem A, Underhill DM. Mechanisms of phagocytosis in macrophages. Annu Rev Immunol 1999;17:593-623.
76. Semple JW, Allen D, Rutherford M, et al. Anti-D (WinRhoSD) treatment of children with chronic autoimmune thrombocytopenic purpura stimulates transient cytokine/chemokine production. Am J Hematol 2002;69:225-7.
77. Malinowska I, Obitko-Pludowska A, Buescher ES, et al. Release of cytokines and soluble cytokine receptors after intravenous anti-D treatment in children with chronic thrombocytopenic purpura. Hematol J 2001;2:242-9.
78. Cooper N, Heddle NM, deHaas M, et al. Intravenous (IV) anti-D and IV immunoglobulin achieve acute platelet increases by different mechanisms: Modulation of cytokine and platelet responses to IV anti-D by FcRIIa and FcRIIIa polymorphisms. Br J Haematol 2004; 124:511-18.
79. Coopamah MD, Freedman J, Semple JW. Anti-D initially stimulates an Fc-dependent leukocyte oxidative burst and subsequently suppresses erythrophagocytosis via interleukin 1 receptor antagonist. Blood 2003;102:2862-7.
80. Crow AR, Song S, Semple JW, et al. A role for IL-1 receptor antagonist or other cytokines in the acute therapeutic effects of IVIG? Blood 2007;109:155-8.
81. Shabani, F, Ziaean G, Branch DR, Denomme GA. Cytokine activation of PBMCs modulate Fc-gamma receptor dependent phagocytosis (abstract). Blood 2002;100(Suppl 2):140b.
82. Raley MJ, Schwacha MG, Loegering DJ. Lysosomotropic agents ameliorate macrophage dysfunction following the phagocytosis of IgG-coated erythrocytes: A role for lipid peroxidation. Inflammation 1997;21;619-28.
83. Wilhelm J, Skoumalova A, Vytasek R, et al. Erythrocyte membranes inhibit respiratory burst and protein nitration during phagocytosis by macrophages. Physiol Res 2005;54:533-9.
84. Vercellotti GM, van Asbeck BS, Jacob HS. Oxygen radical-induced erythrocyte hemolysis by neutrophils: Critical role of iron and lactoferrin. J Clin Invest 1985;76:956-62.
85. Hoepelman IM, Jaarsma EY, Verhoef J, Marx JJM. Effect of iron on polymorphonuclear granulocyte phagocytic capacity: Role of oxidation state and effect of ascorbic acid. Br J Haematol 1988;70:495-500.
86. Loegering DJ, Raley MJ, Reho TA, Eaton JW. Macrophage dysfunction following the phagocytosis of lgG-coated erythrocytes: Production of lipid peroxidation products. J Leuk Biol 1996;59:357-62.
87. Kockx MM, Cromheeke KM, Knaapen MW, et al. Phagocytosis and macrophage activation associated with hemorrhagic microvessels in human atherosclerosis. Arterioscler Thromb Vasc Biol 2003;23:440-6.

88. van Asbeck BS, Marx JJ, Struyvenberg A, Verhoef J. Functional defects in phagocytic cells from patients with iron overload. J Infection 1984;8:232-40.
89. Abbott M, Galloway A, Cunningham JL. Haemochromatosis presenting with a double Yersinia infection. J Infection 1986;13:143-5.
90. Boelaert JR, Van Landuyt HW, Valcke YS, et al. The role of desferrioxamine in dialysis-associated mucormycosis: Report of three cases and review of the literature. Clin Nephrol 1988;29:261-6.
91. Bullen JJ, Spaulding PB, Ward CG, Gutteridge JMC. Hemochromatosis, iron, and septicemia caused by Vibrio vulnificus. Arch Intern Med 1991;151:1606-9.
92. Christopher G. Escherichia coli bacteremia, meningitis, and hemochromatosis (case report). Arch Intern Med 1985;145:1908.
93. Daly AL, Velazquez LA, Bradley SF, Kauffman CA. Mucormycosis: Association with deferoxamine therapy. Am J Med 1989;87:468-71.
94. Robins-Browne R, Prpic JK. Effects of iron and desferrioxamine on infections with Yersinia enterocolitica. Infect Immun 1985;47:774-9.
95. Windus DW, Stokes TJ, Julian BA, Fenves AZ. Fatal Rhizopus infections in hemodialysis patients receiving deferoxamine. Ann Internal Med 1987;107:678-80.
96. Nisonoff A, Lamoyi E. Implications of the presence of an internal image of the antigen in antiidiotypic antibodies: Possible application to vaccine production. Clin Immunol Immunopathol 1981;21:397-406.
97. Bona CA, Heber-Katz E, Paul WE. Idiotype-anti-idiotype regulation. I. Immunization with a levan-binding myeloma protein leads to the appearance of auto-anti-(anti-idiotype) antibodies and to the activation of silent clones. J Exp Med 1981:153:951-67.
98. Zanetti M, Dovezenski N, Lenert P, Sollazo M, Idiotype in autoimmunity. In: Cerny J, Hiernaux J, eds. Idiotypic network and diseases. Washington, DC: American Society for Microbiology, 1990:175-7.
99. Jerne NK, Roland J, Cazenave PA. Recurrent idiotopes and internal images. EMBO J 1982: 1:243-7.
100. Jerne NK. Towards a network theory of the immune system. Ann Immunol 1974:125: 373-89.
101. Bona CA. Internal image concept revisited. Proc Soc Exp Biol Med 1996;213:32-42.
102. Bronshtein IB, Shuster AM, Gololobov GV, et al. DNA-specific anti-idiotypic antibodies in the sera of patients with autoimmune diseases. FEBS Lett 1992;314:259-63.
103. Boughton BJ, Cooke RM, Smith NA, et al. Autoimmune thrombocytopenia: Anti-glycoprotein IIb/IIIa auto antibodies are reduced after human anti-D immunoglobulin treatment. Autoimmunity 1994;18:141-4.
104. Kumpel BM. In vivo studies of monoclonal anti-D and the mechanism of immune suppression. Transfus Clin Biol 2002;9:9-14.
105. Huang Z-Y, Barreda DR, Worth RG, et al. Differential kinase requirements in human and mouse Fcgamma receptor phagocytosis and endocytosis. J Leuk Biol 2006;80:1553-62.
106. Aslam R, Kim M, Speck ER, et al. Platelet and erythrocyte phagocytosis kinetics are differentially controlled by phosphatase activity within mononuclear cells. Transfusion 2007;7:2161-8.
107. Kumpel BM, Beliard R, Brossard Y, et al. Section 1C: Assessment of the functional activity and IgG Fc receptor utilisation of 64 IgG Rh monoclonal antibodies. Coordinator's report. Transfus Clin Biol 2002;9:45-53.
108. Thomson A, Contreras M, Gorick B, et al. Clearance of Rh D-positive red cells with monoclonal anti-D. Lancet 1990;336:1147-50.
109. Kumpel BM, De Haas M, Koene HR, et al. Clearance of red cells by monoclonal IgG3 anti-D in vivo is affected by the VF polymorphism of Fcgamma RIIIa (CD16). Clin Exp Immunol 2003;132:81-6.
110. Chauhan AR, Bhattacharyya MS, Turakhia N, Daftary G. Efficacy and safety of monoclonal anti-D immunoglobulin in comparison with polyclonal anti-D immunoglobulin in prevention of Rho immunization. J Assoc Physicians India 2002;50:1341-2.
111. Godeau B, Oksenhendler E, Brossard Y, et al. Treatment of chronic autoimmune thrombocytopenic purpura with monoclonal anti-D. Transfusion 1996;36:328-30.
112. Kumpel BM, van de Winkel JG, Westerdaal NA, et al. Antigen topography is critical for interaction of IgG2 anti-red-cell antibodies with Fc gamma receptors. Br J Haematol 1996;94:175-83.
113. Bazin R, Aubin E, Boyer L, et al. Functional in vivo characterization of human monoclonal anti-D in NOD-scid mice. Blood 2002;99:1267-72.

114. Armstrong-Fisher SS, Carter MC, Downing I, et al. Evaluation of a panel of human monoclonal antibodies to D and exploration of the synergistic effects of blending IgG1 and IgG3 antibodies on their in vitro biological function. Transfusion 1999;39:1005-12.
115. Kjaersgaard M, Aslam R, Kim M, et al. Epitope specificity and isotype of monoclonal anti-D antibodies dictate their ability to inhibit phagocytosis of opsonized platelets. Blood 2007; 110:1359-61.
116. Haurum JS. Recombinant polyclonal antibodies: The next generation of antibody therapeutics? Drug Discov Today 2006;11:655-60.
117. Wikén M, Valentin-Jensen AM, Andersen PS, Flegel WA. Binding of the recombinant polyclonal anti-D product rozrolimupab (Sym001) and plasma derived anti-D to RhD variants (abstract). Haematologica 2009;94(Suppl 2): 72.
118. Hjelmström P, Hallén B, Lindenstroem E, Gyaw S. Sym001, the first recombinant polyclonal Rhesus-D specific antibody product, was safe and well-tolerated in a placebo-controlled randomized Phase I trial (abstract). Blood 2008;112(Suppl):1987a.

10

The Clinical Use of Anti-D

C. Ellen van der Schoot, MD, PhD

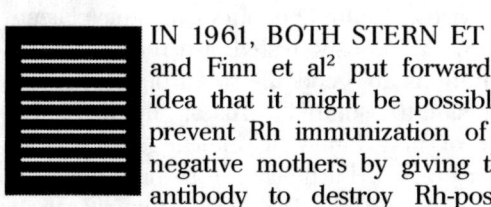

IN 1961, BOTH STERN ET AL[1] and Finn et al[2] put forward the idea that it might be possible to prevent Rh immunization of Rh-negative mothers by giving them antibody to destroy Rh-positive fetal cells. Subsequently, in the mid 1960s, several groups in Europe and North America performed additional experimental studies on the prevention of Rh-immunization.[3-6] At the same time, Clarke et al[3] and Freda et al[4] reported that when D+ red cells were given to D− male volunteers, Rh-immunization could be prevented by the administration of anti-D. In 1965, the first results of a clinical trial on the prevention of Rh immunization in pregnant women was published,[7] and in 1967, the combined results of the British, American, and German trials in pregnant women were reported. None of the 329 women who received anti-D postnatally became immunized, whereas 15% of untreated women had detectable anti-D.[8] Because of these clinical successes, anti-D has been licensed for prophylaxis of Rh disease in North America and Europe since 1968.

The clinical use of anti-D exclusively for the prevention of Rh immunization began to change when, in 1983, Salama et al[9] noticed that intravenous immunoglobulin (IVIG) could induce mild hemolysis when used to treat patients with immune thrombocytopenia (ITP). They postulated that IVIG contained anti-erythrocyte antibodies that elevated platelet counts by sequestering autologous red cells in the spleen and blocking the reticuloendothelial system. Indeed, in 8 out of 10 patients with chronic ITP, which they subsequently treated with anti-D, there was a rise in platelet count.[10] In 1995, the US Food and Drug Administration (FDA) licensed anti-D for treatment of ITP. The present indications for anti-D are listed in Table 10-1.

C. Ellen van der Schoot, MD, PhD, Professor in Experimental Immunohematology, Department of Experimental Immunohematology, Sanquin Research, and Landsteiner Laboratory, Academic Medical Centre, University of Amsterdam, Amsterdam, the Netherlands

The author has disclosed no conflicts of interest.

Table 10-1. Clinical Indications for Anti-D

1. Prevention of Rh allommunization:
   a. After birth of a D+ newborn in a D− woman
   b. Routine antenatal anti-D prophylaxis in D− pregnant women
   c. Certain obstetric conditions in D− pregnant women
   d. After transfusion of D+ red cells to a D− recipient
   e. After transfusion of D+ platelets to a D− female of childbearing potential
2. Treatment of ITP:
   a. Acute ITP in children
   b. Chronic ITP in children and adults
   c. HIV-associated thrombocytopenia

ITP = immune thrombocytopenia; HIV = human immunodeficiency virus.

This chapter will review the clinical usage of anti-D in Rh immunizaition and ITP.

Production, Infectious Risk, and Pharmacology of Anti-D

Anti-D immunoglobulin is produced from pooled plasma of donors with high titers of anti-D, who are repeatedly boostered with D+ red cells. Originally, these donors were mainly women primarily immunized by pregnancy. As a result of the success of the Rh prophylaxis program, however, deliberately immunized men are increasingly being recruited as anti-D donors.

The production process can be either ion-exchange chromatography [eg, Rhophylac (CSL Behring, King of Prussia, PA) and WhinRho SDF (Baxter, Deerfield, IL)] or cold ethanol fractionation [eg, Rhogam (Ortho-Clinical Diagnostics, Raritan, NJ)]. Anti-D prepared by chromatography has greater purity and is therefore less likely to produce adverse reactions. Because anti-D is produced from pools of plasma, only 1% of the IgG is serologically active anti-D, and thus the product contains many other antibodies, including anti-HLA and antibodies to blood group antigens. In addition, small amounts of IgA are present, which may impart a risk of hypersensitivity reactions in IgA-deficient recipients who have formed anti-IgA.

With regard to the infectious safety of anti-D products, although earlier reports demonstrated that anti-D could transmit viruses such as hepatitis C virus,[11,12] anti-D donors and their plasma are now rigorously tested. Currently, anti-D preparations are generally safe from all known transfusion-transmitted viruses, although the threat of new emerging infectious threats is always present. Furthermore, to minimize the risk of transmission of variant Creutzfeld-Jakob disease, plasma used for anti-D production in the United Kingdom is sourced from North America. Because of the emerging infectious risks and shortages of anti-D in some parts of the world, an unlimited supply of monoclonal anti-D would be desirable. To date, however, the reported efficacy of monoclonal anti-D in clinical trials has been generally disappointing; these studies have been extensively reviewed by Kumpel.[13] Nonetheless, it is expected that, eventually, biotechnologically-produced antibodies will be available to replace the polyclonal anti-D produced from pooled human plasma. More knowledge on the working mechanisms of anti-D for the different clinical indications is needed to design optimally engineered anti-D.

The content, or specific activity, of anti-D refers to the World Health Organization's international unit (IU) standard (1 μg anti-D is 5 IU).

When anti-D is given intravenously, the peak plasma concentration is about 2.5 times greater than when given intramuscularly.[14-16] Intramuscular (IM) or intravenous (IV) anti-D are considered to be equally effective to prevent Rh-immunization by fetal red cells. Ten to 14 days after injection, there is no difference in the levels of anti-D in the plasma of women given IV vs IM anti-D.[15] Anti-D is given intravenously for treatment of ITP; however, the same beneficial effect in ITP has been reported after subcutaneous injection of anti-D.[17] For IM administration, the peak plasma concentration is reached after about 2 to 4 days.[14,16] The mean elimination half-life of IgG is 21 days, which has also been found for anti-D.[18] The expected plasma level of anti-D after IM injection of 100 µg of antibody is 10 ng/mL after 1 day and 15 ng/mL after 3 days.[15] The mean residual anti-D IgG at 12 weeks after administration of 300 µg anti-D is 10 µg/L.[16] However, there is considerable variation seen among women, and it is quite possible that plasma levels vary with different preparations of anti-D immunoglobulin.[16,19] Nevertheless, the rule of thumb is similar for all products: 20 µg or 100 IU of anti-D to prevent Rh D immunization by 1 mL of D+ red cells. It can be calculated that under these conditions only about 8% to 15% of D antigens (1000-2000 molecules/red cell) have anti-D bound to them.

Postnatal Immune Prophylaxis

Fetomaternal hemorrhage (FMH) occurring during delivery or pregnancy in a D– woman carrying a D+ fetus can induce Rh immunization. Alloimmunization can lead to hemolytic disease of the fetus and newborn (HDFN) in subsequent pregnancies. HDFN is a disease that, if untreated, can cause perinatal mortality and morbidity with a substantial risk for long-term sequelae. HDFN was for many years the major specific cause of perinatal mortality and morbidity. Since the first description of the disease, the treatment possibilities have substantially improved the prognosis of affected fetuses, provided that the onset of the disease is detected in time. In all developed countries, pregnant women are therefore screened for the presence of antibodies, and immunoprophylaxis with anti-D is one of the most important achievements in the prevention of HDFN. One prophylactic dose of anti-D is given to nonimmunized D– women who have given birth to a D+ child. It is generally recommended to administer IM anti-D as soon as possible after birth, at least within 72 hours after delivery. However, it has been experimentally shown that protection was achieved when anti-D was given up to 13 days after transfusion of D+ red cells.[20]

The percentage of anti-D immunizations decreased to 0.7% to 2.5% in the various countries after the introduction of anti-D immunoprophylaxis.[21] In general, it is assumed that more than 90% reduction of immunization risk is achieved by postnatal prophylaxis. Moreover, it has been suggested that in women who become alloimmunized despite prophylaxis, the level of the antibody response is lowered.[22] Based on the immunization risk and the number of consecutive D+ children, it can be calculated that the dosage needed to prevent Rh immunization is 20 µg. The recommended dose varies between countries, from 500 IU (eg, United Kingdom) and 1000 IU (eg, the Netherlands) to 1500 IU (eg, United States).[21] As outlined above, these dosages will be able to prevent immunization when the FMH does not exceed 5 to 15 mL.[15,23] However, it is known that in 0.2% to 1% of women the FMH is higher, so only 99% to 99.8% of women at risk are protected by the standard dose. Screening tests to recognize larger FMHs are recommended to adjust the dose but not always routinely applied.

Several studies have been undertaken to identify risk factors for immunization caused by larger FMH. In most of these studies, the Kleihauer-Betke (KB) test quantifying fetal red cells in the maternal circulation was applied as a surrogate for immunization. These studies showed varying results and provided little evidence for a correlation between large FMH and the incidence of FMH risk factor events such as caesarean section.[24,25] Recently, however, Koelewijn et al[26] showed that by applying not the KB test, but the actual Rh immunization as an outcome parameter, assisted delivery is a factor significantly correlated with immunization. Of interest, 50% of women making anti-D despite full antenatal and postnatal prophylaxis had a history of traumatic delivery, including caesarean section. Possibly, these cases may have had fetal blood loss into the maternal intraperitoneal cavity, which has been missed by KB tests applied shortly after delivery. Routine administration of extra anti-D might therefore be considered after assisted delivery, but prospective clinical studies are needed to confirm this hypothesis.

One of the controversies of anti-D prophylaxis is whether pregnant women who have a weak D phenotype and/or a partial D phenotype should receive anti-D.[27] Because of the complexity of the D antigen, however, this question cannot be simply answered. Most D+ individuals making anti-D are partial-D category VI, which has a frequency of 0.02% to 0.05% in people of European ethnicity. Therefore, these women should be treated as D− and get prophylaxis. Typing reagents should be selected to prevent labeling them as D+. However, many more Rh variants have been described, and no consensus exists yet how important it is to recognize all these variants in pregnant women, either to correctly administer anti-D because they are at risk for immunization or to withhold anti-D because they have no risk—for example, women with the most commonly occurring weak D types.[28] Conversely, it is not clear how immunogenic fetal red cells with weak D expression are. In addition, whether the anti-D will be able to clear fetal red cells with weak D expression from the maternal circulation is also not clear. Because of the correlation between antigen dose and risk for immunization, a larger FMH will be needed to cause immunization. However, since as little as 30 μL of red cells of common Rh phenotype can be immunogenic, it is generally recommended to administer anti-D whenever fetal D expression has been demonstrated.

Anti-D must be given to all nonimmunized D− women having a spontaneous or therapeutic abortion, regardless of gestational age.[29,30] The risk of sensitization by spontaneous abortion before 12 weeks' gestation is thought to be negligible, but published data are scant.[28] In some countries (eg, United Kingdom, the Netherlands) no prophylaxis is required following spontaneous complete miscarriage before 10 weeks. It is reassuring that, in the Netherlands, spontaneous abortion was not found to be a risk factor in Rh-immunized women.[26]

Although the adherence to guidelines on postnatal prophylaxis is near 100%, women still become immunized because they did not receive immunoprophylaxis as a result of technical or clerical errors. In a Dutch study of new anti-D immunizations detected in 21,000 D− women (all para-1, having their first delivery in the Netherlands), in 20 of the 113 (17.5%) newly immunized women, the first child was erroneously typed as D− (n = 12) or the mother erroneously as D+ (n = 8).[26]

Antenatal Prophylaxis

Routine Antenatal Anti-D Prophylaxis

Women can also become immunized by fetal red cells circulating in the maternal circulation during pregnancy, especially in the last trimester, where spontaneous silent FMH might occur. Bowman et al[15] demonstrated a FMH of >1 mL between 30 and 39 weeks of gestation in 146 out of 1895 women (8%). For these women, postnatal prophylaxis might be too late. Indeed, in several studies it has been shown that routine antenatal anti-D prophylaxis (RAADP) further reduced the immunization prevalence. The dosage and timing of the anti-D Ig administration in these studies varied: a single dose of 1500 IU in week 34, or two doses in week 28 and week 34 of 250 IU, 500 IU, or 1500 IU.[31-37] More recently, RAADP with a single dose of 1000 IU in week 30 has been introduced in the Netherlands.[38] This regimen was employed to ensure a high procedural feasibility: only one extra administration of anti-D of the same dose as was used postnatally. Besides differences in timing and doses, supportive studies for antenatal prophylaxis also showed considerable heterogeneity in patient selection, outcome measures (predominantly proxy outcomes are used—ie, immunizations after birth or in the next pregnancy rather than the occurrence of HDFN), and results. From these studies, including one quasi-experimental study,[32] it can be concluded that a dosage of at least 2 × 500 IU anti-D Ig (in weeks 28 and 34) reduces the remnant risk of anti-D immunization by 50% to 80% (summarized by Jones et al[39]). However, in all studies reported in the literature, the number of included women was small and no randomized trials have been conducted.

The effect of the Dutch schedule of a single dose of 1000 IU was established in a nationwide study over a 3-year duration, including 21,000 pregnant para-1 women who gave birth to a D+ child in their first pregnancy just before or after the introduction of RAADP.[38] In this study for all immunized individual patients, data on previous prophylaxis were carefully collected. The prevalence of anti-D immunization at first trimester screening in the next pregnancy decreased from 671/100,000 [95% confidence interval (CI) = 499-843] in women with only postnatal anti-D after the first delivery to 310/100,000 (95% CI = 213-407) in women who received postnatal and antenatal anti-D, showing that the immunization risk is halved. Remarkably, no difference was observed in late immunizations detected at the 30th week of pregnancy. In the Dutch study, the observed sensitization risk in women receiving full prophylaxis (0.31%) was similar to the risk observed in a meta-analysis.[39] This might suggest that the single dose of 1000 IU at 30 weeks is equally effective as the schemes analyzed in these meta-analyses (2 × 500 IU at 28 and 34 weeks or a single dose of 1500 IU at the 28th week). But it should be emphasized that most of the other studies were community-based studies in which women were included in the intervention group who did not receive complete antenatal and postnatal prophylaxis.[40] In studies reporting a "true" sensitization rate in women who received antenatal prophylaxis, the immunization risk was lower[37] or even 0%.[36] However, these studies are too small to draw conclusions on the comparison of the different dosages.

The Dutch study was the first to study the effect of full prophylaxis on the incidence of subsequent severe HDFN.[38] The introduction of RAADP halved the incidence of subsequent severe HDFN from 230/100,000 to 104/100,000 women at risk (ie, D− women with a previous D+ child). An interesting observation was that although RAADP did not influence the incidence of late immunizations (detected only at the 30th week of pregnancy), the risk for severe HDFN caused by these "late" D antibodies was significantly lower after administration of antenatal and postnatal prophylaxis compared to the risk in women with only postnatal prophylaxis (3% vs 28%; $p = 0.02$). These data suggest that, at least in a subgroup of patients, the addition of antenatal prophylaxis has a long-lasting suppressive effect on the strength of the immune response. Possibly, women who encounter the RhD antigen for the first time in the presence of anti-D (which occurs during their first pregnancy), and who become immunized later, have an attenuated immune response.

It has even been suggested that RAADP given only during the first pregnancy provides some continuing long-term protection against immunization in subsequent pregnancies, but no strong clinical data are available to support this hypothesis.[34,40] However, some experimental data are in favor of the hypothesis of a protracted effect. For example, Mollison et al described a decreased response rate to repeated red cell injections in subjects who had previously been administered anti-D-coated red cells compared with those who received unmodified red cells.[41] A similar observation has been shown by Kumpel et al[42] when investigating the protective effect of monoclonal anti-D antibodies in 24 healthy volunteers. Only six of these volunteers had accelerated clearance of red cells after repeated subsequent unprotected challenging, which is lower than expected. Moreover, in one of these responders the level of anti-D was too low to detect serologically, and in the other five responders the levels of anti-D tended to decrease rapidly, unlike responses in individuals immunized by pregnancy or transfusion.

At present RAADP is administered to all D− women. It can be calculated that, in a population of European ethnicity, approximately 40% of D− women will carry a D− fetus and thus receive anti-D prophylaxis unnecessarily. Until recently, the only method of determining the fetal RhD type was by invasive procedures, such as amniocentesis or chorionic villus sampling, to obtain fetal cells for genetic analysis. These procedures carry a risk of miscarriage of up to 0.3% and may also lead to immunization in themselves. With the demonstration that maternal plasma and serum contain cell-free fetal DNA,[43] it became possible to determine fetal RHD genotype noninvasively.[44,45] In recent years, several groups have developed fully automated noninvasive RHD genotyping assays and have shown that it is indeed feasible and reliable to guide antenatal prophylaxis by these assays.[46-48]

Obstetric Conditions

Anti-D is also administered to nonimmunized D− women during pregnancy following an event that might allow fetal red cells to enter the maternal circulation. These events include ectopic pregnancy, invasive prenatal diagnosis (amniocentesis, chorionic villus sampling, cordocentesis), external version of the fetus, blunt abdominal trauma, or fetal death. Because of the lack of evidence, opinion is divided about the need to administer anti-D where there is uterine bleeding in the first trimester of a viable pregnancy.[30] Doses of anti-D given during pregnancy vary between countries, although mostly lower doses (50-100 μg) are administered in the first trimester, and then standard doses of 200 to 300 μg later in pregnancy.[21]

After Transfusion of D+ Blood Components

Because the D− antigen is highly immunogenic, transfusion of D+ blood to D− recipients should be avoided. However, where ABO-mismatched transfusions can be fatal, Rh typing is of less concern for immediate patient safety. Therefore, in emergency situations or during blood shortages, D+ red cells have been given to D− patients. Rarely, mismatched transfusions occur erroneously. Remarkably, the observed incidence of alloimmunization after mismatched transfusion is much lower (20%-30%)[49,50] than would be expected from earlier studies on healthy volunteers, in which 80% of subjects given D+ red cells became immunized.[51-53] This lower immunization risk might be the result of immune suppression caused by stress or underlying disease in some of the patients.[54,55]

For ethical reasons, the effectiveness of anti-D to prevent immunization after mismatched transfusion in patients has not been systematically studied, and all knowledge comes from case reports (almost exclusively of females of childbearing potential) and from studies of healthy volunteers. As mentioned earlier, a dose of 20 μg of anti-D protects against 1 mL of D+ red cells, and Pollock et al[56] have shown that this dose (given as 5-10 IM injections) was tolerable and successful in preventing immunization in 20 volunteers after transfusion of 500 mL of mismatched D+ blood. Nowadays preparations for IV administration are available, and when more than 1500 μg has to be given per injection site, intravenous administration is advised to diminish patient discomfort and to achieve a more rapid effect.[57] For the IV route, only 12 μg of anti-D is needed per 1 mL of D+ RBCs (or 2 mL of whole blood).[57] Too rapid a rate of destruction of large numbers of red cells must be avoided. In case of transfusion of more than 2 units of D+ blood, exchange transfusions should be considered. Several case reports of inadvertently mismatched transfused patients demonstrate that prevention of Rh immunization can be achieved using anti-D (reviewed by Ayache and Herman[58]), but, as mentioned above, the actual efficacy cannot be established.

Platelets do not express the D− antigen, but red cell contamination can be present in platelet concentrates. It is therefore advised to give

D− females of childbearing potential, or younger, Rh-matched platelet concentrates or to consider the administration of anti-D after an occasional mismatched platelet transfusion. However, most platelet concentrates are given to immunocompromised hematology/oncology patients, who are less susceptible to immunization. Indeed, the incidence of immunization by D+ platelet concentrates is very low and mainly seen in patients not suffering from hematologic malignancies.[55,59] Because the contamination with red cells in platelet concentrates is low (less than 2 mL), low doses of anti-D without risk of adverse effects is sufficient.

Treatment of Primary Immune Thrombocytopenia

Efficacy of Anti-D in Treatment of ITP

Primary ITP is an acquired autoimmune disorder defined by isolated thrombocytopenia and the exclusion of other causes of thrombocytopenia. ITP can be classified based on age (adult onset and childhood onset) and based on duration [acute or chronic (>6 months)].[60] Children typically present with a sudden onset a few weeks after an infectious illness, and in more than 70% of children the disease is self limiting. By contrast, ITP in adults has an insidious onset and has a chronic course. Patients with platelet counts below 20,000/μL may have a significant risk of fatal bleedings, mostly intracranial hemorrhage. The main mechanism of platelet destruction in ITP is the clearance of autoantibody-coated platelets by Fcγ receptor (FcγR)-expressing cells, mainly in the spleen or liver. This is supported by the observation that platelet counts in ITP could be increased by infusion of a monoclonal FcγRIII antibody.[61] In addition, cytotoxic T cells may have a role in platelet destruction,[62] and it is now generally accepted that platelet production may also be impaired in ITP.[63]

Corticosteroid therapy is the first-line treatment of ITP (reviewed by Godeau et al[64]). A short-term response is observed in more than two-thirds of patients, but only in approximately 30% is the response durable. IVIG is also a first-line treatment for patients with critical bleeding in whom the platelet count has to be rapidly increased and in patients not responding to corticosteroid therapy. In addition, it is well recognized that anti-D can be used in D+ patients with ITP to increase platelet counts.

Originally, it was observed that the rise in platelet counts 24 hours after anti-D administration was slower than after IVIG infusion,[65,66] but later studies showed that higher doses of anti-D (75 μg/kg) resulted in platelet kinetics similar to that with IVIG treatment.[67] Anti-D dose-response effects can be observed in individual patients,[68] and some patients require higher doses of anti-D (100 μg/kg) in order to achieve adequate platelet counts.[69] Scaradavou et al[66] performed an extensive study on 261 patients (124 children and 137 adults) who were treated with to 25 or 50 μg/kg of anti-D on day 1 and, if there was no response, repeated doses on days 3 and 4. A total of 189 patients (72%) responded to anti-D with an increase in platelet count ≥20,000 at day 7. The effect of anti-D lasted more than 21 days in 50% of the responders. All patient and age groups (acute, chronic, and human immunodeficiency syndrome-related ITP) responded. Andrew[70] also reported high response rates to anti-D in children.

In a subsequent study, it was shown that in patients treated with a higher dose of 75 μg/kg/day, the duration of the response could be increased to 46 days.[67] Unlike IVIG, anti-D Ig is less effective in splenectomized patients,[66] but there have been limited reports to suggest that some splenectomized patients with ITP do respond to anti-D treatment.[71] In a randomized clinical trial in adults with newly diagnosed ITP, intermittent anti-D has been compared with current routine care (glucocorticoid treatment followed by splenectomy).[72] Although anti-D deferred splenectomy for a short period, splenectomy could not be avoided. Alternative treatment strategies such as rituximab (a monoclonal CD20 antibody that eliminates B cells[73]) and especially the thrombopoietin receptor agonists eltrombopag and romiplostin[74] are far more promising in this respect.

A few small randomized trials in children compared the efficacy of anti-D and IVIG.[65,75,76] IVIG and 75 µg/kg anti-D were found to be equally effective in acute and chronic ITP in children.[75,76]

In conclusion, anti-D can be considered as a good alternative for IVIG. The cost of anti-D is substantially lower, and administration of anti-D requires a shorter infusion time (minutes). Because it is produced from a much smaller donor size, its safety profile should also be favorable. The use of anti-D is, however, restricted to D+ patients because, as expected, no effect was seen in D− patients.[68,77] Oksenhendler et al[77] have shown that in D− thrombocytopenic patients polyclonal anti-c can exert a similar therapeutic effect.

It should be mentioned that some authors have doubted the lack of effect in D− patients and suggested that other antibodies present in anti-D are mediating the effect in ITP.[78] These authors refer to Evans' syndrome, a severe autoimmune hemolytic anemia that occurs with severe ITP. The destruction of sensitized red cells does not prevent the destruction of sensitized platelets in this disease. Furthermore, a monoclonal anti-D that labeled the red cells better than that observed in ITP patients who were successfully treated with polyclonal anti-D did not lead to an increase in platelet count in six out of seven patients.[79]

Because of the potential for shortages of anti-D for immunoprophylaxis and because volunteers have to be immunized for the production of anti-D, many clinicians prefer the use of IVIG above anti-D.[78] However, different working mechanisms may underlie the beneficial effects of IVIG and anti-D, and thus some nonresponders to IVIG might benefit from anti-D treatment.[80,81] Related to this, Bussel et al[82] recently showed that the majority of patients who failed to respond to high-dose oral corticosteroids and/or IVIG did respond to combination IV therapy with IVIG, methylprednisolone, and anti-D.[82]

Adverse Effects of Anti-D in ITP Treatment

Anti-D induces extravascular hemolysis, an expected adverse reaction that is consistent with the presumed mechanism of action. Hemoglobin decreases by an average of 1.6 g/dL, with its nadir occurring 6 to 7 days after transfusion.[66,68] For patients with a hemoglobin level <100 g/L, it is therefore recommended to lower the initial dose of anti-D. In the first 4 years after licensing of anti-D for its use in ITP, the FDA reported 15 unexpected cases of hemoglobinemia and/or hemoglobinuria.[83] The temporal association between anti-D administration and the onset of symptoms suggested a causal relationship. Additional case reports of acute hemolysis were published, but given the large number of patients treated with anti-D, the frequency appeared to be low.[84] Diffuse intravascular coagulation (DIC) is a potential complication of hemoglobinemia. Indeed, in 2005, Gaines et al[82] reported six cases of DIC associated with "acute hemolysis" following anti-D treatment for ITP, five of which involved fatalities.[85] Because of these reports, the United Kingdom has suspended the use of anti-D for the treatment of ITP.

The mechanism for acute hemolysis occurring in a small number of patients after IV anti-D therapy for ITP is not known.[86,87] The onset, symptoms, and complications are compatible with the intravascular hemolysis of acute hemolytic transfusion reactions. However, anti-D cannot activate complement. Only a single D antibody can bind to each D antigen, which is deeply buried in the membrane, and the D antigens are too far apart from one another on the red cell surface to activate complement. Nevertheless, some C1q binding has been shown on cells heavily coated with anti-D, but C1r and C1s are not activated.[88] Anti-D is made from pooled plasma, and many other antibodies, including other blood group specificities, are present.[89] It might be possible that these antibodies initiate the hemolysis. However, Gaines et al could not detect any incompatibility in vitro with a hemolysin assay, including in the red cells of a patient who experienced acute hemolysis after anti-D administration.[90] Therefore, possibly, antibodies against non-red-cell antigens might initiate complement activation and cause bystander lysis of red cells.

Conclusion

In summary, anti-D has been highly successful at preventing Rh immunization in the setting of HDFN as well as in the treatment of ITP. Future studies aimed at understanding its adverse effects, its mechanism of action, and the design of a potential replacement, are awaited.

References

1. Stern K, Goodman HS, Berger M. Experimental isoimmunization to hemoantigens in man. J Immunol 1961;87:189-98.
2. Finn R, Clarke CA, Donohoe WT, et al. Experimental studies on the prevention of Rh haemolytic disease. Br Med J 1961;1:1486-90.
3. Clarke CA, Donohoe WTA, McConnell RB, et al. Further experimental studies in the prevention of Rh-haemolytic disease. Br Med J 1963; 1:979-84.
4. Freda VJ, Gorman JG, Pollack W. Successful prevention of experimental Rh sensitization in man with an anti-Rh gamma 2-globulin antibody preparation: A preliminary report. Transfusion 1964;4:26-32.
5. Preisler O, Schneider J. Attempts at preventing the sensitization of RH-negative women by antibody-containing sera. Geburtshilfe Frauenheilkd 1964;24:124-31.
6. Zipursky A, Israels LG. The pathogenesis and prevention of Rh immunization. Can Med Assoc J 1967;97:1245-57.
7. Clarke CA, Sheppard PM. Prevention of Rhesus haemolytic disease. Lancet 1965;2:343.
8. Freda VJ, Gorman JG, Pollack W, et al. Prevention of Rh isoimmunization. Progress report of the clinical trial in mothers. JAMA 1967;199:390-4.
9. Salama A, Mueller-Eckhardt C, Kiefel V. Effect of intravenous immunoglobulin in immune thrombocytopenia: Competitive inhibition of reticuloendothelial system function by seques-tration of autologous red blood cells? Lancet 1983;2:193-5.
10. Salama A, Kiefel V, Amberg R, Mueller-Eckhardt C. Treatment of autoimmune thrombocytopenic purpura with rhesus antibodies [anti-Rho(D)]. Blut 1984;49:29-35.
11. Power JP, Lawlor E, Davidson F, et al. Hepatitis C viraemia in recipients of Irish intravenous anti-D immunoglobulin. Lancet 1994;344:1166-7.
12. Smith DB, Lawlor E, Power J, et al. A second outbreak of hepatitis C virus infection from anti-D immunoglobulin in Ireland. Vox Sang 1999;76:175-80.
13. Kumpel BM. Efficacy of RhD monoclonal antibodies in clinical trials as replacement therapy for prophylactic anti-D immunoglobulin: More questions than answers. Vox Sang 2007;93:99-111.
14. Smith GN, Griffith B, Mollison D, Mollison PL. Uptake of IgG after intramuscular and subcutaneous injection. Lancet 1972;1:1208-12.
15. Bowman JM, Pollock JM. Failures of intravenous Rh immune globulin prophylaxis: An analysis of the reasons for such failures. Transfus Med Rev 1987;1:101-12.
16. Bichler J, Schöndorfer G, Pabst G, Andresen I. Pharmacokinetics of anti-D IgG in pregnant Rh D− negative women. BJOG 2003;110:39-45.
17. Meyer O, Kiesewetter H, Hermsen M, et al. Replacement of intravenous administration of anti-D by subcutaneous administration in patients with autoimmune thrombocytopenia. Pediatr Blood Cancer 2006;47(Suppl):721-2.
18. Eklund J, Hermann M, Kjellman H, Pohja P. Turnover rate of anti-D IgG injected during pregnancy. Br Med J 1982;284:854-5.
19. MacKenzie IZ, Roseman F, Findlay J, et al. The kinetics of routine antenatal prophylactic intramuscular injections of polyclonal anti-D immunoglobulin. BJOG 2006;113:97-101.
20. Samson D, Mollison PL. Effect on primary Rh-immunization of delayed administration of anti-Rh. Immunology 1975;28:349-57.
21. Engelfriet CP, Reesink HW, Judd WJ, et al. Current status of immunoprophylaxis with anti-D immunoglobin. Vox Sang 2003;85:328-37.
22. Tovey DLA, Robinson AE. Reduced severity of Rh-haemolytic disease after anti-D immunoglobulin. Br Med J 1975;4:320-2.
23. Huchet J, Defossez Y, Brossard Y. Detection of transplacental hemorrhage during the last trimester of pregnancy. Transfusion 1988;28:506.

24. Ness PM, Baldwin ML, Niebyl JR. Clinical high-risk designation does not predict excess fetal-maternal hemorrhage. Am J Obstet Gynecol 1987;156:154-8.
25. Salim R, Ben Shlomo I, Nachum Z, et al. The incidence of large fetomaternal hemorrhage and the Kleihauer-Betke test. Obstet Gynecol 2005;105:1039-44.
26. Koelewijn JM, de Haas M, Vrijkotte TG, et al. Risk factors for RhD immunisation despite antenatal and postnatal anti-D prophylaxis. BJOG 2009;116:1307-14.
27. Garratty G. Do we need to be more concerned about weak D antigens? Transfusion 2005;45:1547-51.
28. Matthews CD, Matthews AE, Gilbey BE. Antibody development in rhesus-negative patients following abortion. Lancet 1969;2:318-9.
29. Simonovits I, Timár I, Bajtai G. Rate of Rh immunization after induced abortion. Vox Sang 1980;38:161-4.
30. Urbaniak SJ. Consensus conference on anti-D prophylaxis, April 7 and 8, 1997: Final consensus statement. Royal College of Physicians of Edinburgh/Royal College of Obstetricians and Gynaecologists. Transfusion 1998;38:97-9.
31. Tovey LA, Townley A, Stevenson BJ, Taverner J. The Yorkshire antenatal anti-D immunoglobulin trial in primigravidae. Lancet 1983;2:244-6.
32. Bowman JM, Chown B, Lewis M, Pollock JM. Rh isoimmunization during pregnancy: Antenatal prophylaxis. CMAJ 1978;118:623-7.
33. Trolle B. Prenatal Rh-immune prophylaxis with 300 micrograms immune globulin anti-D in the 28th week of pregnancy. Acta Obstet Gynecol Scand 1989;68:45-7.
34. Thornton JG, Page C, Foote G, et al. Efficacy and long term effects of antenatal prophylaxis with anti-D immunoglobulin. Br Med J 1989;298:1671-5.
35. Lee D, Rawlinson VI. Multicentre trial of antepartum low dose anti-D immunoglobulin. Transfus Med 1995;5:15-9.
36. Mayne S, Parker JH, Harden TA, et al. Rate of RhD sensitisation before and after implementation of a community based antenatal prophylaxis programme. Br Med J 1997;315:1588.
37. MacKenzie I, Bowell P, Gregory H, et al. Routine antenatal rhesus D immuoglobulin prophylaxis: The results of a prospective 10 year study. Br J Obstet Gynaecol 1999;106:492-7.
38. Koelewijn JM, de Haas M, Vrijkotte TG, et al. One single dose of 200 microg of antenatal RhIG halves the risk of anti-D immunization and hemolytic disease of the fetus and newborn in the next pregnancy. Transfusion 2008;48:1721-9.
39. Jones ML, Wray J, Wight J, et al. A review of the clinical effectiveness of routine antenatal anti-D prophylaxis for rhesus-negative women who are pregnant. BJOG 2004;111:892-902.
40. MacKenzie IZ, Roseman F, Findlay J, et al. Clinical validation of routine antenatal anti-D prophylaxis questions the modelling predictions adopted by NICE for Rhesus D sensitisation rates: Results of a longitudinal study. Eur J Obstet Gynecol Reprod Biol 2008;139:38-42.
41. Mollison PL, Frame M, Ross ME. Differences between Rh(D) negative subjects in response to Rh(D) antigen. Br J Haematol 1970;19:257-66.
42. Kumpel BM, Goodrick MJ, Pamphilon DH, et al. Human Rh D monoclonal antibodies (BRAD-3 and BRAD-5) cause accelerated clearance of Rh D+ red blood cells and suppression of Rh D immunization in Rh D− volunteers. Blood 1995;86:1701-9.
43. Lo YMD, Corbetta N, Chamberlain PF, et al. Presence of fetal DNA in maternal plasma and serum. Lancet 1997;350:485-7.
44. Faas BH, Beuling EA, Christiaens GC, et al. Detection of fetal RhD-specific sequences in maternal plasma. Lancet 1998;352:1196.
45. Lo YM, Hjelm NM, Fidler C, et al. Prenatal diagnosis of fetal RhD status by molecular analysis of maternal plasma. N Engl J Med 1998;339:1734-8.
46. Finning K, Martin P, Summers J, et al. Effect of high throughput RHD typing of fetal DNA in maternal plasma on use of anti-RhD immunoglobulin in RhD negative pregnant women: Prospective feasibility study. Br Med J 2008;336:816-8.
47. Van der Schoot CE, Soussan AA, Koelewijn J, et al. Non-invasive antenatal RHD typing. Transfus Clin Biol 2006;13:53-7.
48. Müller SP, Bartels I, Stein W, et al. The determination of the fetal D status from maternal plasma for decision making on Rh prophylaxis is feasible. Transfusion 2008;48:2292-301.
49. Frohn C, Dumbgen L, Brand JM, et al. Probability of anti-D development in D− patients receiving D+ RBCs. Transfusion 2003;43:893-8.

50. Yazer MH, Triulzi DJ. Detection of anti-D in D– recipients transfused with D+ red blood cells. Transfusion 2007;47:2197-201.
51. Gunson HH, Stratton F, Cooper DG, Rawlinson VI. Primary immunization of Rh-negative volunteers. Br Med J 1970;1:593-5.
52. Pollack W, Ascari WQ, Crispen JF, et al. Studies on Rh prophylaxis. II. Rh immune prophylaxis after transfusion with Rh-positive blood. Transfusion 1971;11:340-4.
53. Urbaniak SJ, Robertson AE. A successful program of immunizing Rh-negative male volunteers for anti-D production using frozen/thawed blood. Transfusion 1981;21:64-9.
54. Baldwin ML, Ness PM, Scott D, et al. Alloimmunization to D antigen and HLA in D-negative immunosuppressed oncology patients. Transfusion 1988;28:330-3.
55. Cid J, Ortin X, Elies E, et al. Absence of anti-D alloimmunization in hematologic patients after D-incompatible platelet transfusions. Transfusion 2002;42:173-6.
56. Pollack W, Ascari WQ, Kochesky RJ, et al. Studies on Rh prophylaxis. Relationship between doses of anti-Rh and size of antigenic stimulus. Transfusion 1971;11:333-9.
57. Parker J, Wray J, Gooch A, et al for the British Committee for Standards in Haematology. Guidelines for the use of prophylactic anti-D immunoglobulin. (June 2008) London: British Committee for Standards in Haematology, 2008. [Available at http://www.bcshguidelines.org/pdf/Anti-D_070606.pdf (accessed February 28, 2010).]
58. Ayache S, Herman JH. Prevention of D sensitization after mismatched transfusion of blood components: Toward optimal use of RhIG. Transfusion 2008;48:1990-9.
59. Atoyebi W, Mundy N, Croxton T, et al. Is it necessary to administer anti-D to prevent RhD immunization after the transfusion of RhD-positive platelet concentrates? Br J Haematol 2000;111:980-3.
60. Cines DB, Blanchette VS. Immune thrombocytopenic purpura. N Engl J Med 2002;346:995-1008.
61. Clarkson SB, Bussel JB, Kimberly RP, et al. Treatment of refractory immune thrombocytopenic purpura with an anti-Fc gamma-receptor antibody. N Engl J Med 1986;314:1236-9.
62. Olsson B, Andersson PO, Jernås M, et al. T-cell-mediated cytotoxicity toward platelets in chronic idiopathic thrombocytopenic purpura. Nat Med 2003;9:1123-4.
63. Ballem PJ, Segal GM, Stratton JR, et al. Mechanisms of thrombocytopenia in chronic autoimmune thrombocytopenic purpura. Evidence of both impaired platelet production and increased platelet clearance. J Clin Invest 1987;80:33-40.
64. Godeau B, Provan D, Bussel J. Immune thrombocytopenic purpura in adults. Curr Opin Hematol 2007;14:535-56.
65. Blanchette V, Imbach P, Andrew M, et al. Randomised trial of intravenous immunoglobulin G, intravenous anti-D, and oral prednisone in childhood acute immune thrombocytopenic purpura. Lancet 1994;344:703-7.
66. Scaradavou A, Woo B, Woloski BM, et al. Intravenous anti-D treatment of immune thrombocytopenic purpura: Experience in 272 patients. Blood 1997;89:2689-700.
67. Newman GC, Novoa MV, Fodero EM, et al. A dose of 75 microg/kg/d of i.v. anti-D increases the platelet count more rapidly and for a longer period of time than 50 microg/kg/d in adults with immune thrombocytopenic purpura. Br J Haematol 2001;112:1076-8.
68. Bussel JB, Graziano JN, Kimberly RP, et al. Intravenous anti-D treatment of immune thrombocytopenic purpura: Analysis of efficacy, toxicity, and mechanism of effect. Blood 1991;77:1884-93.
69. Varma M, Beautyman EJ, Grossbard ML. Optimal response to 100 microg/kg anti-Rh(D) in two patients who had suboptimal responses to 75 microg/kg anti-Rh(D). Am J Hematol 2009;84:124.
70. Andrew M, Blanchette VS, Adams M, et al. A multicenter study of the treatment of childhood chronic idiopathic thrombocytopenic purpura with anti-D. J Pediatr 1992;120:522-7.
71. Ramadan KM, El-Agnaf M. Efficacy and response to intravenous anti-D immunoglobulin in chronic idiopathic thrombocytopenic purpura. Clin Lab Haematol 2005;27:267-9.
72. Cooper N, Woloski BM, Fodero EM, et al. Does treatment with intermittent infusions of intravenous anti-D allow a proportion of adults with recently diagnosed immune thrombocytopenic purpura to avoid splenectomy? Blood 2002;99:1922-7.
73. Godeau B, Porcher R, Fain O, et al. Rituximab efficacy and safety in adult splenectomy candidates with chronic immune thrombocytopenic purpura: Results of a prospective multicenter phase 2 study. Blood 2008;112:999-1004.

74. Nurden AT, Viallard JF, Nurden P. New-generation drugs that stimulate platelet production in chronic immune thrombocytopenic purpura. Lancet. 2009;373:1562-9.
75. Tarantino MD, Young G, Bertolone SJ, et al. Acute ITP Study Group. Single dose of anti-D immune globulin at 75 microg/kg is as effective as intravenous immune globulin at rapidly raising the platelet count in newly diagnosed immune thrombocytopenic purpura in children. J Pediatr 2006;148:489-94.
76. El Alfy MS, Mokhtar GM, El-Laboudy MA, Khalifa AS. Randomized trial of anti-D immunoglobulin versus low-dose intravenous immunoglobulin in the treatment of childhood chronic idiopathic thrombocytopenic purpura. Acta Haematol 2006;115:46-52.
77. Oksenhendler E, Bierling P, Brossard Y, et al. Anti-RH immunoglobulin therapy for human immunodeficiency virus-related immune thrombocytopenic purpura. Blood 1988;71:1499-502.
78. Engelfriet CP, Reesink HW, Bussel J, et al. The treatment of patients with autoimmune thrombocytopenia with intravenous IgG-anti-D.Vox Sang 1999;76:250-5.
79. Godeau B, Oksenhendler E, Brossard Y, et al. Treatment of chronic autoimmune thrombocytopenic purpura with monoclonal anti-D. Transfusion 1996;36:328-30.
80. Cooper N, Heddle NM, Haas M, et al. Intravenous (IV) anti-D and IV immunoglobulin achieve acute platelet increases by different mechanisms: Modulation of cytokine and platelet responses to IV anti-D by FcgammaRIIa and FcgammaRIIIa polymorphisms. Br J Haematol 2004;124:511-8.
81. Bussel JB, Kaufmann CP, Ware RE, Woloski BM. Do the acute platelet responses of patients with immune thrombocytopenic purpura (ITP) to IV anti-D and to IV gammaglobulin predict response to subsequent splenectomy? Am J Hematol 2001;67:27-33.
82. Boruchov DM, Gururangan S, Driscoll MC, Bussel JB. Multiagent induction and maintenance therapy for patients with refractory immune thrombocytopenic purpura (ITP). Blood 2007;110:3526-31.
83. Gaines AR. Acute onset hemoglobinemia and/or hemoglobinuria and sequelae following Rh(o)(D) immune globulin intravenous administration in immune thrombocytopenic purpura patients. Blood 2000;95:2523-9.
84. Boughton BJ, Chakraverty R, Baglin TP, et al. The treatment of chronic idiopathic thrombocytopenia with anti-D (Rho)immunoglobulin: Its effectiveness, safety and mechanism of action. Clin Lab Haematol 1988;10:275-84.
85. Gaines AR. Disseminated intravascular coagulation associated with acute hemoglobinemia or hemoglobinuria following Rh(0)(D) immune globulin intravenous administration for immune thrombocytopenic purpura. Blood 2005;106:1532-7.
86. Tarantino MD, Bussel JB, Cines DB, et al. A closer look at intravascular hemolysis (IVH) following intravenous anti-D for immune thrombocytopenic purpura (ITP). Blood 2007;109:5527.
87. Garratty G. What is the mechanism for acute hemolysis occurring in some patients after intravenous anti-D therapy for immune thrombocytopenic purpura? Transfusion 2009;49:1026-31.
88. Hughes-Jones N, Ghosh S. Anti-D-coated Rh-positive red cells will bind the first component of the complement pathway, C1q. FEBS Lett 1981;128:318-20.
89. Rushin J, Rumsey DH, Ewing CA, Sandler SG. Detection of multiple passively acquired alloantibodies following infusions of IV Rh immune globulin. Transfusion 2000;40:551-4.
90. Gaines AR, Lee-Stroka H, Byrne K, et al. Investigation of whether the acute hemolysis associated with Rh(D) immune globulin intravenous (human) administration for treatment of immune thrombocytopenic purpura is consistent with the acute hemolytic transfusion reaction model. Transfusion 2009;49:1050-8.

11

Monoclonal Antibodies in Hematology

Roberto Stasi, MD, PhD; Fenella Willis, MD, FRCP, FRCPath;
Ruth Pettengell, MD; Muriel S. Shannon, MD; and
Edward C. Gordon-Smith, MD

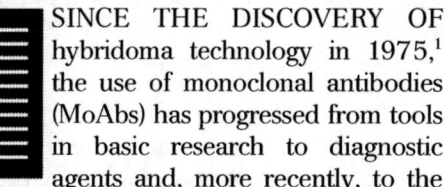SINCE THE DISCOVERY OF hybridoma technology in 1975,[1] the use of monoclonal antibodies (MoAbs) has progressed from tools in basic research to diagnostic agents and, more recently, to the status of bona fide therapeutic agents in various clinical areas, such as oncology, autoimmunity, and cardiovascular disease. Initial therapeutic antibodies were simple murine analogues, which contributed to the early lack of success. It has since been shown that these antibodies 1) have a short half-life in vivo because of the development of human mouse antibodies (HAMA), 2) have limited penetration into tumor sites, and 3) inadequately recruit host effector functions.[2] It is therefore not surprising that the only real success of murine therapeutic MoAbs was muromonab (Orthoclone OKT3, Ortho Biotech, Raritan, NJ), a CD3 antibody that induced strong immunosuppression needed to help control the rejection of renal grafts.[3]

To overcome the limitations of mouse MoAbs, several technical issues had to be addressed using new strategies. While hybridoma technology has been replaced by recombinant DNA technology, transgenic mice, and phage display, chimeric and humanized antibodies have generally replaced murine antibodies in modern therapeutic antibody applications.[4] Four major antibody generations have been developed and are characterized by progressive reduction of the xenogeneic protein (Fig 11-1): murine (100% mouse protein), chimeric (34% mouse protein), humanized (5%-10% mouse protein), and human (100% human protein).[5]

Roberto Stasi, MD, PhD, Consultant Hematologist; Fenella Willis, MD, FRCP, FRCPath, Consultant Haematologist; Ruth Pettengell, MD, Senior Lecturer in Haematology and Honorary Consultant in Oncology; Muriel S. Shannon, MD, Consultant Haematologist; and Edward C. Gordon-Smith, MD, Emeritus Professor of Haematology, Department of Haematology, St George's Hospital, London, United Kingdom

The authors have disclosed no conflicts of interest.

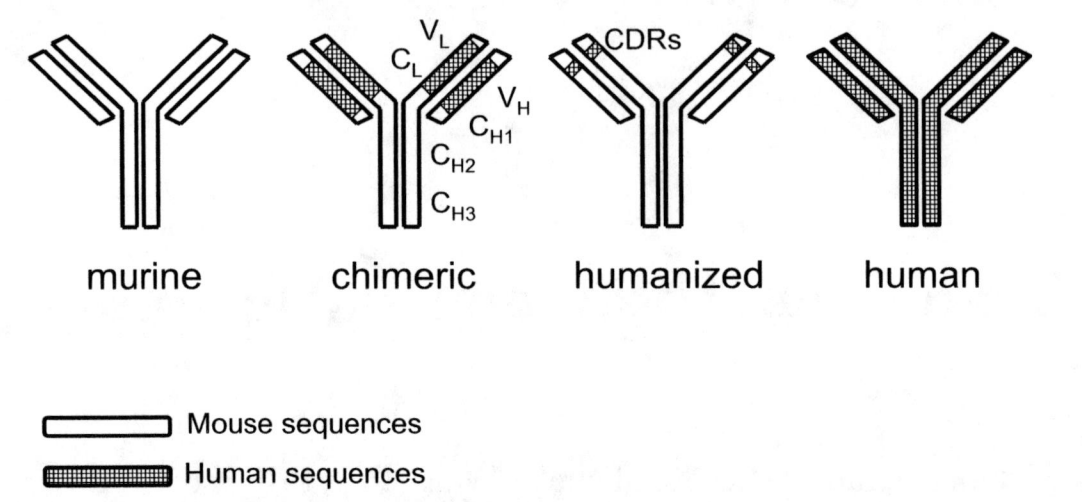

Figure 11-1. Sequence of antibody generations developed for clinical purposes. Murine monoclonal antibodies (MoAbs) originate from hybridoma technology following immunization of mice or, less commonly, rats. Cloning of mouse variable genes into human constant-region genes generates chimeric antibodies: mouse V_L to human C_L and mouse V_H to human C_{H1}-C_{H2}-C_{H3} for light and heavy chains, respectively. Humanized antibodies are created by grafting the antigen-binding loops, known as complementarity-determining regions (CDRs), from a mouse MoAb into a human and onto human constant and variable domain frameworks; however, additional changes in the framework regions have, in several cases, been shown to be crucial in maintaining identical antigen specificity. Fully human antibodies are routinely obtained from very large, single-chain variable fragments (scFvs) or Fab phage display libraries. High-affinity human antibodies have also been obtained from transgenic mice that contain some, or preferably many, human immunoglobulin genes and genetically disrupted endogenous immunoglobulin loci. Immunization elicits the production of human antibodies recoverable using standard hybridoma technology.

The evolution in generation of MoAbs (ie, moving away from murine antibodies toward humanized or human antibodies) has drastically reduced (although not completely abrogated) immunogenicity, improved pharmacokinetics, and improved antibody-dependent cellular cytotoxicity (ADCC) with human mononuclear cells.

Another major advance has been the modification of unconjugated, or "naked," monoclonal antibodies for delivery of a toxin, radioisotope, cytokine, or other active molecule (immunoconjugates). Furthermore, it is now possible to design bispecific antibodies that can bind with their Fab regions both to target antigen and to a conjugate or effector cell. In fact, every intact antibody can bind to cell receptors or other proteins with its Fc region.

This chapter will review the use of currently marketed monoclonal antibodies and immunoconjugates in clinical hematology: rituximab, alemtuzumab, eculizumab, gemtuzumab ozogamicin, ibritumomab tiuxetan, and tositumomab. Regarding the description of the therapeutic efficacy of these agents, emphasis has been given to data from randomized Phase III trials.

Rituximab

Rituximab is a chimeric murine/human MoAb produced by recombinant technology. It contains the complementarity-determining regions of the murine anti-CD20 antibody 2B8 in conjunction with human kappa and IgG1 heavy-chain constant-region sequences. The vector was cloned into Chinese hamster ovarian cells as the production source of immunoglobulin.[6] Rituximab is composed of two heavy chains of 451 amino acids and two light chains of 213 amino acids with a molecular weight of 145 kD. It binds specifically to CD20, a cell-surface antigen specific to B cells,[7] with an affinity of approximately 8.0 nM, which is similar to the parent murine antibody, 2B8.[6] With the exception of plasma cells, the CD20 molecule is present on all normal B cells after the pro-B-cell state[7] and on >90% of non-Hodgkin lymphoma (NHL) cells and ~14% of chronic lymphocytic leukemia (CLL) malignant B cells.[8] CD20 regulates cell cycle initiation and, possibly, functions as a calcium channel.

The proposed mechanisms for the elimination of B cells by rituximab (Fig 11-2) include complement-dependent cytotoxicity (CDC),[9] ADCC,[10] and signaling-induced apoptosis[6] as well as synergistic effects with corticosteroids,[11] chemotherapeutic agents, and radiation therapy.[12] Engagement of Fc receptors (FcγRs) on effector cells appears to be an important component of the in-vivo antitumor activity of rituximab. Using Fc-deficient mice that cannot express FcγRIII, the stimulatory Fc receptor,

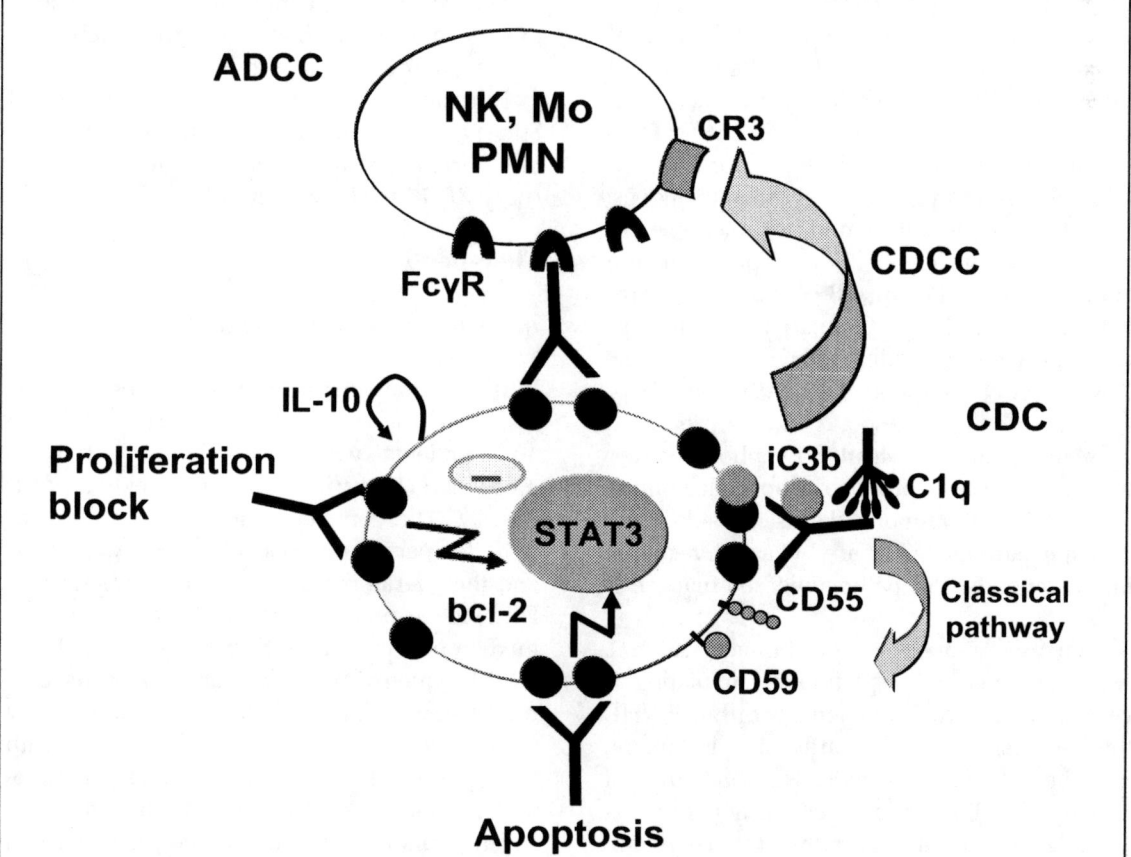

Figure 11-2. Principal mechanisms of B-cell depletion induced by rituximab. The cytotoxic effects of rituximab on CD20-positive malignant B cells appear to involve complement-dependent cytotoxicity (CDC), complement-dependent cellular cytotoxicity (CDCC), antibody-dependent cellular cytotoxicity (ADCC), and induction of apoptosis.

NK = natural killer (cell); Mo = monocyte; PMN = polymorphonuclear (cell); FcγR = Fc gamma receptor; IL-10 = interleukin-10.

Clynes et al demonstrated that the efficacy of rituximab in mouse xenograft models required engagement by the antibody of this receptor.[13] Furthermore, retrospective studies have indicated that certain polymorphisms of the IgG Fc receptor may affect the activation and killing function of cytotoxic cells and predict response to rituximab in patients with follicular lymphoma.[14] However, most of the resistance developed against rituximab by malignant cells is reported to be through complement regulatory proteins such as CD55 and CD59 on target cells.[15] This finding may suggest that complement-mediated B-cell depletion is the main mechanism involved in the rituximab effect on malignant B cells.[16,17]

B-cell depletion has been used in clinical practice not only to eradicate malignant B-cell clones but also to modulate the deranged mechanisms of autoimmune disorders. In a healthy immune system, B cells are tolerant of autoantigens and will bind only to alloantigens. B cells acquire this immune tolerance to autoantigens during their development in the marrow, where immature B cells that recognize autoantigens undergo apoptosis or change their antigen specificity. Additionally, B cells that recognize soluble autoantigens in the periphery loose their ability to respond and are prevented from migrating to follicular lymphoid tissues, where they would produce a normal immune response.[18] Autoimmune diseases result when such mechanisms fail or are bypassed, resulting in the generation of pathogenic, self-reactive B cells.[19,20]

Rituximab induces a rapid (usually within 1 week) and marked depletion of circulating B cells in the majority of patients with B-cell NHL that persists for 3 to 6 months after treatment, until hematopoietic stem cells (which do not express CD20) effect recovery of lymphopenia 9 to 12 months after treatment.[21] There are some indications that prolonging the administration of rituximab beyond induction therapy would continue to suppress the B-cell population and, thus, prevent the re-emergence of deranged B-cell clones.[22] The same pattern of B-cell depletion and recovery is observed in autoimmune diseases such as immune thrombocytopenia[23] (ITP, previously referred to as idiopatic thrombocytopenic purpura; Fig 11-3) and rheumatoid arthritis.[24]

The half-life of rituximab in NHL elimination is proportional to dose, and wide ranges reflect variable tumor burden and changes in CD20-positive B-cell populations with repeated doses. At the standard dose of 375 mg/m^2 weekly for 4 consecutive weeks, the mean half-life of rituximab was 3.2 days (range = 1.3 to 6.4 days) following the first dose, and 8.6 days (range = 3.5 to 17 days) following the fourth dose.[25,26] In RA, where rituximab is given at the dose of 1000 mg every other week for two doses (roughly equivalent to the standard four-dose regimen when applied to a 1.73-m^2 adult), the mean terminal half-life of rituximab after the second dose was 19 to 22 days.[27]

Rituximab has been approved in the United States and Europe since 1997 for the treatment of different forms of B-cell NHL and since February 2006 for treatment of RA.

Therapeutic Efficacy

Indolent Non-Hodgkin Lymphoma

Rituximab was first licensed on the basis of the results of the pivotal Phase II trial, in which 166 patients with relapsed indolent NHL received 375 mg/m^2 rituximab weekly for four doses.[28] The complete response (CR) rate was 6%, the partial response (PR) rate was 42%, and the overall response (OR) rate was 48%.[28] Durable responses were achieved despite a median of 3 prior therapies (range = 1-10).

Subsequent Phase III trials comparing chemotherapy with rituximab vs chemotherapy alone were conducted in adult patients with both previously untreated and relapsed indolent or mantle cell NHL. In a meta-analysis of seven randomized trials involving 1943 patients,[29] patients treated with rituximab-containing regimens, as compared to those treated with the same regimens not containing rituximab, had a significantly higher overall response rate [relative risk of obtaining a tumor response = 1.21; 95% confidence interval (CI) = 1.16 to1.27], improved disease control (haz-

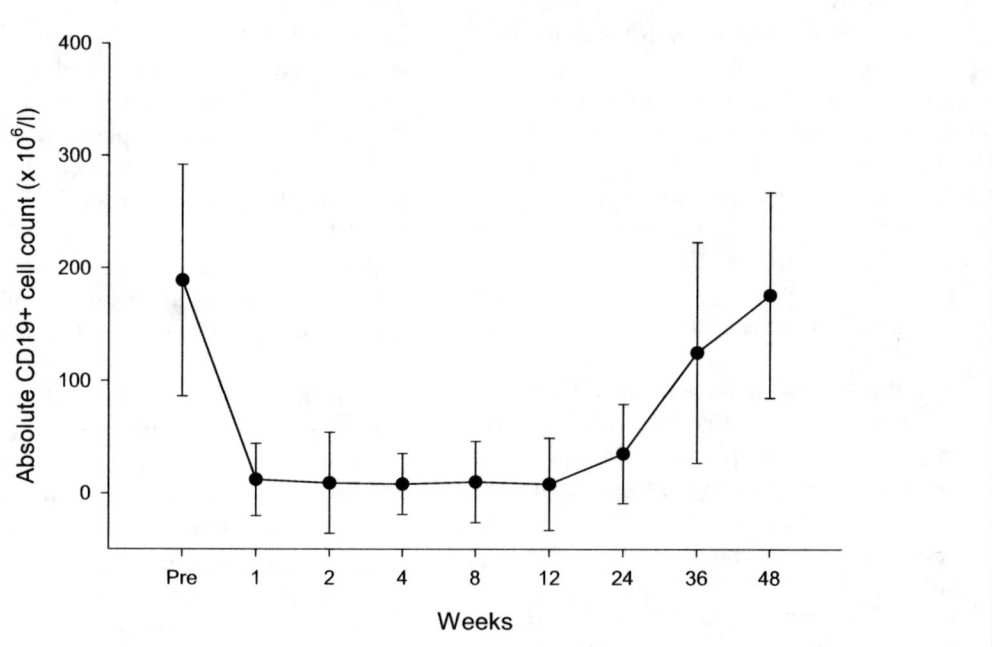

Figure 11-3. CD19+ lymphocyte (B-cell) counts over the course of rituximab treatment and during follow-up in 25 patients with chronic immune thrombocytopenia. Each data point represents the mean (±SD) CD19+ cell count at a particular time (Stasi et al, unpublished data).

ard ratio of developing a disease-associated event = 0.62; 95% CI = 0.55 to 0.71), and better overall survival (OS) [hazard ratio (HR) for mortality = 0.65; 95% CI = 0.54 to 0.78].

The rituximab dose in these trials was the recommended 375 mg/m². The chemotherapy regimens administered with rituximab as frontline therapy included cyclophosphamide, doxorubicin, vincristine, and prednisone (CHOP)[30]; mitoxantrone, chlorambucil and prednisone[31]; cyclophosphamide, vincristine and prednisone[32]; and cyclophosphamide, doxorubicin, etoposide, and prednisone.[33] Those used as second-line treatment for relapsed or refractory follicular NHL included fludarabine, cyclophosphamide, and mitoxantrone[34] as well as CHOP.[35] Where reported, immunochemotherapy regimens were administered in six or eight cycles; rituximab was generally administered on the first day of each chemotherapy cycle. Tumor responses and disease progression were determined using the standardized criteria for NHL (as defined by the International Workshop).[36]

No available data from randomized trials have addressed the issue of maintenance rituximab following first-line rituximab/chemotherapy. The Primary Rituximab and Maintenance (PRIMA) trial of rituximab maintenance vs observation alone after a variety of immunochemotherapy regimens in previously untreated indolent NHL has completed accrual, and results are expected shortly. Nevertheless, a recent meta-analysis has addressed the value of maintenance therapy with single-agent rituximab, 375 mg/m² (four once-weekly doses repeated every 6 months or a single infusion every 2-3 months, for up to 2 years or until relapse).[37] Five trials including 1143 adult patients with follicular lymphoma were included, with data on OS available for 985 patients. Those treated with maintenance rituximab had statistically significantly better OS than patients in the observation arm or patients treated at relapse (HR for death = 0.60; 95% CI = 0.45 to 0.79). Significantly, only patients with refractory or relapsed (ie, previously treated) follicular lymphoma had a survival benefit with maintenance rituximab therapy (HR for death = 0.58; 95% CI = 0.42 to 0.79), whereas previously untreated patients did not (HR for death = 0.68; 95% CI = 0.37 to 1.25).

Chronic Lymphocytic Leukemia

Two of the largest trials ever conducted in patients with CLL show that the addition of rituximab to fludarabine plus cyclophosphamide significantly improves outcomes. One of the trials, known as CLL8,[38] used the new combination as first-line treatment for previously untreated patients; the other trial, known as REACH (Rituximab Plus Chemotherapy in Relapsed/Refractory Chronic Lymphocytic Leukemia),[39] used it as second-line treatment in relapsed or refractory patients.

The CLL8 study was conducted in 817 patients with previously untreated CLL and good physical fitness, as defined by a cumulative illness rating scale score. Patients were randomized to 1 of 2 groups: six courses of fludarabine, 25 mg/m^2 intravenously on days 1 to 3 plus cyclophosphamide, 250 mg/m2 intravenously on days 1 to 3, every 28 days (the FC group); and both drugs plus rituximab (375 mg/m^2 intravenously) on day 0 at the first cycle and 500 mg/m2 on day 1 for all subsequent cycles, every 28 days (the FCR group).

Progression-free survival (PFS) at 2 years was 76.6% among patients in the FCR group and 62.3% among patients in the FC group (p <0.003). The overall response rate was significantly higher in the FCR group than in the FC group (95% vs 88%). Patients in the FCR groups also showed an improved CR rate compared with those in the FC group (52% vs 27%). There was a trend toward an OS benefit in the FCR group (91% vs 88% at 2 years; p = 0.18), but this was not significant. Hematologic toxicities were more common among patients in the FCR group, with severe hematologic toxicity occurring in 55% of patients in the FCR group and 39% in the FC group. There were significant differences observed for neutropenia (33.6% for FCR and 20.9% for FC; p = 0.0001) and leukocytopenia (24% for FCR and 12.1% for FC; p <0.0001), but not for thrombocytopenia (7.4% for FCR and 10.8% for FC; p = 0.09) or anemia (5.4% for FCR and 6.8% for FC; p = 0.42). However, the incidence of severe infections was similar between the two groups (18.8% for FCR and 14.8% for FC).

The REACH trial involved 552 patients with relapsed or refractory CLL who had received an average of 1 previous treatment. The drugs were given as outlined for the CLL8 trial. PFS was 30.6 months in the FCR group and 20.6 months in the FC group. The OR rate was significantly higher in the FCR than in the FC group (70% vs 58%). This was because of the superior CR rates in the FCR group compared with those in the FC group (24 % vs 13%). No new or unexpected toxicity was seen, and the FCR combination showed a favorable risk/benefit profile. Adverse events were seen in 80% of patients in the FCR group and 74% in the FC group, and serious adverse events were seen in 50% and 48%, respectively. The median OS in the FC group was 53 months, but it has not been reached yet in the FCR group; 80% of patients were still alive at the time of data analysis.

Aggressive NHL

The combination of rituximab, 375-mg/m^2 intravenous infusions, with a CHOP or a CHOP-like regimen, administered in six to eight cycles, was compared to chemotherapy alone as the first-line treatment in patients with advanced-stage, diffuse, large B-cell NHL or mantle-cell lymphoma (MCL) in several Phase III trials. In elderly patients with previously untreated advanced, diffuse, large B-cell lymphoma (DLBCL), rituximab plus CHOP (R-CHOP) was superior to CHOP in achieving a complete response (CR = 76% vs 63%) and in improving 5-year OS (58% vs 45%).[40,41]

A US Intergroup study also compared R-CHOP and CHOP in older patients (≥60 years old).[42] Patients were initially assigned to R-CHOP or CHOP, and responders received either no additional treatment or maintenance rituximab for 2 years. Whether rituximab was part of induction therapy or maintenance after CHOP, it significantly improved failure-free survival (the time from random assignment to relapse, nonprotocol treatment, or death). However, its continuing use after R-CHOP did not produce any substantial benefit.

The benefits of R-CHOP also extend to younger adults with DLBCL who have a good prognosis. The MabThera International Trial, designed by cooperative groups from 18 countries, was stopped early when it demonstrated the superiority of R-CHOP (or CHOP-like chemotherapy) over CHOP-like chemotherapy alone in that patient population.[43] At median follow-up of 34 months, event-free survival (EFS), PFS, and OS were significantly better in patients who received rituximab plus CHOP or CHOP-like chemotherapy than in those who received only chemotherapy. Only 21% of patients failed after chemotherapy plus rituximab, compared with 41% who failed after chemotherapy alone, suggesting that the proportion of young patients who need salvage treatment could be halved with rituximab. One of the CHOP-like chemotherapies, CHOEP (CHOP plus etoposide), was superior to CHOP with regard to EFS, but the comparison of R-CHOP and R-CHOEP showed no significant difference in EFS or OS. R-CHOP is therefore preferable to R-CHOEP because it has fewer toxic effects and is a 1-day regimen. Thus, the addition of rituximab to CHOP has been associated with improvements in OS and in EFS or PFS, without increased toxicity, in all patient groups studied (no data have been published on younger patients at high risk). The addition of rituximab to CHOP is now considered the standard of care for treatment of DLBCL with curative intent.

In addition, CHOP-14 (CHOP cycles given every 14 days) was compared with R-CHOP-14 in elderly patients with intermediate-to-aggressive B-cell NHL. In the RICOVER-60 (Rituximab with CHOP over 60) trial, elderly patients with stages I-IV DLBCL received six or eight cycles of CHOP-14 with granulocyte colony-stimulating factor support and with or without rituximab.[44] Radiotherapy was included for patients who had initial bulky disease and/or extranodal involvement. Using six cycles of CHOP-14 (6 × CHOP-14) as the comparator, EFS was significantly better in both rituximab arms, but OS was significantly better only with 6 × R-CHOP-14. These results suggest that addition of chemotherapy beyond six cycles, at least in elderly patients, is not justified.

Recruitment for a Phase III trial comparing R-CHOP-14 vs R-CHOP-21 is now complete, with 1080 patients (median age = 61 years) randomized.[45] A preliminary analysis indicates that R-CHOP-14 can be delivered as effectively as R-CHOP-21, with comparable levels of acute toxicity, but no data on survival outcomes are available yet. A similar Phase III study in elderly individuals by the French group GELA is still ongoing.

Other Lymphoproliferative Disorders

In a randomized, open-label, multicenter, Phase III trial, 64 evaluable patients with previously untreated lymphoplasmacytic lymphoma (LPL) were randomly assigned to R-CHOP (n = 34) or CHOP (n = 30).[46] In all, 48 of the 64 LPL patients fulfilled the criteria of Waldenström macroglobulinemia (WM). R-CHOP resulted in significantly higher OR rates (94% vs 67%; p = 0.0085) in the LPL patients and in the WM subgroup (91% vs 60%; p = 0.0188). R-CHOP also induced a significantly longer time-to-treatment failure, with a median of 63 months for R-CHOP vs 22 months in the CHOP arm in the LPL patients (p = 0.0033) and in the WM subgroup (p = 0.0241).

Rituximab has shown activity in other CD20-positive lymphoproliferative disorders, including B-cell acute lymphoblastic leukemia.[47] The risk/benefit ratio of adding rituximab to conventional therapies for these malignancies is being evaluated in ongoing Phase III trials.

Off-Label Uses

This section focuses on the three autoimmune hematologic diseases that account for most of the published literature on off-label use of rituximab: primary ITP, autoimmune hemolytic anemia (AIHA), and thrombotic thrombocytopenic purpura (TTP). The results in less common autoimmune disorders are summarized in recent reviews.[48,49]

Primary Immune Thrombocytopenia. A systematic review of Phase II studies using rituximab for the treatment of adults with chronic ITP included 19 eligible reports on efficacy (313 patients).[50] The pooled response rate (platelets $\geq 50 \times 10^9/L$) was 62.5%, the CR rate (platelets $\geq 150 \times 10^9/L$) was 46.3%, and the median duration of response was 10.5 months. In most studies, there were two patterns of response: the majority of responders (approximately 72%) responded to rituximab within 4 weeks, whereas the rest did not achieve a complete response until several weeks or even months after the start of rituximab therapy.[51] These distinct patterns of response suggest that rituximab may operate through at least two separate mechanisms. The rituximab response in early responders is too rapid to be explained by the depletion of autoantibodies. Instead, it has been proposed that in these patients, opsonized B cells block the macrophage Fc-receptor function, reducing the sequestration of platelets in the spleen.[23,52] Further, it has been speculated that the late and sustained responses are more likely to result from a reduction in autoantibody levels. However, the lack of direct correlation between platelet antibody levels and clinical response suggests that additional mechanisms involving T cells may also be at work.[53,54]

Although most studies using rituximab in ITP employed the same dose as is used to treat lymphoma (375 mg/m^2 weekly for 4 weeks), more recent reports suggest that treatment with four once-weekly doses of 100 mg (fixed-dose) rituximab can produce the same results.[55,56]

The use of rituximab as upfront therapy in patients with newly diagnosed ITP was investigated in a prospective randomized study.[57] The addition of rituximab to a therapeutic pulse of dexamethasone significantly improved the long-term rate of sustained response (platelets $>50 \times 10^9/L$ at 6 months) at 85 percent, more than double the rate of dexamethasone alone (39%). Even after failure of dexamethasone alone in 27 patients (defined as platelets $<20 \times 10^9/L$ within 6 months), salvage therapy with rituximab and dexamethasone was effective with a sustained response in more than half of the latter group.

Autoimmune Hemolytic Anemia. AIHA is classified as either warm AIHA or cold AIHA, depending upon the temperature at which the autoantibodies show maximal binding. Cold AIHA is subdivided into cold agglutinin syndrome (CAS) and paroxysmal cold hemoglobinuria. In rare cases, patients can have both warm and cold autoantibodies. In eight studies in warm AIHA, the use of rituximab produced a clinical response in 62 of 76 patients (82%).[58-65] Responses were assessed based on a reduction in reticulocyte count, absence of hemolysis, decreased need of transfusion, and normalization of hemoglobin, neutrophil, and platelet counts. Patients typically received three to four infusions at a dose of 375 mg/m^2 at weekly intervals, often in combination with other therapies. The association of AIHA with CLL did not affect the response rate to rituximab.[60,64] In this setting, one particularly effective protocol combined dexamethazone and cyclophosphamide with rituximab, leading to a response in 8 of 8 patients.[64]

With regard to CAS, a positive clinical response to rituximab was observed in 62% of 105 patients in four studies. A clinical response was defined as improvements in hemoglobin levels and serum IgM levels.

Both in warm AIHA and in CAS, rituximab was used according to the lymphoma protocol. No serious adverse events were reported.

Thrombotic Thrombocytopenic Purpura. Most cases of TTP are caused by a deficiency in a plasma metalloprotease, ADAMTS13 (<u>a</u> <u>d</u>isintegrin <u>a</u>nd <u>m</u>etalloproteinase with <u>t</u>hrombospondin motifs), which cleaves a specific peptide bond in plasma von Willebrand factor. The ADAMTS13 deficiency in patients with sporadic TTP usually results from the presence of inhibitory IgG autoantibodies, which have been detected in 70% to 80% of such patients.[66]

In five studies, rituximab therapy was effective in 60 of 61 patients (98%).[67-71] The objective parameters to measure response included improvements in hemoglobin levels, platelet counts, lactate dehydrogenase (LDH) elevation, ischemic signs, and need for plasma exchange. One study reported a decrease in ADAMTS13 titers after rituximab therapy.[67]

Patients with long-standing TTP appeared to respond as well to rituximab treatment as those being treated during their first acute episode. In addition, in two prospective trials, patients treated with rituximab during an acute refractory episode of TTP and those receiving rituximab for severe relapsing TTP achieved complete responses.[67,70] Patients receiving rituximab were refractory to at least one of the following: plasma exchange, corticosteroids, vincristine, splenectomy, immunosuppressive agents, or intravenous immunoglobulin. Most patients were treated with rituximab at lymphoma doses, and all patients received plasma exchange concurrently, at least until disease symptoms stabilized. However, how long plasma exchange should be delayed after rituximab treatment is a controversial issue. Some have recommended delaying plasma exchange for 72 hours after rituximab treatment to maximize the effect of the drug[72]; others maintain that an interval of 24 hours between rituximab treatment and plasma exchange is adequate.[73,74]

Safety

Greater than 80% of patients with NHL experience infusion-related reactions.[75] These generally occur during the first infusion, and the majority are classified as mild or moderate. Commonly reported symptoms include fever, chills, rigors, and general flu-like symptoms. Other reported symptoms include nausea, pruritus, angio-edema, asthenia, and hypotension. In rare instances, severe and fatal infusion-related reactions have occurred in lymphoma patients, which may be attributed to hypoxia, pulmonary infiltrates, adult respiratory distress syndrome, myocardial infarction, ventricular fibrillation, cardiogenic shock, or tumor lysis syndrome. Risk factors for serious infusion reactions in lymphoma patients include high tumor burden, high circulating-lymphocyte counts, and concurrent cardiovascular or pulmonary disease.[75] Rapid infusions of rituximab (90-minute infusion schedule: 20% of the dose administered in the first 30 minutes, and the remaining 80% administered over 60 minutes) with corticosteroid premedication appear to abrogate severe infusion reactions.[76,77] Also, the use of low-dose rituximab in autoimmune cytopenias has produced minimal infusion-related side effects.[55,78]

Approximately 30% of rituximab-treated NHL patients acquire some type of infection; however, infections are severe in only 1% to 2% of patients.[75] In randomized Phase III trials in rheumatoid arthritis, the infection rate was 35% to 41%,[24,79,80] with serious infections occurring in 1.2% to 3.7% of patients. A review of the use of rituximab in other autoimmune disorders found that, in 25 studies involving 389 patients, the incidence of serious infections varied from 2.8% to 45% (mean = 12.5%).[49] However, patients were frequently on concomitant immunosuppressive therapies, which also enhanced or contributed to susceptibility to infection. In this regard, a few cases of progressive multifocal leukoencephalopathy have been reported for US Food and Drug Administration (FDA)-approved or off-label use of rituximab in patients receiving or having received other immunosuppressive therapies.[81] Finally, reactivation of the hepatitis B virus is considered to be associated with immunosuppression caused by rituximab treatment. Among patients with aggressive lymphoma treated with R-CHOP who tested negative for hepatitis B surface antigen and positive for antibodies to hepatitis B core antigen, 25% developed hepatitis B virus reactivation.[82] Increase of hepatitis C virus RNA levels during or after rituximab-combination chemotherapy has also been described,[63,83] although the clinical significance of these findings are uncertain.

The incidence of human anti-chimeric antibodies (HACA) is very low in patients with NHL and does not influence the efficacy or toxicity of rituximab therapy.[75] On the other hand, in some patients with autoimmune disease, studies have reported the appearance of significantly high titers of HACA and reported that the presence of HACA was associated with failure to deplete B cells.[49]

Serum sickness, characterized by fever, rash, and arthralgias, can occur in a minority of patients, particularly in those with autoimmune conditions who receive rituximab and develop HACA. The rates of serum sickness ranged from 6% to 20% in patients receiving rituximab for pediatric chronic ITP or Sjögren syndrome.[84]

The following tests are recommended before initiating rituximab therapy: complete blood count with differential and CD19 counts; aspartate aminotransferase and alanine aminotransferase; hepatitis B and C virus; human immunodeficiency virus; electrocardiogram; the tuberculin test; and chest x-ray. These tests will identify patients with subclinical infections that could flare with use of rituximab and patients with borderline cardiac function that would be more likely to experience severe infusion-related adverse events. Also, no vaccine should be administered just before administration of the drug. It is unclear whether the immune response to vaccine after rituximab has been administered is sufficient. Therefore, when vaccinations are contemplated, these should be performed at least 1 month before drug administration. After therapy has been administered, the number of CD19+ cells can be monitored every 3 months to follow the return of B-cell counts. Some investigators use this marker to help them decide when to retreat. It is still unclear how often rituximab should be administered in patients with autoimmune diseases.

Alemtuzumab

Alemtuzumab (Campath-1H, Genzyme Corp, Cambridge, Massachusetts) is a humanized rat monoclonal antibody (rat IgG2b) directed against the CD52 antigen, a glycosylphosphatidylinositol (GPI)-anchored glycoprotein with an exceptionally short peptide sequence of only 12 amino acids and a single, complex, N-linked oligosaccharide. CD52, whose function is yet unknown,[85] is highly expressed on both normal and malignant lymphocytes (B and T cells) and is also found on monocytes, macrophages, and eosinophils, in addition to the male reproductive tract.[85] Because CD52 antigen is not expressed on CD34+ hematopoietic progenitor cells, alemtuzumab does not interfere with early hematopoietic progenitor cell development.[86]

After binding to CD52-bearing cells, alemtuzumab may cause cell death through host-effector mechanisms such as CDC,[87,88] ADCC,[89,90] or apoptosis.[91] Alemtuzumab shares the lympholytic activity of murine IgM and IgG2b predecessors but is significantly less immunogenic, thereby facilitating its use clinically.[92]

In a population study in patients with B-cell CLL (B-CLL), alemtuzumab displayed nonlinear time- and concentration-dependent pharmacokinetics.[93] Because of the large interpatient variability, which was probably reflective of differences in tumor burden among patients, no single estimate of half-life could be reported. When antigen concentration is high, plasma half-life is short (hours) because the MoAb binds to its epitope and is subsequently rapidly cleared from the blood. However, as the antigen is depleted, clearance from the plasma decreases and plasma half-life increases. As the MoAb accumulates, a new steady state is reached. Eventually, when the target is either totally depleted or saturated, the clearance of the MoAb will be at its slowest and half-life will be at its longest, approaching the half-life of endogenous IgG (~21 days).[93] A direct relationship between maximal trough concentrations and clinical outcomes was observed, with increasing alemtuzumab exposure resulting in a greater probability of positive tumor response.[94]

Alemtuzumab was initially approved by the FDA in 2001 under accelerated approval regulations for treatment of fludarabine-refractory B-CLL. Conversion to regular approval and expanded labeling for use as single-agent treatment for B-CLL was granted in 2007.

Therapeutic Efficacy

Alemtuzumab was initially approved for the treatment of patients with CLL who had failed both alkylating agents and fludarabine therapy based on the results of the pivotal Phase II study, in which 93 patients with fludarabine-relapsed or refractory disease were treated with intravenous alemtuzumab, 30 mg three times weekly for up to 12 weeks.[95] The median OS was 32 months among responding patients and 16 months for the entire cohort. Alemtuzumab was effective in clearing CLL from the peripheral blood and marrow compartments but induced lower responses in patients with bulky lymphadenopathy (>5-cm lymph-node diameter). The reason for this is not clear but may be related to decreased penetration of the antibody in bulky lymph nodes or mechanisms protecting against antibody-mediated killing at that site. Alemtuzumab has considerable efficacy in patients with high-risk cytogenetic profiles and is capable of inducing responses even at a molecular level in patients with relapsed and/or refractory CLL regardless of 17p deletion or TP53 mutation status.[96]

Subcutaneous administration of alemtuzumab produces similar efficacy in patients with relapsed/refractory CLL compared with intravenous alemtuzumab.[97]

Efficacy of alemtuzumab as first-line treatment was demonstrated in an open-label, international, multicenter, randomized trial of 297 patients with previously untreated, Rai stage I to IV B-CLL with progressive disease.[98] Patients in the alemtuzumab arm received intravenous alemtuzumab, 30 mg three times weekly for up to 12 weeks. The results from this study showed significantly superior response rates for alemtuzumab compared with chlorambucil (OR rate = 83% vs 56%; p <0.0001; and CR rate = 24% vs 2%; p <0.0001).

A Phase II trial investigated the activity and toxicity of subcutaneous alemtuzumab, 30 mg three times weekly (following dose escalation from 3 mg), as a first-line therapy in 41 patients with symptomatic CLL, with an extended treatment period of up to 18 weeks.[99] The OR rate among 38 evaluable patients was 87% (CR = 19%; PR = 68%), and no apparent difference in response rates was observed among patients with advanced-stage disease (OR = 81%; CR = 22%). However, CR was observed only among patients with minimal (<2-cm nodes) or no lymphadenopathy, and up to 18 weeks of therapy may be required to maximize response in the marrow (45% OR at 12 weeks vs 100% at 18 weeks). In a long-term follow-up analysis of the patients who responded to alemtuzumab therapy in this trial, the median time to treatment failure was 28 months (range = 4 to 102+ months).[100]

The potential use of alemtuzumab in combination with chemotherapy in CLL is actively being explored. After promising Phase II trials, a randomized, prospective, Phase III study is currently under way comparing the efficacy and safety of fludarabine and alemtuzumab (FluCam regimen) with fludarabine alone in patients with relapsed/refractory CLL.[101]

Alemtuzumab has shown activity and beneficial effects in a number of off-label settings, including other lymphoproliferative diseases such as T-cell NHL (including peripheral T-cell lymphomas), stem cell transplantation, and autoimmune disorders. A recent review has summarized the results in these conditions.[101] Currently, two registration trials are ongoing in Japan to evaluate the role of alemtuzumab in stem cell transplantation.

Safety

Toxicities occurring with alemtuzumab monotherapy are categorized as infusion-related, hematologic, and infectious events, and guidelines are available for their prevention and management.[102] In studies involving patients with relapsed/refractory CLL, the most common adverse events were infusion-related toxicities (eg, fever, rigors, nausea, dyspnea, hypotension), which were primarily grade 1 or 2 and resolved with continued therapy.[95] Infusion-related reactions associated with subcutaneous administration were reduced (except for local injection site reactions), and severe reactions were rare.[97] Hematologic toxicities with either routes of administration were generally transient and included thrombocytopenia (grade 3 or 4 in 27% to 50% of patients) and neutropenia (grade 3 or 4 in 34% to 67%).[101] Infectious events are common in patients with refractory CLL and occur as a result of decreased immune function associated with CLL itself as well as immunosuppression induced by prior therapeutic regimens. Grade 3 or 4 infections were reported in 24% to 35% of patients with relapsed and/or refractory CLL treated with alemtuzumab.[101] Cytomegalovirus (CMV) reactivation occurs in 10% to 30% of patients with relapsed and/or refractory disease treated with alemtuzumab, but deaths related to CMV are rare.[95] The consensus guidelines on the management of patients treated with alemtuzumab stress the importance of screening or monitoring for CMV reactivation and initiating therapy promptly with ganciclovir or its equivalent upon confirmation of reactivation.[102]

As expected, infusion-related reactions were common with first-line intravenous alemtuzumab therapy, but most reactions were mild, with grade 3 or 4 reactions in only 14% of patients.[98] The most commonly treated grade 3 or 4 emergent adverse events were hematologic toxicities, with grade 3 or 4 neutropenia and thrombocytopenia reported in 42% and 18% of patients respectively. The incidence of febrile neutropenia, however, was only 5% with intravenous alemtuzumab, which was comparable to the 3% incidence observed in the chlorambucil arm. Grade 3 or 4 infectious events occurred in 16% of patients (grade 3 in 15%) treated with alemtuzumab, with an additional 2% experiencing grade 3 or 4 CMV infection. The overall incidence of symptomatic CMV reactivation was 11%.

In the Phase II study of first-line therapy with subcutaneous alemtuzumab, infusion-related reactions (except for fever and local injection site reactions) were substantially reduced compared with intravenous delivery.[99] Reduced infusion reactions may be attributed to slower rate of absorption and accumulation in plasma. The incidence of severe hematologic toxicities with subcutaneous alemtuzumab was similar to that seen with intravenous administration of alemtuzumab, and no patients developed febrile neutropenia.

While intravenous and subcutaneous delivery of alemtuzumab appear to induce similar response rates (although there has been no formal trial showing the equivalency of the two routes of administration), the toxicity profile is clearly improved with the subcutaneous administration, which is now preferred in many centers.

Eculizumab

Eculizumab (5G1.1) is a IgG2/IgG4-kappa humanized murine monoclonal antibody that binds with high affinity to the complement protein C5, which ultimately prevents the assembly of the membrane attack complexes.[103] The IgG2/IgG4 hybrid constant region of eculizumab includes the CH1 and hinge regions of human IgG2 fused to the CH2 and CH3 regions of human IgG4 and lacks the ability to bind Fc receptor and to activate complement.[104] Inhibition of the complement cascade at the level of C5 conserves the patient's ability to generate early components of complement, particularly C3b. These early components of complement are necessary for the opsonization of microorganisms and clearance of immune complexes.[105] Terminal complement-mediated intravascular haemolysis is inhibited in patients with paroxysmal nocturnal hemoglobinuria (PNH) treated with eculizumab.[106]

Pharmacokinetic data were obtained from 40 patients receiving the FDA-approved dosage regimen. A standard one-compartment model was used to determine the population pharmacokinetics in patients receiving multiple doses of eculizumab. At week 26, the mean observed peak serum concentration was 194 ±76 µg/mL and the mean observed trough concentration 97 ±60 µg/mL. Studies have demonstrated that maintaining peak and trough levels of eculizumab >35 µg/mL were necessary in order to block serum hemolytic activity.[107,108] The clearance of eculizumab for a 70-kg patient with PNH using the model described has been reported at 22 mL/hour with a volume of distribution of 7.7 L. The half-life was reported as 272 hours (mean ± standard deviation).[109] No pharmacokinetic data are available for patients with renal hepatic impairment or for pediatric or geriatric patients.

Eculizumab was approved by the FDA and by the European Medicines Agency in 2007 for the treatment of PNH. Because it is estimated that 1 in 1 million people are diagnosed with PNH, eculizumab is considered an orphan drug by the FDA.

Therapeutic Efficacy

The safety and efficacy of eculizumab in patients with PNH were tested in a randomized, double-blind, placebo-controlled trial called TRIUMPH (Transfusion Reduction Efficacy and Safety Clinical Investigation Using Eculizumab in Paroxysmal Nocturnal Hemoglobinuria).[110] Patients aged 18 years and older were eligible if they fulfilled the following inclusion criteria: 1) had received at least four transfusions in the preceding year, 2) had at least 10% PNH type III erythrocytes (ie, erythrocytes that are completely deficient of GPI-anchored proteins CD55 and CD59), 3) had a platelet count of at least 100,000/mm^3, and 4) had LDH levels ≥1.5 × the upper limit of normal (as a marker of hemolysis). All patients received vaccinations against *Neisseria meningitidis*. Patients received intravenous eculizumab, 600 mg, or placebo every week for 4 weeks; intravenous eculizumab, 900 mg, or placebo the following week; and then intravenous eculizumab, 900 mg, or placebo every 2 weeks until week 26. A total of 43 patients were randomly assigned to receive eculizumab, and 44 were assigned to placebo. In 42 of 43 eculizumab patients, serum hemolytic activity was completely blocked by the dose of 900 mg every 2 weeks. Type III erythrocytes increased from 28.1 ±2.0% at baseline to 56.9 ±3.6% at 26 weeks in the eculizumab group. In the placebo group, type III erythrocytes remained the same (35.7 ±2.8% at baseline to 35.5 ±2.8% at 26 weeks; p <0.001 for eculizumab vs placebo at 26 weeks). During the study, a median of 0 units of Red Blood Cells was administered in the eculizumab group, as compared with 10 units in the placebo group (p <0.001). Clinically significant improvements were also found in the quality of life.

The results of a second Phase III study called SHEPHERD (Safety and Efficacy of the Terminal Complement Inhibitor Eculizumab in Patients with Paroxysmal Nocturnal Hemoglobinuria) have confirmed the results of the previous trial.[111] In addition, pooled data from three clinical trials demonstrated that eculizumab treatment decreased the overall thromboembolism rate in patients with PNH.[112]

Safety

The safety profile of eculizumab was established in the two Phase III trials.[110,111] Eculizumab was well tolerated, with an adverse-event profile comparable to placebo. The most frequent adverse events with eculizumab were headache, nasopharyngitis, back pain, and nausea. Antibody formation was detected in three patients receiving eculizumab in clinical trials; however, this did not affect the efficacy of the drug.[109] Patients should be monitored for serious hemolysis for at least 8 weeks after discontinuation of eculizumab because treatment increases the number of PNH erythrocytes.

Eculizumab carries a black-box warning for the potential increased risk of meningococcal infections and requires patients to receive the meningococcal vaccine at least 2 weeks before starting treatment for PNH.

Gemtuzumab Ozogamicin

Gemtuzumab ozogamicin (GO) is a humanized IgG4 anti-CD33 monoclonal antibody (hP67.6) conjugated to N-acetyl-gamma calicheamicin dimethyl hydrazide, a derivative of calicheamicin (Fig 11-4).[113] Calicheamicin is a naturally occurring hydrophobic enediyne antibiotic that was isolated from the actinomycete *Micromonospora echinospora calichensis*.[114] The anti-tumor

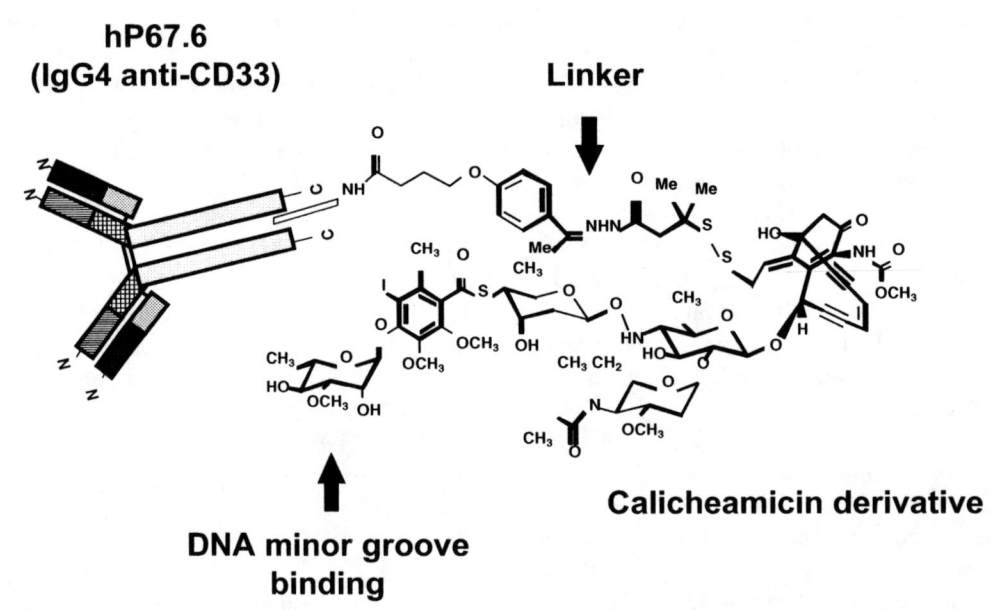

Figure 11-4. Schematic structure of gemtuzumab ozogamicin (GO). GO is composed of a humanized monoclonal antibody (hP67.6) joined to N-acetyl-gamma calicheamicin dimethyl hydrazide via 4-(4-acetylphenoxy)butanoic acid, a bifunctional linker.

mechanism of calicheamicin is thought to occur when it binds to the minor groove in the DNA and produces site-specific double-strand breaks by forming p-benzene diradical.[115] The CD33 antigen is a 67-kD sialic-acid-dependent adhesion protein that is specific for myeloid cells. CD33 is expressed in approximately 90% of acute myeloid leukemia (AML) cases, as defined by the presence of the antigen on greater than 20% of the leukemic blasts but not on normal CD34+ pluripotent hematopoietic stem cells or nonhematopoietic tissues.[116]

In-vitro data indicate that when GO binds the CD33 antigen, the complex is rapidly internalized.[117,118] Upon internalization, the calicheamicin derivative is released inside the lysosomes of the myeloid cell by acid hydrolysis. The released calicheamicin derivative binds to DNA in the minor groove, resulting in DNA double-strand breaks and cell death by apoptosis.

Pharmacokinetic parameters of the immunoconjugate were reported for patients with AML recruited for Phase I and II clinical trials,[119] and they are characterized by separate assays of the antibody portion of the conjugate as well as calicheamicin (total and unconjugated) in plasma. The elimination half-life of the hP67.6 antibody was highly variable after intravenous administration of the 9 mg/m^2 dose and ranged from 67 ±37 hours to 88 ±58 hours from dose period 1 to dose period 2.[120] The mean C_{max} of hP67.6 antibody following the first dose for patients who received 9 mg/m^2 GO was 3.0 mg/L, with values that ranged from 0.4 to 18.3 mg/L. The C_{max} increased to 3.6 mg/L (0.3 to 10.6 mg/L) after the second dose, and the increase was believed to be caused by a decrease in clearance by CD33-positive blast cells, a result of the reduced tumor burden following the first dose.[119]

Marketing approval of GO was granted in May 2000 by the FDA under the accelerated approval regulations.[120] GO was indicated for the treatment of patients with CD33-positive AML in first relapse who are 60 years of age or older and who are not considered candidates for cytotoxic chemotherapy. The approval of GO by the FDA was conditional on the conduct of studies of regimens combining it with standard anti-AML chemotherapy in patients with de novo AML.[120]

Therapeutic Efficacy

GO monotherapy in patients with AML in first relapse was first investigated in three pivotal Phase II multicenter trials in North America and Europe (studies 0903B1-201-US/CA, 0903B1-202-EU, and 0903B1-203-US/EU). Because of the similarity in study designs, objectives, patient demographics, and dosing schedules, data from the three studies were pooled to attain a larger efficacy population (277 patients). The initial report[121] was followed by a detailed subset analysis[122] and a final report.[123] The main inclusion criteria included CD33+ AML patients in first relapse (>5% leukemic blasts as determined by central flow cytometry laboratory tests). Patients with a median age of 61 years received GO, 9 mg/m^2, as a 2-hour intravenous infusion in two doses separated by 2 weeks. Further consolidation therapy [hematopoietic stem cell transplantation (HSCT) or other chemotherapy] was allowed 30 days after the marrow-clearing of blasts, indicating remission.

Using the 1988 criteria of the National Cancer Institute[124] (protocol-defined criteria), 13% of patients achieved a CR, and 13% a CRp (defined as all the criteria for CR except recovery to 100,000 platelets/µL). However, an additional analysis performed using the 2003 International Working Group (IWG) criteria[125] showed CR and CRp rates of 15% and 19%, respectively (Professor Sergio Amadori, personal communication). GO was found to be equally effective in patients 60 years old or over (OR = 26%) and in younger patients (OR = 34%). Furthermore, the adverse effects were similar in the two age groups. The duration of first complete remission (less than or more than 1 year) and cytogenetics (poor, intermediate, or high risk) had no effect on the rate of response to GO. The median OS was 4.8 months (5.3 months and 4.5 months for patients <60 and ≥60 years old, respectively). The early death rate (death within 28 days) was 16%. Median survival for responders (CR + CRp) was 12.5 months, in part a reflection of consolidation therapy, because it was 18.1 months for those receiving consolidation vs 11.0 months for those receiving no consolidation.

Remission durations ranged between 4.5 (CRp patients) and 6.4 months (CR patients). A significant difference in remission duration was observed between patients younger than 60 years old and patients aged 60 years and older (p = 0.008). This was possibly affected by postremission treatment options, especially HSCT.

A number of Phase II studies (in relapsed/refractory cases and in patients with previously untreated AML) have assessed the feasibility of treatment protocols integrating GO and chemotherapy (Table 11-1).[126-136] The results of these trials are quite heterogeneous, reflecting not only the variable activity of the regimens used but also the different characteristics of the patient populations.

The Medical Research Council AML15 study randomly assigned patients <60 years of age to receive induction chemotherapy with or without GO/consolidation or with or without GO. A preliminary analysis on 1115 patients[137] indicated that the use of GO (3 mg/m^2 on day 1) results in a significant reduction in relapse risk (37% vs 52% at 3 years; p = 0.01) and improvement in disease-free survival (DFS) (51% vs 40% at 3 years; p = 0.008). A subset analysis showed that GO is beneficial for patients with favorable or intermediate-risk cytogenetics but not for those with adverse cytogenetics. Subsequent follow-up has even shown a significant OS benefit in the favorable and intermediate groups.[138] Other Phase III studies that incorporate GO as part of standard induction chemotherapy in newly diagnosed patients with AML are ongoing.

Safety

In the pivotal Phase II studies, adverse events were categorized as either infusion-related (those that occurred on the day of GO adminis-

Table 11-1. Phase II Studies of GO-Based Combination Chemotherapy in AML

Reference	No. of Patients	Median Age in Years (Range)	AML Status	Chemotherapy Agents (Besides GO)	CR/CRp (%)	Induction Deaths (%)	Incidence of Veno-Occlusive Disease (%)	Median Overall Survival
Cortes et al[126]	17	55 (20-70)	AML, relapsed	Topotecan, Ara-C	12	29	5.9	8.2 weeks
Alvarado et al[127]	14	61 (34-74)	AML, relapsed	Idarubicin, Ara-C	21/21	43	14.3	8 weeks
Apostilodou et al[128]	11	37 (16-67)	AML, relapsed	Ara-C, DNX, CSA	9/9	18	0	3 months
Tsimberidou et al[129]	59	57 (27-76)	AML, untreated	Fludarabine, Ara-C, CSA	46/2	25	6.8	8 months
Tsimberidou et al[130]	32	53 (18-78)	AML, relapsed	Fludarabine, Ara-C, CSA	28/6	NR	9.4	5.3 months
Kell et al[131]	64	46.5 (18-59)	AML, untreated	DNR, Ara-C, 6-TG Or Fludarabine, Ara-C, Idarubicine	84	9	10.9	78% at 8 months

Study	n	Age (range)	Status	Regimen	CR/CRp (%)	Induction death (%)	Median DFS
Amadori et al[132]	57	68 (71-73)	AML, untreated	Mitoxantrone, Ara-C, VP-16	35/19	14	8.8	10.4 months
Piccaluga et al[136]	9	63 (50-71)	5, untreated 2, relapsed	Ara-C	55	0	0	6 months
Chevallier et al[133]	17	54 (21-68)	13, relapsed 4, refractory	Mitoxantrone, Ara-C	70/6	11.7	5.8	11 months
Clavio et al[134]	46	66 (60-80)	Untreated	Fludarabine, Ara-C, Idarubicin	52.1	2.1	0	8 months
Specchia et al[135]	21	52 (36-68)	10, relapsed 11, refractory	Mitoxantrone, Ara-C	9.5/9.5	19.0	0	7 months for CR/CRp

AML = acute myeloid leukemia; GO = Gemtuzumab ozogamicin; AML = acute myeloid leukemia; CR = complete remission; CRp = complete remission with incomplete platelet recovery; MDS = myelodysplastic syndrome; Ara-C = cytosine arabinoside; DNX = liposome-encapsulated daunorubicin; CSA = cyclosporine A; DNR = daunorubicin; 6-TG = 6-thioguanine; VP-16 = etoposide; NR = not reported.

tration) or those that occurred during the remainder of the treatment period.[123] The incidence of infusion-related symptoms was significantly lower on repeat administration: 30% of patients experienced grade 3 or 4 infusion-related events after the first dose, whereas only 10% experienced such events after the second dose (p <0.0001). Preventive therapy with corticosteroids in addition to acetaminophen and diphenhydramine has been reported to eliminate or greatly reduce infusion-related toxicities.[139]

Myelosuppression was reported in virtually all patients and was expected because CD33 is expressed on normal myeloid cells beyond the progenitor cell stage. Grade 3 or 4 neutropenia occurred in 98% of patients. Patients with CR and CRp had recovery of their absolute neutrophil count (ANC) to 500/μL in medians of 40 days and 43 days, respectively, from the first dose of GO. There was no significant difference in the median time to ANC recovery to 500/μL between younger and older patients. The incidence of grade 3 or 4 thrombocytopenia was 99%. Patients who achieved CR or CRp had recovery of platelet counts to 25,000/μL in medians of 36 days and 51 days, respectively, from the first dose of GO.

Extrahematological grade 3 or 4 toxicity was manifested primarily by elevations of liver transaminases (18%) or hyperbilirubinemia (29%). Liver toxicity was usually transient and required no medical intervention. However, some patients developed liver sinusoidal injury manifesting features similar to veno-occlusive disease or sinusoidal obstruction syndrome (SOS) of the liver. McKoy et al reviewed safety reports for GO included in reports of clinical trials and observational studies, interim reports from the FDA-mandated Prospective Observational Registry, and the FDA's Adverse Event Reporting System.[140] Among adult AML patients who received GO in clinical trials, stem cell transplantation (SOS) incidence was 3% at doses 6 mg/m², if administered as monotherapy or in combination with nonhepatotoxic agents, vs 28%, if administered with thioguanine, and 15%, when administered as monotherapy at a dose of 9 mg/m². Observational studies identified SOS rates between 15% and 40% if an SCT is performed within 3 months of GO administration.

Ibritumomab Tiuxetan

Ibritumomab tiuxetan (Fig 11-5) is the immunoconjugate resulting from a stable thiourea covalent bond between the monoclonal antibody ibritumomab and the linker-chelator tiuxetan: [N-[2-bis(carboxymethyl)amino]-3-(p-isothiocyanatophenyl)-propyl]-[N-[2-bis(carboxymethyl)amino]-2-(methyl)-ethyl]glycine.[141] This linker-chelator provides a high-affinity, conformationally restricted chelation site for indium-111 (^{111}In) or yttrium-90 (^{90}Y). Ibritumomab is an anti-CD20 mouse IgG1-kappa monoclonal antibody (IDEC-2B8).[141] The radioimmunoconjugate kills CD20+ cells by the effects of the ionizing radiation (mostly beta emission) as well as by the direct effects of the MoAb via ADCC, CDC, and apoptosis.[141,142]

In the United States, a course of therapy involves administering a dose of unlabeled rituximab on the first day of therapy to saturate nontumor CD20 sites and to facilitate the biodistribution of the radioimmunoconjugate. This is not included in the European license. Because ^{90}Y is a beta emitter and cannot be used for imaging, a tracer amount of ^{111}In-labeled ibritumomab is administered to assess the biodistribution and to ensure the appropriate localization of the isotope. About a week later, a low dose of rituximab is administered, followed by the administration of 0.4 mCi of intravenous ^{90}Y-labeled ibritumomab tiuxetan per kilogram of body weight for patients with a baseline platelet count >150 × 10^9/L or 0.3 mCi for patients with platelets between 100 and 150 × 10^9/L. The radiolabelled ibritumomab dose may be adjusted for platelet count. Patients who have marked cytopenias or compromised marrow are not candidates for therapy with this agent because of the risk of excessive hematologic toxic effects.[143]

In 2002, ibritumomab tiuxetan was the first radioimmunotherapy (RIT) drug approved by the FDA with an indication for the treatment of

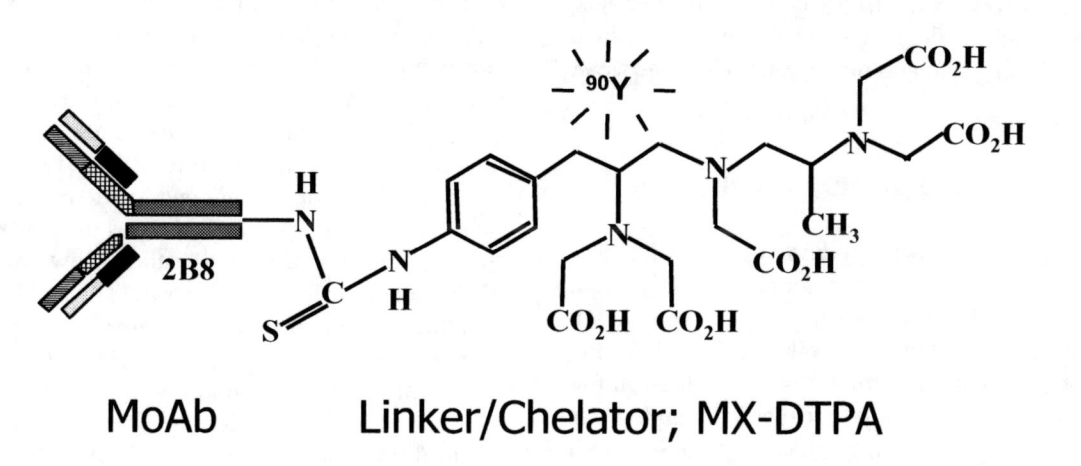

Figure 11-5. Schematic structure of ^{90}Y ibritumomab tiuxetan. A murine IgG1-kappa MoAb (IDEC-2B8) is covalently linked to the high-energy, pure-β-emitting ^{90}Y nuclide (2.3 MeV) by the chelator tiuxetan (MX-DTPA). MoAb = monoclonal antibody; MX-DTPA = methlbenzyl-diethylenetriaminepentaacetic acid.

patients with relapsed or refractory low-grade, follicular, or transformed B-cell NHL, including patients that are refractory to rituximab.

Therapeutic Efficacy

A Phase III randomized study compared ^{90}Y ibritumomab tiuxetan with a control immunotherapy, rituximab, in 143 patients with relapsed or refractory low-grade, follicular, or transformed CD20+ NHL.[144] The OR rate was 80% for the ^{90}Y ibritumomab tiuxetan group vs 56% for the rituximab group (p = 0.002). CR rates were 30% and 16% in the ^{90}Y ibritumomab tiuxetan and rituximab groups, respectively (p = 0.04). An additional 4% achieved an unconfirmed CR in each group. Durable responses of ≥6 months were 64% vs 47% (p = 0.03).

Several single-arm studies have demonstrated that upfront ibritumomab tiuxetan administered either alone or with chemotherapy to previously untreated indolent NHL patients produces OR rates of 90% to 100% and durable remissions.[145,146]

In one Phase III trial, 414 patients in either partial or complete remission after a variety of chemotherapy induction regimens (chlorambucil; cyclophosphamide, vincristine, and prednisone; CHOP; and fludarabine or rituximab combinations) were randomly assigned to either consolidation with RIT (consisting of two doses of rituximab, 250 mg/m^2, followed by ^{90}Y-ibritumomab tiuxetan) or no consolidation.[147] RIT dramatically improved the median PFS in the total patient population (36.5 vs 13.3 months with no RIT; p <0.0001), and this advantage was observed regardless of whether patients were in partial remission (29.3 vs 6.2 months with no RIT; p <0.0001) or complete remission (53.9 vs 29.5 months with no RIT; p = 0.015) at the time of consolidation. Nearly all subgroups of patients seemed to benefit regardless of prognostic score (Follicular Lymphoma International Prognostic Index score) or chemotherapy induction regimen. Furthermore, RIT consolidation converted 77% of patients who were in partial remission after induction chemotherapy to complete remission after RIT.

Safety

The RIT consolidation regimen with ibritumomab tiuxetan was well tolerated aside from expected reversible cytopenias [National Cancer Institute Common Toxicity Criteria (version

2) grade 3 or 4 neutropenia in 67% of patients, with grade 3 or 4 infections in 8%]. The incidence of human anti-mouse antibodies was <2%.

^{131}I-Tositumomab

Tositumomab, formally known as anti-B1, is a murine IgG2a-l monoclonal antibody that binds to CD20. Iodine-131 (^{131}I), which has a half-life of 8 days, is covalently linked by the iodogen method to the tyrosine residues on the monoclonal antibody. Because ^{131}I emits γ as well as β radiation, it can be used for both dosimetry and treatment. In contrast to ^{90}Y-ibritumomab tiuxetan, the therapeutic dose of tositumomab is based on dosimetry.[142] Patient-specific dosing is necessary because of the inter-patient differences in spleen size, tumor burden, and the metabolism and renal excretion of ^{131}I. Iodine concentrate (Lugol's solution) is given before treatment to block uptake of ^{131}I in the thyroid. On day 1, 450 mg of cold tositumomab followed by 5 mCi of ^{131}I-tositumomab is given. Dosimetry is performed on day 1 and repeated within 2 to 4 days and 6 to 7 days after the dose. Patients receive a dose of ^{131}I-tositumomab calculated to deliver 75 cGy to the whole body for patients who have a platelet count >150 × 10^9/L, or 65 cGy for patients with platelets between 100 and 150 × 10^9/L. The therapeutic dose is given within 7 to 14 days of the dosimetric dose and consists of 450 mg of unconjugated tositumomab followed by the calculated dose of ^{131}I-tositumomab.

Marketing approval for the therapeutic regimen was granted by the FDA in 2003, yet it remains unavailable outside clinical trials in Europe. The product is indicated for the treatment of CD20+ relapsed or refractory low-grade, follicular or transformed NHL, including patients with rituximab refractory disease.

Therapeutic Efficacy

The pivotal Phase III study employed a "patient-as own-control" design, the primary end point being a comparison of the number of patients that had a longer response to their last chemotherapy (>30 days) and the number of patients who had a longer duration of response after ^{131}I-tositumomab.[148] The entry criteria included previous exposure to at least two previous chemotherapy regimens, with relapse or failure to respond within 6 months of their last therapy; all patients had either "low-grade" (60%) or transformed disease (38%). Given that this population was refractory to chemotherapy, patient demographics report a median of four previous chemotherapies, with 71% not responding to their last therapy. The OR rate to ^{131}I-tositumomab was 65%, and the CR rate was 20%. This compared favorably to the OR rate of 28% and CR rate of 3% following their last chemotherapy. Of the patients, 74% had a longer duration of response to ^{131}I-tositumomab compared with their last chemotherapy regimen (28% equivalent duration), with a median duration of response that was almost twice as long (6.5 months for ^{131}I-tositumomab vs 3.5 months for last chemotherapy) and a median PFS of 8.4 months for ^{131}I-tositumomab responders. In multivariate analysis, tumor burden (<500 g) and nontransformed disease were significantly associated with a higher response rate, and low burden was the only variable associated with longer duration of response. The most recent update to this trial reports that 7 of the 12 patients who entered complete remission remain so between 4.9 and 7.2 years following therapy.[149]

^{131}I-tositumomab has been the subject of a further Phase III study in the relapsed/refractory setting to determine the relative contribution of the radioisotope to the regimen based on the observation that unlabelled tositumomab alone resulted in some tumor regressions.[150] Not unsurprisingly, response rates were superior in those patients that received the radioimmunoconjugate (55% vs 19%; p = 0.002), with a significantly higher CR rate (33% vs 8%; p = 0.012) and time to progression (6.3 months vs 5.5 months; p = 0.035). Nineteen patients whose disease failed to respond or progress to treatment with unlabeled tositumomab were crossed over into the

RIT arm, and only three of these had responded with no complete remission; 68% went on to have a response, with 42% entering complete remission.

The potential value of ^{131}I-tositumomab used as initial treatment of advanced-stage follicular B-cell NHL has been explored in a Phase II, single-group, open-label, single-center study.[151] Responses were observed in 95% of patients, including 75% who had complete remissions. At 5 years, 59% of the patients were free from progression of the disease; the median PFS was 6.1 years. This regimen has also been administered after chemotherapy, resulting in durable responses and conversion of partial remission to complete remission without serious toxic effects.[152]

Safety

When assessed by differing methods, grade 4 neutropenia was relatively infrequent, at about 16%, with grade 4 thrombocytopenia seen in only about 3% of the 677 patients assessed.[153] It is critically important to recognize that the time to count nadirs (3-6 weeks) is substantially longer for RIT with tositumomab and ^{131}I-tositumomab therapy than with typical chemotherapy. In general, hematopoietic toxicity is more severe the more extensive the prior therapy.

Other toxicities include that of free radioiodine. Patients are given thyroid blockade with a saturated solution of potassium iodide to prevent the development of hypothyroidism. However, elevated thyroid-stimulating hormone (TSH) levels have been observed in a fraction of patients. Some patients had preexisting elevated TSH before treatment was started. Of the 995 patients evaluated for the safety data product approval process, 9.5% developed elevated TSH levels at 2 years after treatment, whereas the incidence was 17.4% at 4 years after treatment.[154] Development of HAMAs was uncommon in patients who had been treated previously with chemotherapy and was observed in 10% of the 995 patients evaluated for safety for FDA approval.

Conclusions and Future Directions

Over the last decade, monoclonal antibody therapy has transformed the treatment of lymphoid malignancies and many hematologic autoimmune disorders. Optimizing the use of the existing agents and developing new agents will be critical to continuing these advances.

At this time, remarkable efforts are produced to improve on the rituximab molecule. Attempts include modifications that permit binding to a better epitope, binding more tightly to CD20, increasing activation of ADCC, and facilitating apoptosis. The product furthest along in clinical development is ofatumumab, a fully human IgG1-kappa monoclonal antibody that targets a novel epitope of CD20.[155] Preclinical studies indicate that ofatumumab is associated with greater CDC than rituximab, presumably because of a slower rate of dissociation from its antigen ("off rate") and greater interaction with the complement component C1q.[156] Other humanized CD20 antibodies, veltuzumab and ocrelizumab, have produced promising preliminary results.[157] It is likely that these new antibodies will be first developed to occupy the therapeutic niches where rituximab is used in an off-label setting.

Clinical success with CD20 antibodies has led to further investigation and discovery of other potential targets of lymphoma cells, including antibodies against CD22, CD23, CD40, CD52, and CD80. These agents have been used both as solitary therapy and in combination with other MoAbs and nontargeted treatments.[157]

The value of certain B-cell-depletion therapies for immune modulation also needs to be further delineated. In particular, long-term observations of protective immunity are needed to further evaluate the rate of infections.

Finally, development of new antibodies to target myeloid malignancies are expected in the next few years, whereas optimization of anti-CD33 therapy with GO should be accomplished with ongoing trials.

References

1. Kohler G, Milstein C. Continuous cultures of fused cells secreting antibody of predefined specificity. Nature 1975;256:495-7.
2. Stern M, Herrmann R. Overview of monoclonal antibodies in cancer therapy: Present and promise. Crit Rev Oncol Hematol 2005; 54:11-29.
3. Ortho Multicenter Transplant Study Group. A randomized clinical trial of OKT3 monoclonal antibody for acute rejection of cadaveric renal transplants. N Engl J Med 1985;313:337-42.
4. Hudson PJ, Souriau C. Engineered antibodies. Nat Med 2003;9:129-34.
5. Roskos LK, Davis GC, Schwab GM. The clinical pharmacology of therapeutic monoclonal antibodies. Drug Develop Res 2004;61:108-20.
6. Reff ME, Carner K, Chambers KS, et al. Depletion of B cells in vivo by a chimeric mouse human monoclonal antibody to CD20. Blood 1994;83:435-45.
7. Stashenko P, Nadler LM, Hardy R, Schlossman SF. Characterization of a human B lymphocyte-specific antigen. J Immunol 1980;125:1678-85.
8. Plosker GL, Figgitt DP. Rituximab: A review of its use in non-Hodgkin's lymphoma and chronic lymphocytic leukaemia. Drugs 2003; 63:803-43.
9. van Meerten T, van Rijn RS, Hol S, et al. Complement-induced cell death by rituximab depends on CD20 expression level and acts complementary to antibody-dependent cellular cytotoxicity. Clin Cancer Res 2006;12:4027-35.
10. Lefebvre ML, Krause SW, Salcedo M, Nardin A. Ex vivo-activated human macrophages kill chronic lymphocytic leukemia cells in the presence of rituximab: Mechanism of antibody-dependent cellular cytotoxicity and impact of human serum. J Immunother 2006;29:388-97.
11. Rose AL, Smith BE, Maloney DG. Glucocorticoids and rituximab in vitro: Synergistic direct antiproliferative and apoptotic effects. Blood 2002;100:1765-73.
12. Cvetkovic RS, Perry CM. Rituximab: A review of its use in non-Hodgkin's lymphoma and chronic lymphocytic leukaemia. Drugs 2006; 66:791-820.
13. Clynes RA, Towers TL, Presta LG, Ravetch JV. Inhibitory Fc receptors modulate in vivo cytoxicity against tumor targets. Nat Med 2000;6: 443-6.
14. Weng WK, Levy R. Two immunoglobulin G fragment C receptor polymorphisms independently predict response to rituximab in patients with follicular lymphoma. J Clin Oncol 2003; 21:3940-7.
15. Golay J, Zaffaroni L, Vaccari T, et al. Biologic response of B lymphoma cells to anti-CD20 monoclonal antibody rituximab in vitro: CD55 and CD59 regulate complement-mediated cell lysis. Blood 2000;95:3900-8.
16. Treon SP, Mitsiades C, Mitsiades N, et al. Tumor cell expression of CD59 is associated with resistance to CD20 serotherapy in patients with B-cell malignancies. J Immunother 2001;24:263-71.
17. Ziller F, Macor P, Bulla R, et al. Controlling complement resistance in cancer by using human monoclonal antibodies that neutralize complement-regulatory proteins CD55 and CD59. Eur J Immunol 2005;35:2175-83.
18. Samuels J, Ng YS, Coupillaud C, et al. Human B cell tolerance and its failure in rheumatoid arthritis. Ann N Y Acad Sci 2005;1062:116-26.
19. Edwards JC, Cambridge G. Prospects for B-cell-targeted therapy in autoimmune disease. Rheumatology (Oxford) 2005;44:151-6.
20. Anderton SM, Fillatreau S. Activated B cells in autoimmune diseases: The case for a regulatory role. Nat Clin Pract Rheumatol 2008;4: 657-66.
21. Maloney DG, Grillo-Lopez AJ, White CA, et al. IDEC-C2B8 (rituximab) anti-CD20 monoclonal antibody therapy in patients with relapsed low-grade non-Hodgkin's lymphoma. Blood 1997;90:2188-95.
22. Ghielmini M, Schmitz SF, Cogliatti SB, et al. Prolonged treatment with rituximab in patients with follicular lymphoma significantly increases event-free survival and response duration compared with the standard weekly × 4 schedule. Blood 2004;103:4416-23.
23. Stasi R, Pagano A, Stipa E, Amadori S. Rituximab chimeric anti-CD20 monoclonal antibody treatment for adults with chronic idiopathic thrombocytopenic purpura. Blood 2001;98:952-7.
24. Edwards JC, Szczepanski L, Szechinski J, et al. Efficacy of B-cell-targeted therapy with ritux-

imab in patients with rheumatoid arthritis. N Engl J Med 2004;350:2572-81.
25. Maloney DG, Liles TM, Czerwinski DK, et al. Phase I clinical trial using escalating single-dose infusion of chimeric anti-CD20 monoclonal antibody (IDEC-C2B8) in patients with recurrent B-cell lymphoma. Blood 1994;84:2457-66.
26. Tobinai K, Kobayashi Y, Narabayashi M, et al. Feasibility and pharmacokinetic study of a chimeric anti-CD20 monoclonal antibody (IDEC-C2B8, rituximab) in relapsed B-cell lymphoma. The IDEC-C2B8 Study Group. Ann Oncol 1998;9:527-34.
27. Breedveld F, Agarwal S, Yin M, et al. Rituximab pharmacokinetics in patients with rheumatoid arthritis: B-cell levels do not correlate with clinical response. J Clin Pharmacol 2007;47:1119-28.
28. McLaughlin P, Grillo-Lopez AJ, Link BK, et al. Rituximab chimeric anti-CD20 monoclonal antibody therapy for relapsed indolent lymphoma: Half of patients respond to a four-dose treatment program. J Clin Oncol 1998;16:2825-33.
29. Schulz H, Bohlius JF, Trelle S, et al. Immunochemotherapy with rituximab and overall survival in patients with indolent or mantle cell lymphoma: A systematic review and meta-analysis. J Natl Cancer Inst 2007;99:706-14.
30. Hiddemann W, Kneba M, Dreyling M, et al. Frontline therapy with rituximab added to the combination of cyclophosphamide, doxorubicin, vincristine, and prednisone (CHOP) significantly improves the outcome for patients with advanced-stage follicular lymphoma compared with therapy with CHOP alone: Results of a prospective randomized study of the German Low-Grade Lymphoma Study Group. Blood 2005;106:3725-32.
31. Herold M, Haas A, Srock S, et al. Rituximab added to first-line mitoxantrone, chlorambucil, and prednisolone chemotherapy followed by interferon maintenance prolongs survival in patients with advanced follicular lymphoma: An East German Study Group Hematology and Oncology Study. J Clin Oncol 2007;25:1986-92.
32. Marcus R, Imrie K, Solal-Celigny P, et al. Phase III study of R-CVP compared with cyclophosphamide, vincristine, and prednisone alone in patients with previously untreated advanced follicular lymphoma. J Clin Oncol 2008;26:4579-86.
33. Salles G, Mounier N, de Guibert S, et al. Rituximab combined with chemotherapy and interferon in follicular lymphoma patients: Results of the GELA-GOELAMS FL2000 study. Blood 2008;112:4824-31.
34. Forstpointner R, Dreyling M, Repp R, et al. The addition of rituximab to a combination of fludarabine, cyclophosphamide, mitoxantrone (FCM) significantly increases the response rate and prolongs survival as compared with FCM alone in patients with relapsed and refractory follicular and mantle cell lymphomas: Results of a prospective randomized study of the German Low-Grade Lymphoma Study Group. Blood 2004;104:3064-71.
35. van Oers MH, Klasa R, Marcus RE, et al. Rituximab maintenance improves clinical outcome of relapsed/resistant follicular non-Hodgkin lymphoma in patients both with and without rituximab during induction: Results of a prospective randomized phase 3 intergroup trial. Blood 2006;108:3295-301.
36. Cheson BD, Horning SJ, Coiffier B, et al. Report of an international workshop to standardize response criteria for non-Hodgkin's lymphomas. NCI Sponsored International Working Group. J Clin Oncol 1999;17:1244.
37. Vidal L, Gafter-Gvili A, Leibovici L, et al. Rituximab maintenance for the treatment of patients with follicular lymphoma: Systematic review and meta-analysis of randomized trials. J Natl Cancer Inst 2009;101:248-55.
38. Hallek M, Fingerle-Rowson G, Fink A-M, et al. Immunochemotherapy with fludarabine (F), cyclophosphamide (C), and rituximab (R) (FCR) versus fludarabine and cyclophosphamide (FC) improves response rates and progression-free survival (PFS) of previously untreated patients (pts) with advanced chronic lymphocytic leukemia (CLL) (abstract). American Society of Hematology Annual Meeting Abstracts 2008;112:325.
39. Robak T, Moiseev SI, Dmoszynska A, et al. Rituximab, fludarabine, and cyclophosphamide (R-FC) prolongs progression free survival in relapsed or refractory chronic lymphocytic leukemia (CLL) compared with FC alone: Final results from the international randomized Phase III REACH trial. American Society of Hematology Annual Meeting Abstracts 2008;112:lba-1.
40. Coiffier B, Pfreundschuh M, Stahel R, et al. Aggressive lymphoma: Improving treatment

outcome with rituximab. Anticancer Drugs 2002;13(Suppl 2):S43-50.
41. Feugier P, Van Hoof A, Sebban C, et al. Long-term results of the R-CHOP study in the treatment of elderly patients with diffuse large B-cell lymphoma: A study by the Groupe d'Etude des Lymphomes de l'Adulte. J Clin Oncol 2005;23:4117-26.
42. Habermann TM, Weller EA, Morrison VA, et al. Rituximab-CHOP versus CHOP alone or with maintenance rituximab in older patients with diffuse large B-cell lymphoma. J Clin Oncol 2006;24:3121-7.
43. Pfreundschuh M, Trumper L, Osterborg A, et al. CHOP-like chemotherapy plus rituximab versus CHOP-like chemotherapy alone in young patients with good-prognosis diffuse large-B-cell lymphoma: A randomised controlled trial by the MabThera International Trial (MInT) Group. Lancet Oncol 2006; 7:379-91.
44. Pfreundschuh M, Schubert J, Ziepert M, et al. Six versus eight cycles of bi-weekly CHOP-14 with or without rituximab in elderly patients with aggressive CD20+ B-cell lymphomas: A randomised controlled trial (RICOVER-60). Lancet Oncol 2008;9:105-16.
45. Cunningham D, Smith P, Mouncey P, et al. A Phase III trial comparing R-CHOP 14 and R-CHOP 21 for the treatment of patients with newly diagnosed diffuse large B-cell non-Hodgkin's lymphoma (abstract). J Clin Oncol 2009;27:abstr 8506.
46. Buske C, Hoster E, Dreyling M, et al. The addition of rituximab to front-line therapy with CHOP (R-CHOP) results in a higher response rate and longer time to treatment failure in patients with lymphoplasmacytic lymphoma: Results of a randomized trial of the German Low-Grade Lymphoma Study Group (GLSG). Leukemia 2009;23:153-61.
47. Claviez A, Eckert C, Seeger K, et al. Rituximab plus chemotherapy in children with relapsed or refractory CD20-positive B-cell precursor acute lymphoblastic leukemia. Haematologica 2006;91:272-3.
48. Garvey B. Rituximab in the treatment of autoimmune haematological disorders. Br J Haematol 2008;141:149-69.
49. Gurcan HM, Keskin DB, Stern JN, et al. A review of the current use of rituximab in autoimmune diseases. Int Immunopharmacol 2009;9:10-25.
50. Arnold DM, Dentali F, Crowther MA, et al. Systematic review: Efficacy and safety of rituximab for adults with idiopathic thrombocytopenic purpura. Ann Intern Med 2007;146:25-33.
51. Cooper N, Stasi R, Cunningham-Rundles S, et al. The efficacy and safety of B-cell depletion with anti-CD20 monoclonal antibody in adults with chronic immune thrombocytopenic purpura. Br J Haematol 2004;125:232-9.
52. Taylor RP, Lindorfer MA. Drug insight: The mechanism of action of rituximab in autoimmune disease—the immune complex decoy hypothesis. Nat Clin Pract Rheumatol 2007; 3:86-95.
53. Stasi R, Del Poeta G, Stipa E, et al. Response to B-cell depleting therapy with rituximab reverts the abnormalities of T-cell subsets in patients with idiopathic thrombocytopenic purpura. Blood 2007;110:2924-30.
54. Stasi R, Cooper N, Del Poeta G, et al. Analysis of regulatory T-cell changes in patients with idiopathic thrombocytopenic purpura receiving B cell-depleting therapy with rituximab. Blood 2008;112:1147-50.
55. Provan D, Butler T, Evangelista ML, et al. Activity and safety profile of low-dose rituximab for the treatment of autoimmune cytopenias in adults. Haematologica 2007;92:1695-8.
56. Zaja F, Battista ML, Pirrotta MT, et al. Lower dose rituximab is active in adults patients with idiopathic thrombocytopenic purpura. Haematologica 2008;93:930-3.
57. Zaja F, Baccarani M, Mazza P, et al. A prospective randomized study comparing rituximab and dexamethasone vs dexamethasone alone in ITP: Results of final analysis and long term follow up (abstract). Blood 2008;112:1.
58. Shanafelt TD, Madueme HL, Wolf RC, Tefferi A. Rituximab for immune cytopenia in adults: Idiopathic thrombocytopenic purpura, autoimmune hemolytic anemia, and Evans syndrome. Mayo Clin Proc 2003;78:1340-6.
59. D'Arena G, Califano C, Annunziata M, et al. Rituximab for warm-type idiopathic autoimmune hemolytic anemia: A retrospective study of 11 adult patients. Eur J Haematol 2007;79:53-8.
60. D'Arena G, Laurenti L, Capalbo S, et al. Rituximab therapy for chronic lymphocytic leukemia-associated autoimmune hemolytic anemia. Am J Hematol 2006;81:598-602.

61. Narat S, Gandla J, Hoffbrand AV, et al. Rituximab in the treatment of refractory autoimmune cytopenias in adults. Haematologica 2005;90:1273-4.
62. Quartier P, Brethon B, Philippet P, et al. Treatment of childhood autoimmune haemolytic anaemia with rituximab. Lancet 2001;358: 1511-13.
63. Zecca M, Nobili B, Ramenghi U, et al. Rituximab for the treatment of refractory autoimmune hemolytic anemia in children. Blood 2003;101:3857-61.
64. Gupta N, Kavuru S, Patel D, et al. Rituximab-based chemotherapy for steroid-refractory autoimmune hemolytic anemia of chronic lymphocytic leukemia. Leukemia 2002;16:2092-5.
65. Rao A, Kelly M, Musselman M, et al. Safety, efficacy, and immune reconstitution after rituximab therapy in pediatric patients with chronic or refractory hematologic autoimmune cytopenias. Pediatr Blood Cancer 2008;50:822-5.
66. Lammle B, Kremer Hovinga JA, George JN. Acquired thrombotic thrombocytopenic purpura: ADAMTS13 activity, anti-ADAMTS13 autoantibodies and risk of recurrent disease. Haematologica 2008;93:172-7.
67. Scully M, Cohen H, Cavenagh J, et al. Remission in acute refractory and relapsing thrombotic thrombocytopenic purpura following rituximab is associated with a reduction in IgG antibodies to ADAMTS-13. Br J Haematol 2007;136:451-61.
68. Sallah S, Husain A, Wan JY, Nguyen NP. Rituximab in patients with refractory thrombotic thrombocytopenic purpura. J Thromb Haemost 2004;2:834-6.
69. Reddy PS, Deauna-Limayo D, Cook JD, et al. Rituximab in the treatment of relapsed thrombotic thrombocytopenic purpura. Ann Hematol 2005;84:232-5.
70. Fakhouri F, Vernant JP, Veyradier A, et al. Efficiency of curative and prophylactic treatment with rituximab in ADAMTS13-deficient thrombotic thrombocytopenic purpura: A study of 11 cases. Blood 2005;106:1932-7.
71. Heidel F, Lipka DB, von Auer C, et al. Addition of rituximab to standard therapy improves response rate and progression-free survival in relapsed or refractory thrombotic thrombocytopenic purpura and autoimmune haemolytic anaemia. Thromb Haemost 2007;97:228-33.
72. Boctor FN, Smith JA. Timing of plasma exchange and rituximab for the treatment of thrombotic thrombocytopenic purpura. Am J Clin Pathol 2006;126:965; author reply 965-6.
73. Hull MJ, Eichbaum QG. Efficacy of rituximab and concurrent plasma exchange in the treatment of thrombotic thrombocytopenic purpura. Clin Adv Hematol Oncol 2006;4:210-14; discussion 217-18.
74. Darabi K, Berg AH. Rituximab can be combined with daily plasma exchange to achieve effective B-cell depletion and clinical improvement in acute autoimmune TTP. Am J Clin Pathol 2006;125:592-7.
75. Kimby E. Tolerability and safety of rituximab (MabThera). Cancer Treat Rev 2005;31:456-73.
76. Sehn LH, Donaldson J, Filewich A, et al. Rapid infusion rituximab in combination with corticosteroid-containing chemotherapy or as maintenance therapy is well tolerated and can safely be delivered in the community setting. Blood 2007;109:4171-3.
77. Tuthill M, Crook T, Corbet T, et al. Rapid infusion of rituximab over 60 min. Eur J Haematol 2009;82:322-5.
78. D'Arena G, Scalzulli PR, Nobile M, et al. Attenuated doses of rituximab for the treatment of adults with autoimmune cytopenias. Am J Hematol 2008;83:686-7.
79. Emery P, Fleischmann R, Filipowicz-Sosnowska A, et al. The efficacy and safety of rituximab in patients with active rheumatoid arthritis despite methotrexate treatment: Results of a Phase IIB randomized, double-blind, placebo-controlled, dose-ranging trial. Arthritis Rheum 2006;54:1390-400.
80. Cohen SB, Emery P, Greenwald MW, et al. Rituximab for rheumatoid arthritis refractory to anti-tumor necrosis factor therapy: Results of a multicenter, randomized, double-blind, placebo-controlled, Phase III trial evaluating primary efficacy and safety at twenty-four weeks. Arthritis Rheum 2006;54:2793-806.
81. Calabrese LH, Molloy ES. Progressive multifocal leucoencephalopathy in the rheumatic diseases: Assessing the risks of biological immunosuppressive therapies. Ann Rheum Dis 2008;67(Suppl 3):iii64-5.
82. Yeo W, Chan TC, Leung NW, et al. Hepatitis B virus reactivation in lymphoma patients with prior resolved hepatitis B undergoing anticancer therapy with or without rituximab. J Clin Oncol 2009;27:605-11.

83. Ennishi D, Terui Y, Yokoyama M, et al. Monitoring serum hepatitis C virus (HCV) RNA in patients with HCV-infected CD20-positive B-cell lymphoma undergoing rituximab combination chemotherapy. Am J Hematol 2008;83: 59-62.
84. Todd DJ, Helfgott SM. Serum sickness following treatment with rituximab. J Rheumatol 2007;34:430-3.
85. Hale G. The CD52 antigen and development of the CAMPATH antibodies. Cytotherapy 2001;3:137-43.
86. Gilleece MH, Dexter TM. Effect of Campath-1H antibody on human hematopoietic progenitors in vitro. Blood 1993;82:807-12.
87. Hale G, Bright S, Chumbley G, et al. Removal of T cells from bone marrow for transplantation: A monoclonal antilymphocyte antibody that fixes human complement. Blood 1983;62: 873-82.
88. Xia MQ, Hale G, Waldmann H. Efficient complement-mediated lysis of cells containing the CAMPATH-1 (CDw52) antigen. Mol Immunol 1993;30:1089-96.
89. Hale G, Clark M, Waldmann H. Therapeutic potential of rat monoclonal antibodies: Isotype specificity of antibody-dependent cell-mediated cytotoxicity with human lymphocytes. J Immunol 1985;134:3056-61.
90. Dyer MJ, Hale G, Hayhoe FG, Waldmann H. Effects of CAMPATH-1 antibodies in vivo in patients with lymphoid malignancies: Influence of antibody isotype. Blood 1989;73:1431-9.
91. Mone AP, Cheney C, Banks AL, et al. Alemtuzumab induces caspase-independent cell death in human chronic lymphocytic leukemia cells through a lipid raft-dependent mechanism. Leukemia 2006;20:272-9.
92. Frampton JE, Wagstaff AJ. Alemtuzumab. Drugs 2003;63:1229-43; discussion 1245-6.
93. Mould DR, Baumann A, Kuhlmann J, et al. Population pharmacokinetics-pharmacodynamics of alemtuzumab (Campath) in patients with chronic lymphocytic leukaemia and its link to treatment response. Br J Clin Pharmacol 2007; 64:278-91.
94. Elter T, Molnar I, Kuhlmann J, et al. Pharmacokinetics of alemtuzumab and the relevance in clinical practice. Leuk Lymphoma 2008;49: 2256-62.
95. Keating MJ, Flinn I, Jain V, et al. Therapeutic role of alemtuzumab (Campath-1H) in patients who have failed fludarabine: Results of a large international study. Blood 2002;99:3554-61.
96. Stilgenbauer S, Dohner H. Campath-1H-induced complete remission of chronic lymphocytic leukemia despite p53 gene mutation and resistance to chemotherapy. N Engl J Med 2002;347:452-3.
97. Stilgenbauer S, Winkler D, Buhler A, et al. Subcutaneous alemtuzumab (MabCampath) in fludarabine-refractory CLL (CLL2H trial of the GCLLSG) (abstract). Blood 2007;110:3120.
98. Hillmen P, Skotnicki AB, Robak T, et al. Alemtuzumab compared with chlorambucil as first-line therapy for chronic lymphocytic leukemia. J Clin Oncol 2007;25:5616-23.
99. Lundin J, Kimby E, Bjorkholm M, et al. Phase II trial of subcutaneous anti-CD52 monoclonal antibody alemtuzumab (Campath-1H) as first-line treatment for patients with B-cell chronic lymphocytic leukemia (B-CLL). Blood 2002; 100:768-73.
100. Karlsson C, Norin S, Kimby E, et al. Alemtuzumab as first-line therapy for B-cell chronic lymphocytic leukemia: Long-term follow-up of clinical effects, infectious complications and risk of Richter transformation. Leukemia 2006;20:2204-7.
101. Gribben JG, Hallek M. Rediscovering alemtuzumab: Current and emerging therapeutic roles. Br J Haematol 2009;144:818-31.
102. Keating M, Coutre S, Rai K, et al. Management guidelines for use of alemtuzumab in B-cell chronic lymphocytic leukemia. Clin Lymphoma 2004;4:220-7.
103. Thomas TC, Rollins SA, Rother RP, et al. Inhibition of complement activity by humanized anti-C5 antibody and single-chain Fv. Mol Immunol 1996;33:1389-401.
104. Mueller JP, Giannoni MA, Hartman SL, et al. Humanized porcine VCAM-specific monoclonal antibodies with chimeric IgG2/G4 constant regions block human leukocyte binding to porcine endothelial cells. Mol Immunol 1997;34:441-52.
105. Matis LA, Rollins SA. Complement-specific antibodies: Designing novel anti-inflammatories. Nat Med 1995;1:839-42.
106. Charneski L, Patel PN. Eculizumab in paroxysmal nocturnal haemoglobinuria. Drugs 2008; 68:1341-6.
107. Hillmen P, Hall C, Marsh JC, et al. Effect of eculizumab on hemolysis and transfusion requirements in patients with paroxysmal nocturnal hemoglobinuria. N Engl J Med 2004; 350:552-9.

108. Hill A, Hillmen P, Richards SJ, et al. Sustained response and long-term safety of eculizumab in paroxysmal nocturnal hemoglobinuria. Blood 2005;106:2559-65.
109. Alexion Pharmaceuticals Inc. Soliris (eculizumab) prescribing information. Cheshire, CT: Alexion, 2009. [Available at http://www.soliris.net/Downloads/pdf/soliris.pdf (accessed January 26, 2010)].
110. Hillmen P, Young NS, Schubert J, et al. The complement inhibitor eculizumab in paroxysmal nocturnal hemoglobinuria. N Engl J Med 2006;355:1233-43.
111. Brodsky RA, Young NS, Antonioli E, et al. Multicenter phase 3 study of the complement inhibitor eculizumab for the treatment of patients with paroxysmal nocturnal hemoglobinuria. Blood 2008;111:1840-7.
112. Hillmen P, Muus P, Duhrsen U, et al. Effect of the complement inhibitor eculizumab on thromboembolism in patients with paroxysmal nocturnal hemoglobinuria. Blood 2007;110:4123-8.
113. Hamann PR, Hinman LM, Hollander I, et al. Gemtuzumab ozogamicin, a potent and selective anti-CD33 antibody-calicheamicin conjugate for treatment of acute myeloid leukemia. Bioconjug Chem 2002;13:47-58.
114. Lee MD, Dunne TS, Siegel MM, et al. Calicheamicins, a novel family of antitumor antibiotics 1. Chemistry and partial structure of calicheamicin γ_1^I. J Am Chem Soc 1987;109:3464-6.
115. Zein N, Sinha AM, McGahren WJ, Ellestad GA. Calicheamicin gamma 1I: An antitumor antibiotic that cleaves double-stranded DNA site specifically. Science 1988;240:1198-201.
116. Linenberger ML. CD33-directed therapy with gemtuzumab ozogamicin in acute myeloid leukemia: Progress in understanding cytotoxicity and potential mechanisms of drug resistance. Leukemia 2005;19:176-82.
117. Bernstein ID. Monoclonal antibodies to the myeloid stem cells: Therapeutic implications of CMA-676, a humanized anti-CD33 antibody calicheamicin conjugate. Leukemia 2000;14:474-5.
118. van Der Velden VH, te Marvelde JG, Hoogeveen PG, et al. Targeting of the CD33-calicheamicin immunoconjugate Mylotarg (CMA-676) in acute myeloid leukemia: In vivo and in vitro saturation and internalization by leukemic and normal myeloid cells. Blood 2001;97:3197-204.
119. Dowell JA, Korth-Bradley J, Liu H, et al. Pharmacokinetics of gemtuzumab ozogamicin, an antibody-targeted chemotherapy agent for the treatment of patients with acute myeloid leukemia in first relapse. J Clin Pharmacol 2001;41:1206-14.
120. Bross PF, Beitz J, Chen G, et al. Approval summary: Gemtuzumab ozogamicin in relapsed acute myeloid leukemia. Clin Cancer Res 2001;7:1490-6.
121. Sievers EL, Larson RA, Stadtmauer EA, et al. Efficacy and safety of gemtuzumab ozogamicin in patients with CD33-positive acute myeloid leukemia in first relapse. J Clin Oncol 2001;19:3244-54.
122. Larson RA, Boogaerts M, Estey E, et al. Antibody-targeted chemotherapy of older patients with acute myeloid leukemia in first relapse using Mylotarg (gemtuzumab ozogamicin). Leukemia 2002;16:1627-36.
123. Larson RA, Sievers EL, Stadtmauer EA, et al. Final report of the efficacy and safety of gemtuzumab ozogamicin (Mylotarg) in patients with CD33-positive acute myeloid leukemia in first recurrence. Cancer 2005;104:1442-52.
124. Cheson BD, Cassileth PA, Head DR, et al. Report of the National Cancer Institute-sponsored workshop on definitions of diagnosis and response in acute myeloid leukemia. J Clin Oncol 1990;8:813-19.
125. Cheson BD, Bennett JM, Kopecky KJ, et al. Revised recommendations of the International Working Group for Diagnosis, Standardization of Response Criteria, Treatment Outcomes, and Reporting Standards for Therapeutic Trials in Acute Myeloid Leukemia. J Clin Oncol 2003;21:4642-9.
126. Cortes J, Tsimberidou AM, Alvarez R, et al. Mylotarg combined with topotecan and cytarabine in patients with refractory acute myelogenous leukemia. Cancer Chemother Pharmacol 2002;50:497-500.
127. Alvarado Y, Tsimberidou A, Kantarjian H, et al. Pilot study of Mylotarg, idarubicin and cytarabine combination regimen in patients with primary resistant or relapsed acute myeloid leukemia. Cancer Chemother Pharmacol 2003;51:87-90.
128. Apostolidou E, Cortes J, Tsimberidou A, et al. Pilot study of gemtuzumab ozogamicin, liposomal daunorubicin, cytarabine and cyclosporine regimen in patients with refractory acute myelogenous leukemia. Leuk Res 2003;27:887-91.

129. Tsimberidou A, Estey E, Cortes J, et al. Gemtuzumab, fludarabine, cytarabine, and cyclosporine in patients with newly diagnosed acute myelogenous leukemia or high-risk myelodysplastic syndromes. Cancer 2003;97:1481-7.
130. Tsimberidou A, Cortes J, Thomas D, et al. Gemtuzumab ozogamicin, fludarabine, cytarabine and cyclosporine combination regimen in patients with CD33+ primary resistant or relapsed acute myeloid leukemia. Leuk Res 2003;27:893-7.
131. Kell WJ, Burnett AK, Chopra R, et al. A feasibility study of simultaneous administration of gemtuzumab ozogamicin with intensive chemotherapy in induction and consolidation in younger patients with acute myeloid leukemia. Blood 2003;102:4277-83.
132. Amadori S, Suciu S, Willemze R, et al. Sequential administration of gemtuzumab ozogamicin and conventional chemotherapy as first line therapy in elderly patients with acute myeloid leukemia: A Phase II study (AML-15) of the EORTC and GIMEMA leukemia groups. Haematologica 2004;89:950-6.
133. Chevallier P, Roland V, Mahe B, et al. Administration of mylotarg 4 days after beginning of a chemotherapy including intermediate-dose aracytin and mitoxantrone (MIDAM regimen) produces a high rate of complete hematologic remission in patients with CD33+ primary resistant or relapsed acute myeloid leukemia. Leuk Res 2005;29:1003-7.
134. Clavio M, Vignolo L, Albarello A, et al. Adding low-dose gemtuzumab ozogamicin to fludarabine, Ara-C and idarubicin (MY-FLAI) may improve disease-free and overall survival in elderly patients with non-M3 acute myeloid leukaemia: Results of a prospective, pilot, multi-centre trial and comparison with a historical cohort of patients. Br J Haematol 2007; 138:186-95.
135. Specchia G, Pastore D, Carluccio P, et al. Gemtuzumab ozogamicin with cytarabine and mitoxantrone as a third-line treatment in a poor prognosis group of adult acute myeloid leukemia patients: A single-center experience. Ann Hematol 2007;86:425-8.
136. Piccaluga PP, Martinelli G, Rondoni M, et al. First experience with gemtuzumab ozogamicin plus cytarabine as continuous infusion for elderly acute myeloid leukaemia patients. Leuk Res 2004;28:987-90.
137. Burnett AK, Kell WJ, Goldstone AH, et al. The addition of gemtuzumab ozogamicin to induction chemotherapy for AML improves disease free survival without extra toxicity: Preliminary analysis of 1115 patients in the MRC AML15 trial (abstract). Blood 2006;108:Abstract #13.
138. Burnett AK, Knapper S. Targeting treatment in AML. Hematology Am Soc Hematol Educ Program 2007;2007:429-34.
139. Giles FJ, Cortes JE, Halliburton TA, et al. Intravenous corticosteroids to reduce gemtuzumab ozogamicin infusion reactions. Ann Pharmacother 2003;37:1182-5.
140. McKoy JM, Angelotta C, Bennett CL, et al. Gemtuzumab ozogamicin-associated sinusoidal obstructive syndrome (SOS): An overview from the research on adverse drug events and reports (RADAR) project. Leuk Res 2007;31: 599-604.
141. Chapuy B, Hohloch K, Trumper L. Yttrium 90 ibritumomab tiuxetan (Zevalin): A new bullet in the fight against malignant lymphoma? Biotechnol J 2007;2:1435-43.
142. Witzig TE. Radioimmunotherapy for B-cell non-Hodgkin lymphoma. Best Pract Res Clin Haematol 2006;19:655-68.
143. Wiseman GA, Gordon LI, Multani PS, et al. Ibritumomab tiuxetan radioimmunotherapy for patients with relapsed or refractory non-Hodgkin lymphoma and mild thrombocytopenia: A phase II multicenter trial. Blood 2002; 99:4336-42.
144. Witzig TE, Gordon LI, Cabanillas F, et al. Randomized controlled trial of yttrium-90-labeled ibritumomab tiuxetan radioimmunotherapy versus rituximab immunotherapy for patients with relapsed or refractory low-grade, follicular, or transformed B-cell non-Hodgkin's lymphoma. J Clin Oncol 2002;20:2453-63.
145. Zinzani PL, Tani M, Pulsoni A, et al. Fludarabine and mitoxantrone followed by yttrium-90 ibritumomab tiuxetan in previously untreated patients with follicular non-Hodgkin lymphoma trial: A Phase II non-randomised trial (FLUMIZ). Lancet Oncol 2008;9:352-8.
146. Jacobs SA, Swerdlow SH, Kant J, et al. Phase II trial of short-course CHOP-R followed by 90Y-ibritumomab tiuxetan and extended rituximab in previously untreated follicular lymphoma. Clin Cancer Res 2008;14:7088-94.
147. Morschhauser F, Radford J, Van Hoof A, et al. Phase III trial of consolidation therapy with yttrium-90-ibritumomab tiuxetan compared with no additional therapy after first remission in advanced follicular lymphoma. J Clin Oncol 2008;26:5156-64.

148. Kaminski MS, Zelenetz AD, Press OW, et al. Pivotal study of iodine I 131 tositumomab for chemotherapy-refractory low-grade or transformed low-grade B-cell non-Hodgkin's lymphomas. J Clin Oncol 2001;19:3918-28.
149. Fisher RI, Kaminski MS, Wahl RL, et al. Tositumomab and iodine-131 tositumomab produces durable complete remissions in a subset of heavily pretreated patients with low-grade and transformed non-Hodgkin's lymphomas. J Clin Oncol 2005;23:7565-73.
150. Davis TA, Kaminski MS, Leonard JP, et al. The radioisotope contributes significantly to the activity of radioimmunotherapy. Clin Cancer Res 2004;10:7792-8.
151. Kaminski MS, Tuck M, Estes J, et al. 131I-tositumomab therapy as initial treatment for follicular lymphoma. N Engl J Med 2005;352:441-9.
152. Press OW, Unger JM, Braziel RM, et al. Phase II trial of CHOP chemotherapy followed by tositumomab/iodine I-131 tositumomab for previously untreated follicular non-Hodgkin's lymphoma: Five-year follow-up of Southwest Oncology Group Protocol S9911. J Clin Oncol 2006;24:4143-9.
153. Vose JM. Bexxar: Novel radioimmunotherapy for the treatment of low-grade and transformed low-grade non-Hodgkin's lymphoma. Oncologist 2004;9:160-72.
154. Wahl RL. Tositumomab and (131)I therapy in non-Hodgkin's lymphoma. J Nucl Med 2005; 46(Suppl 1):128S-140S.
155. Teeling JL, Mackus WJ, Wiegman LJ, et al. The biological activity of human CD20 monoclonal antibodies is linked to unique epitopes on CD20. J Immunol 2006;177:362-71.
156. Teeling JL, French RR, Cragg MS, et al. Characterization of new human CD20 monoclonal antibodies with potent cytolytic activity against non-Hodgkin lymphomas. Blood 2004;104:1793-800.
157. Sikder MA, Friedberg JW. Beyond rituximab: The future of monoclonal antibodies in B-cell non-Hodgkin lymphoma. Curr Oncol Rep 2008;10:420-6.

12

Monoclonal Antibody Therapy of Solid Malignancies

Robert O. Dillman, MD, FACP, and Robert K. Oldham, MD, FACP

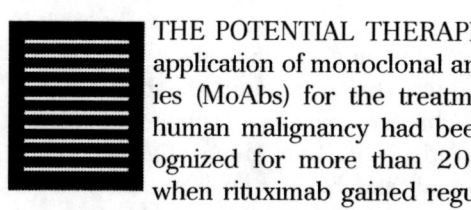

THE POTENTIAL THERAPEUTIC application of monoclonal antibodies (MoAbs) for the treatment of human malignancy had been recognized for more than 20 years when rituximab gained regulatory approval in November 1997 for the treatment of CD20-positive B-cell lymphoma,[1-4] and thus became the first MoAb approved for the treatment of a human malignancy.[5] As of mid-2009, nine MoAb products had US Food and Drug (FDA)-approved marketing indications for the treatment of human malignancies, including four unconjugated MoAbs for the treatment of solid tumors and two unconjugated MoAbs, two radiolabeled MoAbs, and one immunotoxin for the treatment of hematologic malignancies.[6] Most of this chapter focuses on the four MoAb products that are currently in routine clinical use for human solid cancers.

Historical Background for Antibody Therapy

Paul Ehrlich—the German immunologist, bacteriologist, and 1908 Nobel Prize winner—is generally considered the father of antibody therapy. He is recognized as the originator of the term "magic bullets" to describe the potential for antibodies to specifically target bacteria or cancer cells.[7,8] Between 1925 and 1980, numerous clinical studies were reported in which human patients were treated with antisera obtained from animals that had been immunized with human tumors.[9-11] Such trials

---

Robert O. Dillman, MD, FACP, Grace E. Hoag Endowed Chair of Oncology and Executve Medical and Scientific Director, Hoag Cancer Center, Newport Beach, California, and Clinical Professor of Medicine, University of California Irvine, Irvine, California, and Robert K. Oldham, MD, FACP, Director, Hematology-Oncology, Southeast Missouri Hospital, Cape Girardeau, Missouri, and Clinical Professor of Medicine, University of Missouri School of Medicine, Columbia, Missouri

The authors have disclosed no conflicts of interest.

were limited by the quantity of purified antitumor sera available, the purity of such preparations, and the inability to produce identical lots of promising antibody preparations. Some antitumor effects were reported, but mostly in patients with hematologic malignancies. Interpretation of antisera studies was complicated by issues of antibody source, purity, and specificity. Certain toxicities were identified, but it was unclear whether these were caused by impurities, hypersensitivity reactions to foreign proteins, or antitumor effects. Some antisera products, such as antithymocyte globulin, are still in clinical use today.

Before 1975, it was impossible to isolate a specific antibody. In 1975, Hans Kohler and Caesar Milstein described the hybridoma technology to isolate and produce antibodies derived from a single clone of cells; hence, the term monoclonal antibody.[12] They were awarded Nobel Prizes in 1986 for this seminal work. Using this technology, large quantities of reproducible murine MoAb products became available for studies in animal models, and exploratory human trials were carried out during the 1980s. Because of the propensity of melanoma to metastasize to subcutaneous tissue and lymph nodes, many of the first MoAbs directed against solid tumors were derived from immunization with melanoma tissue, and many of the early trials were conducted in patients with metastatic melanoma.[13-24] Other trials were reported in which patients received infusions of MoAbs directed against antigens expressed on colorectal and other gastrointestinal (GI) malignancies[25-29] and cancers of the lung,[30-32] breast,[33,34] prostate,[35,36] and kidney.[37] These studies established safety, tumor targeting, and antitumor effects of various products. Experience with 17 different murine antibodies and three human antibodies in various tumor types demonstrated that most side effects and toxicities were caused by antibody-antigen interactions rather than inherent immunogenicity of the MoAbs themselves.[38-40] However, these studies also established the limitations of murine MoAbs because of pharmacokinetics and human anti-mouse antibodies (HAMA).[41-45] The evidence derived from these trials suggested that larger doses of humanized MoAbs would be superior to murine MoAbs for therapeutic use and that the antigenic target was more important than MoAb interaction with complement and effector cells in producing antitumor benefit.[3,4]

During the 1990s, the DNA from murine hybridomas that were producing promising MoAbs was used to make chimeric or humanized MoAbs using recombinant DNA technology.[46-48] This technology was also used to mass-produce MoAbs in *Escherichia coli*, yeast, and Chinese hamster ovary (CHO) cells.[49-52] In addition, approaches combining complementary DNA libraries derived via polymerase chain reaction (PCR) with transgenic mice have enabled production of completely human MoAbs.[53,54]

The FDA has developed a nomenclature to indicate the construct and target of MoAb products. The suffix *mab* indicates that the product is a monoclonal antibody. The prefix of the name has no specific meaning, but the syllable directly in front of "mab" indicates the source, such as mouse, chimeric, humanized, or human. A second syllable may be added if there is something else linked or attached to the product. The therapeutic MoAbs discussed in this chapter are either chimeric (*-ximab*), humanized (*-zumab*), or human (*-umab*). Thus, trastuzumab and bevacizumab are humanized Moabs, cetuximab is a chimeric MoAb, and panitumumab is completely human. Ipilimumab (MDX-010) and tremelimumab (CP-675, 206; formerly known as ticilimumab) are human MoAbs that that target the CTLA4, a molecule that is important for regulatory T cells.[55] The "lim" syllable indicates that the MoAb targets the immune system. These two products are in Phase III pivotal trials in patients with melanoma.

Mechanisms of Antibody-Mediated Antitumor Effects

There are two major mechanisms by which unconjugated MoAbs are known to produce antitumor effects.[3,4] MoAbs can produce antitumor effects via the immune system secondary to the interaction between the Fc portion of the immunoglobulin molecule and complement proteins or immune effector cells. For such interaction, it is important that large numbers of the target molecule are expressed on the tumor cells and that the MoAb binds with high affinity and avidity. MoAbs also may produce antitumor effects via "regulatory" effects secondary to MoAb binding to a cell surface receptor or a ligand. Ligand/receptor interaction and intracellular signal transduction are crucial for this antitumor mechanism. In addition, MoAbs may alter the microenvironment, resulting in antitumor effects, even if the tumor cell receptor is not the direct target. Three of the MoAbs currently in widespread clinical use target the epidermal growth factor receptor (EGFR)—trastuzumab, cetuximab, and panitumumab—but in vitro they can also interact with human complement or effector cells to produce antitumor effects. The fourth Moab currently in widespread clinical use, bevacizumab, binds to the vascular endothelial growth factor (VEGF) ligand, thereby blocking its interaction with the VEGF receptor (VEGFR) on blood vessels to inhibit angiogenesis.

Epidermal Growth Factor and Its Receptors

The human EGFR family includes four transmembrane receptors, abbreviated as HER1 (human epidermal growth factor receptor 1), HER2, HER3, and HER4 (or Erb-B1, Erb-B2, Erb-B3, and Erb-B4). These are involved in regulation of cell proliferation and survival. EGFRs are expressed or overexpressed in most types of epithelial solid tumors.[56,57] A number of different ligand growth factors can bind to EGFR1, including transforming growth factor beta (TGFβ), epiregulin, betacellulin, and amphiregulin. Ligand-EGFR1 interactions activate the cytoplasmic tyrosine kinase domain of the receptor, which in turn activates intracellular signal transduction that facilitates tumor-cell proliferation and resistance to apoptosis.[58,59] EGFR1 is the target of the commercially available antibodies cetuximab and panitumumab. Heregulin is a known ligand for EGFR3, which, unlike the other heregulin receptors, has no tyrosine kinase activity. Neuroregulins 1, 3, and 4 and epiregulin are ligands for EGFR4. EGFR2, also known as HER2, differs from the other EGFRs in that it has no known ligand. However, it can "dimerize" with other EGFR2 molecules or any of the other EGFR molecules to induce signal transduction that promotes tumor-cell proliferation. HER2 is overexpressed on tumor cells from about 25% of breast cancer patients.[60,61] EGFR2 is the target of trastuzumab, which was developed specifically for breast cancer.

Vascular Endothelial Growth Factor and Its Receptors

The late Judah Folkman is credited with promoting the hypothesis that angiogenesis was critical for tumor proliferation and metastasis.[62] VEGF induces angiogenesis via interaction with VEGFR expressed on blood vessels. Both could be good targets for anticancer therapy.[63,64] Bevacizumab does not bind to VEGFR but binds to VEGF, which is one of a family of proteins that induce angiogenesis and/or lymphoangiogenesis via binding to VEGFR and related receptors. VEGF, the central mediator of tumor angiogenesis, is produced by cells from many tissues, but VEGF messenger RNA is overexpressed in most tumors, and elevated serum levels of VEGF are predictive of poor prognosis. Various preclinical experiments suggested that the VEGF ligand would be a useful anti-cancer target for monotherapy or in combination with other anti-cancer agents.[65-69]

Considerations for Monoclonal Antibody Therapy

Many issues are considered when selecting a MoAb for clinical development for cancer therapy, including its ability to bind to a molecule on tumor cells or the microenvironment, its immunoglobulin class or subclass, and its ability to influence interaction with components of the immune system [Fc receptors (FcRs) and complement]. Clinical trials are needed to determine potential doses, rates of infusion, treatment schedules, toxicity, and antitumor efficacy.

Binding to Cellular Targets

If a given tumor cell does not express the antigen detected by a given monoclonal antibody, there is no basis for monoclonal immune-mediated cytolysis or receptor inhibition for that cell.[3,4] A therapeutic MoAb must readily bind to, and stay attached to, its cellular target antigen, referred to as "affinity" and "avidity." It must also have at least relative specificity for malignant cells over normal cells, or else the target must be more critical for malignant cells. Histochemistry on various tissues is used to determine relative specificity. Testing of multiple tumor tissue specimens is used to determine sensitivity for a particular tumor type. Animal models with antigen-positive tumors are used to verify the extent of in-vivo binding to tumor and normal tissue. These same techniques have been used to verify sensitivity and specificity of MoAb binding in humans with cancer.

Some tumor antigens are shed in large quantities, constituting potential blocking factors to MoAb target cell binding. Such immune complexes might also produce damage to normal tissues and organs as well. Modulation, or down-regulation of receptors, may be desirable for antibodies that act through a regulatory mechanism, perhaps by altering signal transduction. Continued presence of antibody is needed to sustain this effect, which has important implications for duration of therapy. Rapid internalization greatly limits the therapeutic potential of antibodies that effect complement- and/or cell-mediated cytotoxicity but may be useful or a necessary condition for drug or toxin antibody immunoconjugates. As a general rule, modulation is much more common for hematopoietic cell antigens than solid tumor antigens, but it appears that some of the best targets for treatment of solid tumors are antigens that internalize and function as growth factor receptors for tumor cells.

Immunoglobulin Class and Subclass

The preferred strategy is to use chimeric, humanized, or human Ig because of the advantages associated with the human Fc and the more favorable pharmacokinetics with prolonged measurable serum levels of humanized preparations compared to their murine counterparts. Many investigators have chosen a human IgG1 subclass because these are predictably associated with efficient complement-dependent cytotoxicity (CDC) and antibody-dependent cell-mediated cytotoxicity (ADCC).[70] Even with modern commercially available antibodies, there is still the potential for HAMA and/or human anti-chimeric antibodies (HACA) following treatment with a chimeric antibody, and there is potential even for human anti-human antibodies (HAHA) directed against allotypic human antigens on human MoAbs. Human immune responses that result in the production of HAMA, HACA, and HAHA are readily detected by immunoassays that use the therapeutic antibodies in the assays for the treatment of patients. Most of the antibodies in HACA or HAHA are directed to allotypic epitopes and carbohydrates on the Fc portion. Fortunately, the various chimeric and humanized MoAbs that have entered the clinic have been associated with minimal HAMA, HACA, or HAHA. Based on the large clinical experiences with current chimeric and humanized antibodies, it appears that the risk of HACA or HAMA is on the order of only 1% to 2% of all patients treated, and this rarely interferes with treatment.

Tumor Penetration

Unlike some hematopoietic malignancies, solid tumors invariably grow as nodules or masses that can reach a large size. There has been great interest in finding ways to overcome the interstitial pressure effects found in larger tumor lesions, which impair penetration of antibodies into the core areas of such tumors.[71,72] In general, after an intravenous (IV) infusion of a large quantity of MoAb, the heirarchy of binding to antigen-bearing cells is as follows:

circulating blood cells > bone marrow > skin > lymph nodes > small tumor nodules > large tumor masses. MoAbs typically will not cross the blood-brain barrier of a normal brain, but they readily cross this barrier in the setting of vascular tumors, whose growth disrupts it.

There is some preclinical evidence that prior immunotherapy can increase penetration of MoAb into solid tumor nodules, but there have been no clinical trials to confirm this in humans. The issue of whether giving chemotherapy before, after, or during MoAb therapy affects the penetration, therapeutic results, or toxicity is also unresolved.

Tumor lysis syndrome is a constellation of symptoms and complications associated with the rapid cytotoxic death of rapidly proliferating tumor cells.[73,74] It occurs in the setting of large numbers of rapidly proliferating tumor cells, such as in acute leukemia, Hodgkin disease, large B-cell lymphoma, and testicular cancer, when highly effective systemic chemotherapy rapidly destroys large numbers of proliferating cells. This is followed by increases in serum potassium, uric acid, and phosphates released by the destroyed cells, with subsequent hypotension, renal failure, and other medical complications that can be life threatening or lethal. There have been no reports of unconjugated MoAb monotherapy of solid tumors resulting in tumor lysis syndrome. The kinetics of tumor penetration may be one of the reasons this has not been observed.

Interaction with Complement and/or Immune Cells

As part of the immune response, antibodies interact with complement proteins and immune effector cells via carbohydrates that are present on the Fc portion of the immunoglobulin molecule and FcRs on effector cells.[75-77] The interaction between Fc and FcR is influenced by several factors, including the affinity between the antibody isotype and the specific receptor, the composition of the sugar side chain on the Fc portion of the antibody, and inhibitory characteristics of the FcR. There is increasing evidence that these polymorphisms correlate with the clinical efficacy of certain MoAbs, which has led to specific strategies to modify the Fc portion of MoAbs to optimize the antitumor effector functions.[78,79] For both ADCC and CMC, the in-vivo antitumor effect also depends on the host immune system to provide sufficient complement proteins or effector cells to effect cytotoxicity. Therefore, theoretically, in the treatment of solid tumors, the addition of biologic response modifiers may be useful in enhancing MoAb-induced antitumor effects. However, to date, clinical testing of this concept has not yielded dramatic differences between the effects induced by MoAbs alone and MoAbs combined with interferon-gamma,[80-83] interleukin-2 (IL-2),[84-88] interferon-alpha,[89,90] or granulocyte-macrophage colony-stimulating factor (GM-CSF).[91-94]

Infusion Rates

Animal models and Phase I trials typically define a safe infusion rate. Rapid infusions of MoAbs that bind to antigen on circulating blood cells and/or trigger endogenous immune responses leading to cytokine release and cell activation via interactions with Fc receptors can be life threatening.[38-40,95-100] This is a significant safety issue for many MoAbs that are used in the treatment of hematologic malignancies,[95-97] but it is less of a problem for MoAbs used in the treatment of solid tumors because MoAbs that react with circulating blood cells typically are eliminated from further development during the drug development process.[38] In some instances, the interaction between the Fc portion of the MoAb and Fc receptors of circulating immunue cells may trigger the release of cytokines as well. There may also be idiosyncratic immune reactions against certain "foreign" amino acid sequences in some MoAb constructs. Because MoAbs directed against solid tumors typically do not react with circulating cells except via the FcR on leukocytes, infusions are typically associated with much less severe reactions than observed with MoAbs that target a receptor on circulating cells. Pure preparations of humanized MoAbs that do not react with circulating white blood cells via antigen or Fc receptors can be given over a few minutes with no untoward effects.

Antibody Dosing and Schedules

There is a dose/response relationship at low monoclonal antibody doses (<10 mg) because of the volume of distribution, nonspecific uptake and metabolism, and importance of the number of antibody molecules on cell surfaces for complement, reticuloendothelial, or effector cell-mediated effects.[14,17] At higher dose levels that provide antibody excess, these dose-response relationships are no longer an issue. Large quantities of MoAbs are typically needed to penetrate and saturate tumor cells in a large tumor mass. The duration of sustained serum levels probably is important for continuous blockade of the regulatory targets that are associated with survival and proliferation of solid tumor cells. The clinical success of recently approved MoAbs has been associated with delivery of high doses repeated at relatively short intervals, such as every 1 to 2 weeks, which ensures continuous serum levels. It seems likely that there are critical thresholds for dose for sustained antibody levels to produce an antitumor effect. Whether the dose/response relationship is important beyond those threshold levels is unclear, but sustained serum levels are almost certainly related to duration of response in many patients. Because of known antibody-antigen interactions, it has been easy to devise various enzyme-linked immunosorbent assays (ELISA) and radioimmunoassays (RIA) to measure serum levels of MoAb during and following infusions, but these have not been commercialized, so they cannot be used to guide rationale for scheduling.

Toxicity and Side Effects

Toxicity and side effects can be characterized as infusion reactions, acute or delayed hypersensitivity reactions, or nonimmunologic biologic effects. The vast majority of significant adverse events associated with MoAbs are caused by the biologic effects that follow antibody-antigen binding rather than immune reactions to the antibody itself. This explains why most of the toxic effects described for murine MoAbs are also seen with the chimeric, humanized, and human constructs that target the same antigen.

Infusion Reactions

The most predictable side effect is the "infusion reaction" symptom complex that follows MoAb binding to circulating cells and the subsequent release of cytokines.[38-40,95-100] The side effects are similar to those seen with high doses of various cytokines, such as interferon, IL-2, or high doses of GM-CSF. These include fever, rigors/chills, sweats, maculopapular erythematous skin rash, urticaria, pruritus, edema, hypotension, tachycardia, headache, nausea, vomiting, diarrhea, fatigue, elevated hepatic transaminases, throat tightness, pain, thrombocytopenia, dyspnea, bronchospasm, anaphylactic shock, and even death. These side effects can occur from within a matter of minutes to hours after an IV antibody infusion is initiated. This is rarely a problem for MoAbs used to treat solid tumors because of the scarcity of circulating tumor cells in such patients. However, as noted above, because of the binding of MoAb to circulating immune cells via Fc/FcR interaction and/or to endothelial cells, some MoAbs probably cause mild infusion reactions because of the release of cytokines via this interaction.

Acute Hypersensitivity Reactions and Anaphylaxis

MoAb infusions are less often associated with allergic or hypersensitive reactions. Because the first MoAbs were mouse proteins, there was great concern that infusion of these products would be associated with a high frequency of acute anaphylactoid reactions. Fortunately, such complications were rare, and are even less common in association with chimeric and humanized antibodies. Patients with a known history of allergic reaction to rodents or their by-products were typically excluded from trials of murine antibodies. Acute allergic reactions have included anaphylactic shock, less severe anaphylactoid reactions such as bronchospasm, and generalized pruritus and urticaria, and they can be difficult to distinguish from a severe infusion reaction.[98,100] The more severe reactions can be successfully managed with epinephrine. Patients who experience full-blown anaphylaxis during or shortly following an antibody infusion should not be re-treated with the agent, but it is important that a predictable infusion reaction not be confused with such a severe allergic reaction. Dermatologic effects including pruritis, diffuse or focal maculopapular rashes, and urticaria may be seen alone or as part of a full anaphylactic reaction with laryngeal edema, hypotension, and bronchospasm. Pruritus and urticaria alone typically resolve without treatment but may be responsive to diphenhydramine or epinephrine. The chimeric MoAb cetuximab, which is produced in murine plasmacytoma cells, is associated with a higher rate of infusion-associated flu-like symptoms, such as fever, headache, chills, and dyspnea, compared to the human antibody panitumumab that is manufactured in CHO cells.

Immune Complexes and Serum Sickness

There is a potential for complications associated with immune complexes resulting from the binding of MoAb to free circulating antigen or the binding of endogenous antibodies that react with the therapeutic MoAb. Only rarely have symptoms been noted in the presence of the immune complexes formed by the binding of antibody to circulating antigen, probably as a result of the small size of such complexes because the monoclonal antibody binds to only one determinant on the circulating antigen. For this reason, the presence of circulating antigen is not a contraindication to antibody treatment, although the binding to soluble antigen greatly alters the pharmacokinetics of the antibody. However, acute arthralgias, myalgias, nerve palsies, fever, and skin rashes have occasionally been seen in this setting and attributed to the acute immune complex formation.[98,100] Endogenous antibodies against the therapeutic MoAb rarely induce immune complex disease but do increase clearance, thus altering the pharmacokinetics of the MoAb. Classic serum sickness has been seen 2 to 3 weeks following exposure to moderate and high doses of murine MoAb and rarely after chimeric MoAb. A typical symptom complex includes fever, malaise, arthralgias/arthritis, myalgias, maculopapular erythematous skin rash, and fatigue. Proteinuria has been rarely observed in these few patients, and renal insufficiency is extremely rare. Serum sickness can be managed with nonsteroidal, anti-inflammatory agents and corticosteroids in more severe cases.

Side Effects Secondary to Binding to Nonmalignant Tissues

Adverse events may also occur as a consequence of direct effects on noncancerous tissue that also expresses the target antigen. Dermatologic toxicities are predictable complications of agents that interfere with EGFR1 signal transduction, such as cetuximab and panitumumab.[101-103] Trastuzumab, which interferes with EGFR2 signal transduction, is associated with cardiac toxicity.[104-106] Cetuximab and panitumumab both target EGFR1 and have certain toxicities in common that relate to biologic effects associated with blocking EGFR, such as acneiform skin rash and GI symptoms, including abdominal pain, nausea, vomiting, and diarrhea. Bevacizumab has been associated with hemorrhage, vascular thrombosis, hypertension, and proteinuria, presumably all because of effects on blood vessels.[107-109]

Therapeutic Monoclonal Antibodies Commercially Available for Treatment of Solid Tumors

"Magic bullets" became a reality for cancer therapy in November 1997 when the anti-CD20 monoclonal antibody rituximab [Rituxan (Genentech, South San Francisco, CA)] became the first monoclonal antibody product approved by the FDA for the treatment of a malignant disease, namely, B-cell lymphoma.[5] A year later, trastuzumab [Herceptin (Genentech)] became the first MoAb approved for the treatment of a solid tumor when it was granted a marketing indication for breast cancer.[110] In the following decade, three other MoAbs were approved for the treatment of solid tumors. The rest of this chapter focuses on these unconjugated MoAbs (see Table 12-1).

Trastuzumab (Herceptin)

Trastuzumab and HER2

In September 1998, the FDA approved trastuzumab (Herceptin), a humanized MoAb that reacts with the second component of human EGFR, known as HER2. It was approved based on clinical results observed in the treatment of metastatic breast cancer and was the first MoAb approved for the treatment of a solid tumor.[110] It is now in widespread clinical use for the treatment of metastatic breast cancer and in the adjuvant setting. Trastuzumab consists of the idiotopes from the hypervariable region of murine antibody 4D5 united with a human IgG1 kappa antibody that reacts with the p185HER2/neu receptor.[111] The murine construct was humanized by inserting the complementary-determining regions (CDRs) of the murine 4D5 into the constant and variable framework of a consensus human IgG1 to produce rHuMAb 4D5, which was more active in ADCC assays than its mouse counterpart. Trastuzumab is produced using recombinant DNA technology in CHO cells.

HER2 is a 185-kD member of the EGFR tyrosine kinase family of transmembrane receptors. After activation following binding of the EGF ligand to EGFR, it induces autophosphorylation of certain tyrosine residues. Early analysis suggested that a subset of about 25% of breast cancer patients had tumors that overexpressed this receptor.[61] Overexpression of the erbB-2 proto-oncogene results in overexpression of the HER2 receptor on the cell surface and increased cell proliferation.[60] Binding of trastuzumab to the HER2 receptor results in internalization of the receptor and competitive inhibition to binding of EGF ligands to the receptor.[112] This inhibition interferes with phosphorylation and blocks the subsequent signal transduction that facilitates cell proliferation. The human IgG1 Fc constant region on the humanized antibody mediates ADCC in vitro; thus, trastuzumab may also produce antitumor effects via the immune system, although internalization of the receptor may limit this antitumor mechanism. In fact, because of this, early work focused on the potential for immunotoxin immunotherapy approaches rather than for unconjugated monotherapy.[113] However, some investigators suggested a possible role for ADCC, based on the finding that breast cancer samples from patients treated with docetaxel and trastuzumab contained significantly increased numbers of natural killer cells and

Table 12-1. Commercially Available Monoclonal Antibodies for the Treatment of Human Solid Tumors

Generic Name	Commercial Name	Antigen	Antibody Type	Fc/Fv Ig type	Cell Production	Year FDA Approved
Trastuzumab	Herceptin	EGFR2	Humanized	IgG1	CHO	1998
Bevacizumab	Avastin	VEGF	Humanized	IgG1	CHO	2004
Cetuximab	Erbitux	EGFR1	Chimeric	IgG1	MP	2004
Panitumumab	Vectibix	EGFR1	Human	IgG2	CHO	2006

Ig = immunoglobulin; FDA = Food and Drug Administration; EGFR = epidermal growth factor receptor; VEGF = vascular endothelial growth factor; CHO = Chinese hamster ovary; MP = murine plasmacytoma.

increased expression of granzyme B and TiA1 in lymphocytes compared with controls.[114]

The optimal dose and schedule of trastuzumab administration is unknown. Based on the pivotal trial data submitted to the FDA, the recommended initial loading dose is 4 mg/kg administered as a 90-minute infusion followed by a weekly maintenance dose of 2 mg/kg administered as a 30-minute infusion. A 3-week dosing schedule has also been validated.[115,116]

Because HER2 is overexpressed in only about 25% of patients with breast cancer, for appropriate patient selection for treatment, it is necessary to test for high expression of HER2 by immunohistochemistry (IHC) or for overexpression of the HER2-neu gene by fluorescent in-situ hybridization (FISH). Large trials indicate there is poor reproducibility in performance and interpretation of IHC assays for HER2 in laboratories that do not process and analyze large numbers of samples. Even in the best of hands, concordance between IHC and FISH is limited. Many trials have demonstrated lower response rates in IHC 2+ compared to 3+, whereas benefit is almost always seen in patients who are FISH positive. Therefore, most centers use IHC for inititial testing and reserve FISH for patients who are 2+ by IHC. The Dako Herceptest (Genentech) for IHC assay of HER2 was used to determine eligibility in the pivotal trial and is generally considered the most reliable IHC test available.

Many questions have been raised regarding the reliability and reproducibility of the Dako Herceptest, especially when it is performed on paraffin-fixed, rather than fresh, tissues.[117-120] In one analysis, significant numbers of samples that were positive for HER2 by IHC were considered false positives based on negative FISH tests.[118] Comparative studies confirmed wide variation in interobserver reproducibility; confirmed that the two extremes, 0 and 3+, were more reproducible than 1+ and 2+ determinations; and revealed poor discrimination between 2+ and 3+, which contributed the high rate of false positives.[117] In one study, IHC and FISH results from three reference centers were compared for samples from 37 different hospitals for 426 breast carcinomas obtained from patients that were being considered for trastuzumab therapy.[119] Only 2 of 270 (0.7%) IHC 0/1+ tumors were FISH positive, and only 6 of 102 (5.9%) IHC 3+ tumors were FISH negative, suggesting that FISH testing was most valuable for validating that IHC 2+ tumors were really HER2 negative. In a large US adjuvant therapy trial, reference laboratories confirmed that 86% of 2535 registered patients were HER2 positive, but there was only 82% concordance between local and and high-volume central laboratories for IHC and 88% for FISH when the same methodologies were used.[120] For the discordant cases, the central and reference laboratories had 94% agreement for IHC 0, 1+, and 2+ and 95% agreement on those that were FISH. In a large trial by the National Surgical Adjuvant Breast and Bowel Project (NSABP), compared to the central laboratories, concordance rates were 97% for 29 laboratories that interpreted 100 or more HER2 samples per month, but only 76% for 75 laboratories that interpreted fewer than 100 HER2 samples per month.[121]

Clinical Trials with Trastuzumab in Breast Cancer

Numerous clinical trials have confirmed the efficacy of trastuzumab, especially in combination with chemotherapy, for the treatment of HER2-postive breast cancer in the settings of recurrent metastatic disease in previously treated patients, as the inititial treatment for metastatic breast cancer, and as adjuvant therapy.[122] Optimal duration of therapy has not been determined, but most physicians continue trastuzumab maintenance indefinitely or until disease progression, because HER2 is continually being produced by some malignant cells.

Trastuzumab Alone

Various trials have studied trastuzumab as a single agent in the treatment of metastatic breast cancer. In patients with HER2-positive metastatic breast cancer that has relapsed after chemotherapy, available data suggest that trastuzumab alone produces objective response rates of 12% to 33%, depending on the specific patient populations and response definitions.[116,123-127]

In an early Phase II trial of trastuzumab, 46 metastatic breast cancer patients received 250 mg intravenously followed by weekly doses of 100 mg for 9 additional weeks.[123] Patients were eligible if at least 25% of tumor cells expressed HER2 by IHC. There were five responses among 43 evaluable patients. The most frequent toxicity was persistent low-grade fever, which was noted in 15%. This was attributed to immune complexes formed by trastuzumab binding to shed antigen.

The largest trial of trastuzumab as a single-agent was conducted in 222 patients with HER2-positive metastatic breast cancer that had recurred after chemotherapy.[124] Trastuzumab monotherapy was given at an initial dose of 4mg/kg followed by weekly doses of 2 mg/kg. There were eight complete and 26 partial responses, with a median duration of response of 13 months. In the 222 patients who had failed chemotherapy, there were four complete and 21 partial responses for an overall objective response rate of 12% by intent to treat analysis. The median duration of response among the 25 responders was 9 months, and their median survival was 13 months; these are comparable to chemotherapy. In the patient population, 66% had received prior adjuvant chemotherapy, 68% had received two or more chemotherapy regimens for metastatic cancer, and 55 patients (25%) had relapsed after high-dose chemotherapy and autologous stem cell rescue before receiving antibody therapy. The response rate was 14% among patients whose tumors were HER2 2+ or 3+ by IHC, but 20% for patients whose tumors were FISH positive vs 0% for FISH negative. Treatment was generally well tolerated, with 40% of patients experiencing fever during the first infusion. Cardiac dysfunction was noted in 5%, which was usually reversible when treatment was discontinued.

A randomized Phase II trial failed to detect any higher response rate for a higher dose of trastuzumab compared to the standard dose.[125]

In this trial, there was no significant difference in results for an 8-mg/kg loading dose and 4-mg/kg per week maintenance dose vs the standard 4-mg/kg loading dose and 2-mg/kg per week maintenance. The failure to demonstrate any difference between these doses is not surprising in view of the sustained serum levels of trastuzumab that were achieved at the lower dose. In this trial, trastuzumab alone as initial treatment for metastatic breast cancer resulted in seven complete and 23 partial responses, but the response rates were 35% for patients whose tumors were IHC 3+ compared to 0% for tumors that were IHC 2+, and 34% among patients whose tumors were FISH positive compared to 7% for tumors that were FISH negative. This response rate is the highest reported for single-agent trastuzumab in a prospective trial. The most common adverse events attributed to trastuzumab were chills (25%), asthenia (23%), fever (22%), pain (18%), and nausea (14%). Two patients (2%) with histories of cardiac disease experienced reversible cardiac dysfunction.

In another trial, trastuzumab was given at twice the standard dose by the weekly schedule as initial treatment for 8 weeks for patients with HER2-positive metastatic breast cancer who had never received chemotherapy.[126] They reported a response rate of 33% among 52 evaluable patients in a trial that enrolled 61 patients.

It would be more convenient for patients if trastuzumab were given at higher doses and less frequently than weekly. Baselga et al tested an every-3-week schedule of trastuzumab delivery as initial therapy for 105 patients with HER2-positive metastatic breast cancer.[116] The observed response rate was 19% but was 34% for patients whose tumors were IHC 3+ and/or FISH positive for HER2. As with other trastuzumab schedules, the most common treatment-related adverse events were rigors, fever, headache, nausea, and fatigue.

Trastuzumab plus Single-Agent Chemotherapy

In-vitro and animal studies have shown that trastuzumab augments the antitumor cytotoxicity of various chemotherapy agents.[127,128] Phase II clinical trials have studied single-agent chemotherapy combined with trastuzumab for treatment of patients with HER2-positive breast cancer. Trastuzumab has been combined with docetaxel,[114,129-132] paclitaxel,[111,133-136] vinorelbine,[137-144] liposomal doxorubicin,[145,146] cisplatin,[147] gemcitabine,[148] and capecitabine.[149] Administration of trastuzumab does not increase the toxicity of chemotherapy. Response rates of 50% or greater were reported in 18 of the 23 trials. Such response rates appear to be much higher than observed with chemotherapy alone. Although there has never been a prospective comparison of trazutuzumab vs trastuzumab plus chemotherapy, a retrospective analysis of Japanese patients with recurrent breast cancer who were treated with trastusuzmab alone (n = 39) or in combination with chemotherapy (n = 45) found a 65% response rate for monotherapy and an 86% response rate for combination therapy.[150] Time to progression was much longer for patients who received the chemotherapy plus trastuzumab combinations (15.9 vs 5.7 months).

In various breast cancer patient populations, combinations of single-agent chemotherapy plus trastuzumab were associated with response rates ranging from 22% to 78%, with median progression-free survival (PFS) of 6 to 12 months. Many of these reports noted higher response rates in the subsets of patients who had 3+ HER2 expression by IHC and/or overexpression by FISH, as opposed to 2+ IHC HER2 or negative FISH. The addition of trastuzumab was not associated with any additive toxicities other than cardiac disease in association with anthracyclines.

Combination Chemotherapy and Trastuzumab

Phase II clinical trials have used combination chemotherapy plus trastuzumab for treatment of patients with HER2-positive breast cancer. The most frequently tested combinations have been paclitaxel and platinum,[136,151] docetaxel doublets,[152,153] gemcitabine doublets,[154-159] and anthracycline plus taxane doublets.[160-162] Combination chemotherapy has consistently produced higher response rates and longer PFS in clinical trials in patients with metastatic breast cancer, although survival advantages have been harder to establish. Phase II trials of combination chemotherapy plus trastuzumab appear to have produced slightly higher response rates (40% to 98%) than were seen with single agents plus trastuzumab, and the PFS was somewhat longer, with a range from 6 to 16 months.

In a randomized trial, trastuzumab and paclitaxel with or without carboplatin were compared as first-line therapy for 196 women with HER2-overexpressing (2+ or 3+ by IHC) metastatic breast cancer.[136] Treatment consisted of six cycles of trastuzumab, 4 mg/kg loading dose and 2 mg/kg weekly thereafter with paclitaxel, 175 mg/m^2 every 3 weeks, with or without the addition of carboplatin (area under the concentration-vs-time curve, or AUC = 6) every 3 weeks. Endpoints favored the addition of carboplatin based on response rates of 52% vs 36% ($p = 0.04$) and median PFS of 11 vs 7 months (hazard ratio = 0.66; $p = 0.03$). In consecutive Phase II trials, weekly paclitaxel and carboplatin plus trastuzumab appeared superior to an every-3-week schedule of the same agents, with response rates of 81% vs 65%, median PFS of 14 vs 10 months, and median overall survival (OS) of 3.2 vs 2.3 years; it was also associated with less hematologic toxicity.[151]

Similar to what has been seen in other trials with anthracyclines, the combination of epirubicin plus carboplatin was associated with a high rate of significant cardiotoxicity (10/45).[162] The majority of cardiac events occurred late during therapy with trastuzumab alone. Half of the patients were asymptomatic, and all cases of congestive heart failure (CHF) resolved with therapy. In contrast, 15 patients treated with weekly epirubicin, paclitaxel, and trastuzumab did not experience CHF, although three had a greater than 10% reduction in left ventricular ejection fraction.[161] In a trial of 69 patients who received liposomal doxorubicin, paclitaxel, and trastuzumab, no patients developed CHF.[160] In 70 patients treated with dose-dense doxorubicin plus cyclophosphamide followed by paclitaxel and trastuzumab, there was significant cardiotoxicity.[163]

Randomized Trials of Chemotherapy with or without Trastuzumab in Breast Cancer

Randomized trials have compared chemotherapy plus trastuzumab to chemotherapy alone. One of the pivotal trials that led to regulatory approval of trastuzumab compared trastuzumab plus chemotherapy to chemotherapy alone in 469 patients with metastatic disease who had not received prior chemotherapy for metastatic disease.[164] All patients had 2+ or 3+ HER2-positive tumors by IHC on a scale of 0 to 3. An initial 4-mg/kg trastuzumab dose was followed by 2 mg/kg weekly. The first trastuzumab dose was infused intravenously over 90 minutes, but in the absence of significant infusion-related toxicity, subsequent doses were infused intravenously over 30 minutes. Patients who had not received an anthracycline previously were randomized to receive trastuzumab alone or with cyclophosphamide, 600 mg/m^2 intravenously, and doxorubicin, 60 mg/m^2 (AC), or epirubicin intravenously every 3 weeks for six cycles. Patients who had received adjuvant chemotherapy that included an anthracycline were randomized to receive paclitaxel, 175 mg/m^2 intravenously over 3 hours alone every 3 weeks or with trastuzumab. The combination of chemotherapy plus trastuzumab was superior for key endpoints, including response rate (50% vs 32%; p <0.0001), duration of response (9.1 vs 6.1 months), PFS (median = 7.4 vs 4.6 months; p <0.001), OS (death at 1 year = 22% vs 33 %; p = 0.008), and median survival (25.1 vs 20.3 months; p = 0.046), with a 20% reduction of risk of death. The differences were most striking for paclitaxel plus trastuzumab vs paclitaxel alone. The median OS was 22 months for paclitaxel plus trastuzumab vs 18 months for paclitaxel alone (p = 0.17) and 27 months for AC plus trastuzumab vs 21 months for AC alone (p = 0.16).

This trial clearly demonstrated that cardiotoxicity is associated with trastuzumab. Cardiac dysfunction was noted in 11 of 91 patients (12%) who received paclitaxel plus trastuzumab alone compared to only 1 of 95 (1%) who received paclitaxel alone, and in 28 of 143 (20%) who received AC plus trastuzumab compared to 7 of 135 (3%) who received AC alone. Even though trastuzumab does enhance the efficacy of anthracycline-containing regimens, the increased cardiac toxicity that is seen with such combinations has made this an inappropriate treatment strategy.

Another randomized trial compared docetaxel plus trastuzumab to docetaxel alone in patients with metastatic breast cancer who had received no prior chemotherapy.[165] Docetaxel was given every 3 weeks, and trastuzumab was given weekly. This trial confirmed a similar relative advantage for the addition of trastuzumab with roughly a doubling of response rate and PFS as well as better OS (31 vs 23 months; p = 0.032). The trastuzumab arm was associated with more grade 3 and 4 neutropenia (32% vs 22%), more febrile neutropenia (23% vs 17%), and one patient (1%) in the MoAb-containing arm had symptomatic heart failure.

Adjuvant Treatment of Breast Cancer

Based on the positive benefits of trastuzumab in measurable metastatic breast cancer, it was widely assumed that a similar benefit would be confirmed in the adjuvant setting. This has been confirmed by results from three large randomized trials. Because of the cardiotoxicity associated with trastuzumab, patients with active cardiac disease were excluded from these trials. At this time, it is unclear whether it is better to give trastuzumab concurrently with chemotherapy or sequentially following chemotherapy, and it is unclear how long trastuzumab should be continued. However, most expect that trials will confirm that concurrent is better than sequential treatment and that longer duration of adjuvant trastuzumab produces longer PFS. Completed trials have attempted to address whether it is better to give adjuvant trastuzumab for 2 years or 1 year, but it is probable that it is better to give trastuzumab indefinitely if there is reason to believe that the breast cancer has not been completely eliminated.

Three large randomized trials have been reported, at least in preliminary form.[166-170] Two US cooperative group trials were combined for one preliminary analysis.[167] The NSABP trial B-31 compared doxorubicin and cyclophosphamide followed by paclitaxel every 3 weeks with the same regimen plus 52 weeks of trastuzumab beginning with the first dose of paclitaxel. The North Central Cancer Treatment Group (NCCTG) trial N9831 compared three regimens: 1) doxorubicin and cyclophosphamide followed by weekly paclitaxel, 2) the same regimen plus 52 weeks of trastuzumab initiated concomitantly with paclitaxel, and 3) the same chemotherapy regimen followed by 52 weeks of trastuzumab after paclitaxel. For an early analysis at a median follow-up of 2 years, the two similar arms from each trial were combined and compared: doxorubicin plus cyclophosphamide followed by paclitaxel with or without trastuzumab concurrent with paclitaxel.[167] The potential for cardiac toxicity was closely monitored in this trial.[170] The cumulative incidence of cardiac events at 3 years was 10 times higher in the trastuzumab-containing arms vs the control arm, but the frequency of cardiac toxicity was less than 4%. Factors that increased the risk of a significant cardiac dysfunction were older age, lower ejection fraction at study entry, and antihypertensive medications.

The international, multicenter Herceptin Adjuvant (HERA) trial randomized more than 5000 women with HER2-positive-lymph node or high-risk lymph-node-negative breast cancer, comparing 1 or 2 years of trastuzumab given every 3 weeks with observation after completion of locoregional therapy and at least four cycles of neoadjuvant or adjuvant chemotherapy.[166,169] Initial reports compared interim disease-free survival and 1-year OS for the observation arm to the trastuzumab treatment arm.[166,169] In the European trial, 1010 women with node-positive or high-risk node-negative breast cancer were randomized to adjuvant therapy that consisted of three cycles of either docetaxel or vinorelbine, followed by three cycles of fluorouracil, epirubicin, and cyclophosphamide in both groups, with a secondary postchemotherapy randomization for the 232 patients whose tumors were HER2-positive to either observation or trastuzumab for 9 weeks.[168] Because of the use of anthracyclines in these trial designs, patients have been closely monitored for cardiac toxicity, which has been higher in the trastuzumab arms. In the NSABP B-31 trial, 16% of women discontinued trastuzumab therapy because of clinical evidence of myocardial dysfunction or significant decline in left ventricular function. All three of these trials have shown a benefit for the addition of trastuzumab.

Neoadjuvant Treatment of Breast Cancer

Trastuzumab is also being combined with chemotherapy as part of neoadjuvant therapies, with pathologic complete response rates ranging from 13% to 65%.[171-176] After 3 weeks of neoadjuvant treatment with trastuzumab alone, 23% of patients had a partial response before going on to receive 12 more weeks of trastuzumab combined with paclitaxel before surgery.[174] One randomized trial, which was designed to accrue 164 patients, was closed early because of the marked superiority of the trastuzumab-containing arm.[172] Chemotherapy consisted of four cycles of paclitaxel followed by four cycles of 5-fluorouracil (5-FU), epirubicin, and cyclophosphamide, with weekly trastuzumab for all 24 weeks. After 3 years of follow-up, there have been no recurrences in the patients who received neoadjuvant therapy, and they have better PFS (p = 0.041).[173]

Trastuzumab and Hormonal Therapy for Breast Cancer

About half of HER2-positive patients are hormone-receptor positive, and this has led to interest in the interaction "cross-talk" between HER2 and hormone receptors, which appears to increase resistance to hormonal therapies. There is a recent report of a 26% response rate for 31 evaluable patients who were treated with the aromatase inhibitor letrozole in combination with weekly trastuzumab.[177] HER2 positivity was confirmed for 82% (IHC3 positive and/or FISH positive), and 82% had previously been treated with tamoxifen. The median PFS was 6 months.

Trastuzumab in Other Tumor Types

HER2 is sometimes overexpressed in adenocarcinomas other than breast cancer. However, because of the variability in IHC methodology for detecting HER2, many of the higher estimates may be fallacious. So far, there are no tumor types other than breast cancer for which trastuzumab appears to be efficacious, even in trials restricted to patients whose tumors were 2+ or 3+ HER2 positive by IHC. In ovarian cancer, 95 of 837 patients (11%) were HER2 positive, and only 3 of 45 (7%) responded.[178] In non-small-cell lung cancer (NSCLC), 24 of 209 patients (11%) showed HER2-positive tumors by IHC, and only 1 of 24 (4%) had a response.[179] In another NSCLC trial, 13 of 69 patients had HER2-positive tumors by IHC, and none responded to trastuzumab.[180] In hormone-refractory prostate cancer, 0 of 18 HER2-positive patients had a response.[181]

Several exploratory trials have been conducted in which trastuzumab was combined with chemotherapy in HER2-positive patients with tumor types other than breast cancer.[182-187] Very few of the patients enrolled had tumors that were HER2 3+ by IHC. For example, less than 5% of patients in two of the NSCLC trials had tumors that were HER2 3+ by IHC.[182,184] Response rates did not appear to be higher than anticipated for chemotherapy alone, but to determine the true contribution of trastuzumab requires randomized trials. Gatzemeier et al randomized 101 patients with HER2-positive NSCLC to trastuzumab plus gemcitabine and cisplatin or the chemotherapy alone and found no difference in response rate (36% vs 41%) or PFS (6.1 vs 7.0 months), but only six patients had tumors that were 3+ HER2 by IHC, and five of them did have an objective response to treatment.[182] Even though the trials cited above had disappointing results, there are other ongoing trials of trastuzumab with chemotherapy in patient populations selected for overexpression of HER2 by FISH rather than IHC, and it is possible that some of these trials may yield positive results.

Trastuzumab with Other Biologicals

Even though the efficacy of trastuzumab might be enhanced by combining it with other biologic response modifiers, there has been limited exploration of this approach because there are so many efficacious chemotherapy agents with which to combine trastuzumab. Two trials have combined subcutaneous IL-2 with trastuzumab.[87,188] In one trial, there was a response rate of 9% in 45 patients, but more than 10% of patients experienced grade 3 or 4 pulmonary reactions.[188] In the other trial, one of 10 patiens had a clinical response.[87] In both trials, the use of IL-2 was associated with an increase in natural killer cells, but this did not correlate with toxicity or clinical benefit.

Toxicity and Side Effects

The toxicities associated with trastuzumab in pivotal trials are summarized in Table 12-2. Black-box warnings accompanying the label indication address cardiomyopathy and infusion reactions. Trastuzumab infusions can result in serious infusion reactions, including dyspnea and hypoxia, which rarely have been fatal. Most of the time, transfusion reactions are mild and are probably associated with binding to circulating white cells via either cross-reactive antigens or Fc receptors, but they are much milder than seen with rituximab. Typically, symptoms occur during or within 24 hours of trastuzumab infusion. Infusion should be interrupted for patients experiencing dyspnea or clinically significant hypotension, and patients should be monitored until signs and symptoms completely resolve. The basis for the minor infusion reactions that are sometimes seen with initial infusions is not clear, but it may relate to cross-reactivity with an antigen expressed on some circulating cells or a reaction related to binding to Fc on some circulating cells.

The major toxicity associated with trastuzumab is cardiac dysfunction or congestive heart failure that is generally mild and revers-

Table 12-2. Specific Acute Toxicities in Clinical Trials of Trastuzumab Monotherapy in Breast Cancer

Toxicity	Percent of Patients (n = 352)	Toxicity	Percent of Patients (n = 352)
Asthenia/malaise	42	Dyspnea	22
Abdominal pain	22	Rash	18
Fever	36	Rhinitis	14
Nausea	33	Dizzyness	13
Chills/rigors	32	Throat irritation	12
Cough	26	Edema	10
Headache	26	Arthralgia	6
Vomiting	23		

ible.[104-106,170,189,190] Trastuzumab treatment can result in left ventricular dysfunction and congestive heart failure; therefore left ventricular function should be evaluated in all patients before and during treatment. The frequency and severity of left ventricular cardiac dysfunction and/or clinical congestive heart failure is highest in patients who receive trastuzuamb concurrently with anthracycline-containing chemotherapy regimens and is also higher in patients who have recently received anthracycline-containing regimens. If left ventricular dysfunction or clinical heart failure occurs, trastuzumab should be discontinued until cardiac function has improved. Trastuzumab can often be resumed without recurrence of left ventricular dysfunction.

As a single agent, trastuzumab alone was associated with a 4% to 5% frequency of cardiac dysfunction in patients with metastatic disease and in the adjuvant setting.[124] The risk of cardiac toxicity was higher in patients with metastatic breast cancer who received trastuzumab with chemotherapy. Cardiac dysfunction was noted in 11 of 91 patients (12%) who received paclitaxel plus trastuzumab, compared to only 1 of 95 (1%) who received paclitaxel alone; in 28 of 143 (20%) who received AC plus trastuzumab, compared to 7 of 135 (3%) who received AC alone; in 27% for combined therapy vs 8% for anthracycline-based chemotherapy alone; and in 13% for combined therapy vs 1% for paclitaxel alone.[164] The higher rate of cardiotoxicity with the doxorubicin plus trastuzumab combination may be caused in part by increased drug delivery of doxorubicin to cardiac muscle by loose binding between doxorubicin and the MoAb[191] or additive or synergistic cardiotoxic effects of both agents. Other trials have also noted higher rates of cardiotoxicity in patients who have received anthracyclines before or concurrent with trastuzumab.[164,170,192,193] The cardiotoxicity of trastuzumab may relate to HER2 expression on cardiac muscle cells that are involved in tissue repair because absence of the HER2/neu gene in knockout mice is associated with failure to develop an embryonic heart.[194] Results from clinical trials suggest that cardiotoxicity is increased when trastuzumab is administered with or following cardiotoxic agents such as anthracyclines. For this reason it is recommended that trastuzumab not be given in combination with an anthracycline or any other agent that is known to damage the myocardium. Based on the adjuvant trials, when trastuzumab is given after an anthracycline, heart failure rates can be expected to be in the range of 4% to 5% during treatment, but there may be an increased risk that extends beyond treatment.

Summary

The approval of trastuzumab in September 1998 marked the first approval by the US FDA of a therapeutic monoclonal antibody for the treatment of a solid tumor. Because trastuzumab has limited clinical benefit as a single agent, even in patients who overexpress HER2, it is typically administered with chemotherapy agents that have proven benefit in breast cancer, except anthracyclines, which should be avoided because of the increased risk of cardiotoxicity. A decade after its introduction, trastuzumab with chemotherapy is now standard therapy in the neoadjuvant, adjuvant, and metastatic disease settings for breast cancer patients whose tumors are HER2-positive. It is controversial as to whether trastuzumab should be combined with chemotherapy in patients who have previously progressed during trastuzumab treatment with or without chemotherapy. Historically, overexpression of HER2 was associated with a poorer prognosis. Ironically, trastuzumab is so effective that the prognosis for HER2-positive breast cancer patients is now better than for those that are HER2-negative.

Cetuximab (Erbitux)

Cetuximab and the Epidermal Growth Factor Receptor

EGFRs are expressed to some extent on all epithelial tumors. EGFR is frequently overexpressed in cancers of the breast, ovary, bladder, head and neck, prostate, pancreas, and colon. EGFRs are expressed at high levels in about one-third of all epithelial cancers and are associated with accelerated growth.[59] EGFR and its ligands, such as TGFα, have long been recognized as potential targets for antibody-based therapy. EGF ligand/receptor interaction induces tyrosine kinase activity, which in turn enhances cell proliferation capability. Autocrine activation and overexpression of EGFR appears to be crucial for the accelerated growth of many cancers and is associated with increased expression of VEGF.

The murine antibody to EGFR1, called 225, was shown to block receptor function and inhibit cell growth in cultures in nude mouse xenografts.[58] The MoAb bound to the extracellular domain of EGFR, causing internalization of the receptor and antibody and "down-regulation" of the receptor. For this reason, most early development with EGFR antibodies focused on immunoconjugates, especially ricin immunotoxins.[113] Cetuximab, the chimeric form of the antibody, was more effective in the mouse tumor models than the murine antibody, apparently because of a higher affinity for the EGFR target.[195] Internalization of the receptor is slow enough that cetuximab is cytotoxic in vitro in the presence of human effector cells and complement, but its major antitumor mechanism is believed to relate to the receptor blockade, preventing signal transduction that is associated with cellular proliferation. In laboratory tests against tumor cells and in animal models with human tumor xenografts, cetuximab enhanced the chemotherapy effects of many different chemotherapy agents, including platinums, campothecins, taxanes, fluoropyrimidines, and gemcitabine.

The anti-EGFR chimeric MoAb cetuximab [Erbitux (Bristol-Myers Squibb, New York, NY)] was approved in 2004 based on randomized trials in which the agent was combined with the chemotherapy agent irinotecan in the treatment of metastatic colorectal cancer. It is a recombinant chimeric MoAb that includes a murine Fv and human IgG1 kappa constant regions. Unlike most MoAbs, cetuximab is manufactured in murine plasmacytoma cells. This cellular factory results in murine glycosylation, which may increase the risks of allergic reactions in some patients.

Although there is a well-documented association between EGFR2 expression by IHC and FISH and the benefit of trastuzumab therapy, the relationship between EGFR1 expression by IHC and FISH and cetuximab clinical activity is less clear. EGFR1 expressing human tumors was used in animal models to demonstrate the antitumor effects of cetuximab; thus in clinical trials, at least some degree of EGFR1 expression was required. One of the reasons for the variation in EGFR1 expression is that ligand binding and internalization can either block or leave no exposed receptor for binding of an EGFR antibody in the IHC. Gene analysis by FISH may be a better predictor of which patients may benefit from anti-EGFR1 therapy. One group retrospectively analyzed EGFR copy numbers by FISH in paraffin-embedded tumor blocks from 85 chemorefractory colorectal cancer patients who had been treated with cetuximab.[196] Based on their scoring system, the 43 patients who were EGFR positive by FISH had a higher response rate (p = 0.0001) and disease PFS (p = 0.02) than the 42 patients who were EGFR negative by FISH. Another group used both IHC and FISH to analyze paraffin-embedded sections of tumor from 47 patients with metastatic colorectal cancer who had been treated with a cetuximab-chemotherapy regimen.[197] By IHC, 83% had EGFR-positive tumors, but an increase in EGFR gene copy was detected in only 20% of 41 tumors in which this methodology could be performed. Neither EGFR expression (assessed by IHC) nor EGFR gene copy (assessed by FISH) correlated with response rate, PFS, and OS. Unfortunately, in this study the antitumor effects of chemotherapy may have confounded the results.

Clinical Trials with Cetuximab

Colorectal Cancer

The first marketing indication for cetuximab was in colorectal cancer. Although results have been published for single-agent cetuximab in various clinical settings, many of the initial trials with cetuximab, as a single agent and in combination with chemotherapy, were conducted in patients with metastatic colorectal cancer,[198-202] In these trials cetuximab was given at an initial loading dose of 400 mg/m^2 intravenously over 2 hours, then 250 mg/m^2 intravenously over 1 hour weekly. Response rates ranged from 8% to 12% regardless of prior therapy.

Lenz et al treated 346 patients whose metastatic cancer was considered refractory to fluoropyrimidines, irinotecan, and oxaliplatin.[198] EGFR positivity by IHC was an eligibility requirement, but degree of positivity did not correlate with clinical benefit. The most prevalent toxicity was the acneiform rash, which was noted in 83% of patients and was predictive of clinical benefit.

In a study by Jonker et al, 572 patients who had progressed despite 5-FU, irinotecan, and oxaliplatin were randomized to standard-dose cetuximab or observation.[199] Although the objective response rate was only 8%, OS and PFS were better in the cetuximab arm. Severe adverse events of rash and infection were more common in the cetuximab arm. Hypomagnesemia was also more common with cetuximab. Eleven patients discontinued cetuximab because of infusion reactions.

In a large randomized trial designed for regulatory approval, 111 patients whose metastatic colorectal cancer had progressed during or within 3 months after discontinuation of irinotecan were randomized to receive cetuximab alone.[200] Saltz et al treated 57 patients whose metastatic cancers had not responded to prior irinotecan alone or as part of combination chemotherapy.[201] Criteria for treatment included demonstration of EGFR on formalin-fixed, paraffin-embedded tumor tissue by IHC. The most common adverse events were an acneiform skin rash, predominantly on the face and upper chest (86%), and a constellation of asthenia, fatigue, malaise, or lethargy (56%). Three patients were reported to have had a grade 3 allergic reaction; two were withdrawn. Pessino et al treated 39 previously untreated patients with metastatic colorectal cancer, but the response rate was still only 10%.[202]

Numerous trials have examined the combination of irinotecan plus cetuximab. Many of these trials focused on patients who had already experienced progressive disease after treatment with irinotecan. Response rates ranged from 16% to 31% in previously treated patients but as high as 72% in previously untreated patients. Sobrero et al reported a response rate of 16% in 649 patients who had metastatic colorectal cancer previously treated with fluoropyrimidine and oxaliplatin and were randomized to receive cetuximab plus irinotecan.[203] Wilke et al focused on PFS following cetuximab plus irinotecan therapy in patients who had recently failed an irinotecan-containing regimen.[204] In a large randomized trial designed for regulatory approval, a response rate of 23% was observed following cetuximab plus irinotecan in 218 patients whose metastatic colorectal cancer had progressed during or within 3 months after discontinuation of irinotecan.[200] A weekly irinotecan-plus-cetuximab regimen resulted in a 16% response rate in patients whose metastatic colorectal cancer was refractory to oxaliplatin and irinotecan.[205] Gebbia et al treated 60 patients who had received at least two prior therapies and whose metastatic cancer was considered refractory to oxaliplatin and irinotecan.[206] Standard cetuximab dosing was combined with irinotecan, 120 mg/m^2 weekly for 4 out of 6 weeks. Responses were not predicted by EGFR expression. The main grade 3 and 4 toxicities were mostly attributable to the chemotherapy and included nausea (33%), diarrhea (27%), leukopenia (18%), asthenia (13%), and acneiform skin rash (13%). Vincenzi et al treated 55 patients whose metastatic cancer was considered refractory to oxaliplatin and irinotecan.[207] Standard cetuximab dosing was combined with irinotecan, 90 mg/m^2 weekly. Skin toxicity was observed in 89% of patients. The most common grade 3-to-4 adverse events were dermatologic reactions (33%), diarrhea (16%), fatigue (13%), and stomatitis (7%). Fever was noted in 25%, typically in association with the first infusion of cetuximab, but no allergic reactions were recorded. Martín-Martorell reported a 22% response rate with a biweekly irinotecan cetuximab combination.[208] A 31% response rate was noted in Japanese patients who had experienced progressive disease despite various chemotherapy regimens.[209]

More recently, cetuximab has been combined with modern combination therapies such as FOLFOX [folate (leucovorin), 5-fluorouracil, oxaliplatin] and FOLFIRI [folate (leucovorin), 5-fluorouracil, irinotecan] as the initial treatment of patients with metastatic colorectal cancer. Response rates ranged from 34% to 72%. A 47% response rate was observed in 599 patients randomized to treatment with cetuximab plus FOLFIRI.[210] Three FOLFOX regimens produced response rates of 46% to 72%.[211-213] Other investigators have combined the oral fluoropyrimidine capecitabine with irinotecan[214] or oxaliplatin.[215]

The strongest evidence for cetuximab activity in colorectal cancer comes from randomized trials. Cetuximab therapy was associated with longer PFS and OS compared to best supportive care in patients with metastatic colorectal cancer that had progressed after 5-FU, oxaliplatin, and irinotecan.[199] In a regulatory pivotal trial, Cunningham et al randomized 329 patients, who had colorectal cancer that had progressed during or within 3 months after discontinuation of irinotecan, to receive irinotecan plus cetuximab or cetuximab alone using a 2:1 randomization.[200] The combination therapy was associated with a higher response rate (p = 0.007) and longer PFS (p <0.001). Cetuximab plus FOLFIRI was superior to FOLFIRI alone in terms of response rate (47% vs 39%; p = 0.004) and PFS (8.9 vs 8.0 months; p = 0.048).[210] Cetuximab plus FOLFOX was possibly superior to FOLFOX alone in terms of response rate (46% vs 36%; p = 0.064), but there was no improvement in PFS.[211] However, benefit was evident in patients who had an unmutated (ie, "wild-type") K-ras gene.

Another highly anticipated randomized trial examined whether adding cetuximab would enhance capecitabine-oxaliplatin-bevacizumab therapy for metastatic colorectal cancer.[216] It was widely assumed that combining the two antibodies would offer added benefit. To the surprise of most, PFS was actually worse in the patients who received cetuximab, and they experienced more grade 3 or 4 adverse events, mostly because of cetuximab-related cutaneous toxicity. There was no significant difference between the treatment groups in OS or response rates.

Cetuximab is also being explored in rectal cancer. Based on a trial in 40 patients with rectal cancer, preoperative radiotherapy in combination with capecitabine and cetuximab is feasible.[217] A Phase I trial in 20 patients confirmed the feasibility of giving cetuximab in combination with capecitabine, weekly irinotecan, and radiotherapy as neoadjuvant therapy for rectal cancer.[218] Five patients had a pathologic complete remission. In another neoadjuvant trial, 40 patients with locally advanced rectal cancer received neoadjuvant single-agent cetuximab in three doses, followed by weekly cetuximab plus 5-FU and concurrent radiation therapy.[219] Six patients had a dose reduction and/or interruption of treatment; 35 patients completed the neoadjuvant treatment; and three patients had a pathologic complete remission. In another neoadjuvant trial, 60 patients received cetuximab, capecitabine, oxaliplatin, and radiation therapy.[220] Four patients had a complete pathologic response.

Squamous Cell Cancers of the Head and Neck

Cetuximab is approved also for the treatment of squamous cell cancers of the head and neck. Vermorken et al gave single-agent cetuximab at the standard dose and schedule to 109 patients who had recurrent and/or metastatic disease that progressed during platinum chemotherapy.[221] Acneiform skin rash, which occurred in 49%, was the most common toxicity. There was one death caused by an infusion-related allergic reaction. The response rate was similar to that of single-agent cetuximab in colorectal cancer.

Herbst et al treated 130 patients, who did not have an objective response or relapsed within 90 days of completing two cycles of cisplatin/paclitaxel or cisplatin/fluorouracil, with standard cetuximab and cisplatin (75 or 100 mg/m^2 intravenously) every 3 weeks.[222] The most common toxicities were anemia, acneiform skin rash, leukopenia, fatigue/malaise, and nausea/vomiting. Seven patients (5%) experienced a grade 3 or 4 hypersensitivity reaction to cetuximab. Baselga et al treated 96 patients, who were refractory to cisplatin, with standard cetuximab and cisplatin at the same dose and schedule during which progressive disease had occurred.[223] Acneiform rash was the most common toxicity.

Pfister et al treated 22 patients, who had locoregionally advanced disease, with a combination of cisplatin, cetuximab, and 70 Gy of radiotherapy.[224] The trial was closed early because of several adverse events related to infection and cardiac events. Grade 3 or 4 cetuximab-related toxicities included acneiform rash in 10% and hypersensitivity in 5%. With a median follow-up of 52 months, the 3-year OS rate is 76%, the 3-year PFS is 56%, and the 3-year locoregional control rate is 71%.

Bourhis et al treated 53 patients, who had recurrent or metastatic disease, with a combination of cetuximab, cisplatin, or carboplatin and escalating doses of 5-FU as initial therapy.[225] Dermatologic toxicity was the most common adverse event, but the most common grade 3 or 4 adverse events were leucopenia (38%), asthenia (25%), thrombocytopenia (15%), and vomiting (14%). Chan et al treated 59 patients, who had recurrent or metastatic nasopharyngeal cancer that had recurred after cisplatin, with cetuximab and carboplatin.[226] Six patients (10%) experienced serious treatment-related adverse events with cetuximab.

Phase I trials of cetuximab in head and neck cancer suggested that cetuximab could be safely given with radiation therapy and might enhance therapeutic benefit.[227] Bonner et al conducted a multinational trial comparing cetuximab plus radiotherapy to radiotherapy alone in 424 patients with locoregionally advanced disease. It showed a benefit for the addition of cetuximab, including a 26% reduction in death with an increase in survival from 29 to 49 months (p = 0.03).[228] There was no increase in toxicity other than the acneiform rash.

Randomized trials have confirmed that cetuximab enhances chemotherapy in the treatment of head and neck cancer. Burtness et al randomized 117 patients who had recurrent or metastatic disease to receive cisplatin every 4 weeks with weeky cetuximab or placebo.[229] The response rate was higher with the addition of cetuximab, but PFS and OS were not improved. Survival was better for those patients who developed skin rash. Vermorken et al randomized 442 patients with untreated recurrent or metastatic squamous cell carcinoma of the head and neck to receive 5-FU and cisplatin or the same chemotherapy plus cetuximab.[230] The addition of cetuximab enhanced the response rate and PFS.

Cancers Other than Colorectal and Head and Neck Cancers

Although cetuximab has minimal single-agent activity against NSCLC, it appears to increase the benefit derived from chemotherapy. Hanna et al observed a response rate of only 5% for cetuximab alone in 66 patients with metastatic disease that had progressed after previous systemic therapy.[231] Grade 3-to-4 toxicities were uncommon but included acneiform rash (6%), anaphylactic reactions (2%), and diarrhea (2%). Other studies have combined cetuximab with chemotherapy. Borghaei et al treated 53 NSCLC patients with a 28-day cycle of paclitaxel-carboplatin and cetuximab in a multi-institution study.[232] Cetuximab was given at 400 mg/m^2 on day 1, then 250 mg/m^2 with paclitaxel (100 mg/m^2/week for 3 weeks) and carboplatin (AUC = 6) on day 1 of each 28-day cycle. The investigators reported three complete responses and 27 partial responses. Thienelt et al treated 31 previously untreated patients with paclitaxel, carboplatin, and cetuximab.[233] Over 80% of patients experienced dermatologic toxicity, with 13% at grade 3 or 4. Belani et al treated 80 NSCLC patients with docetaxel, carboplatin, and cetuximab.[234] Cetuximab was given at 400 mg/m^2 on day 1 and 250 mg/m^2 on days 8 and 15 plus docetaxel (at a dose of 75 mg/m^2 on day 1) and carboplatin (AUC = 6) on day 1 every 21 days for up to six cycles. Robert et al treated 35 patients with gemcitabine and carboplatin.[235] The most common toxicities attributed to cetuximab were acneiform rash (89%), asthenia (31%), fever/chills (20%), and nausea/vomiting (17.1%).

Randomized trials have demonstrated a benefit for the addition of cetuximab to chemotherapy in advanced NSCLC. The European multicenter FLEX trial (First-line in Lung Cancer with Erbitux) randomized 1125 patients to chemotherapy either alone or with cetuximab.[236] Patients who received cetuximab had a higher response rate and better OS. In a smaller randomized Phase II trial, Rosell et al observed similar benefits for the combination of vinorelbine and cisplatin with cetuximab.[237]

Cetuximab has been combined with chemotherapy in patients with noncolorectal GI malignancies, but up to this point randomized trials have failed to demonstrate an advantage over chemotherapy alone. Response rates of 38% and 34%, respectively, were reported for trials of 1) FOLFOX plus cetuximab as first-line systemic therapy for 38 patients with recurrent or metastatic gastric cancer[238] and 2) FOLFIRI plus cetuximab in 34 patients who had advanced gastric or gastroesophageal junction adenocarcinoma.[239] In the FOLFIRI trial, grade 3-to-4 toxicity included neutropenia (42%), acneiform rash (21%), diarrhea (8%), asthenia (5%), stomatitis (5%), and hypertransaminasemia (5%), with one treatment-related death. A 20% response rate was noted in patients with advanced hepatocellular cancer who were treated with gemcitabine plus oxaliplatin (GEMOX).[240] Grade 3-to-4 toxicities included thrombocytopenia (24%), neutropenia (20%), neurotoxicity (11%), cutaneous toxicity (16%), and anemia (4%).

Several trials have been conducted in patients with locally advanced, recurrent, or metastatic pancreatic cancer. Xiong et al treated 41 untreated patients, who had measurable locally advanced or EGFR-positive metastatic pancreatic cancer, with cetuximab and gemcitabine.[241] The response rate of 12% is similar to what has been reported with gemcitabine alone. Median survival was 7.1 months, and 1-year survival was 32%. The most common grade 3 or 4 adverse events were neutropenia (39.0%), asthenia (22.0%), abdominal pain (22.0%), and thrombocytopenia (17.1%). The GEMOX combination had a much higher response rate (33%),[242] but PFS and OS were similar to that seen with gemcitabine alone. Of more significance, the addition of cetuximab failed to show an advantage over gemcitabine alone in a large randomized trial conducted by the Southwest Oncology Group.[243] A smaller randomized trial failed to show an advantage for the addition of cetuximab to gemcitabine plus cisplatin.[244]

Exploratory trials with cetuximab have been conducted in other malignancies. The combination cetuximab plus carboplatin produced a disappointing response rate of 31% in 29 patients with relapsed platinum-sensitive ovarian or primary peritoneal carcinoma.[245] As initial therapy of 41 patients with advanced-stage ovarian, primary peritoneal, or fallopian tube cancer, the combination of cetuximab, paclitaxel, and carboplatin had a median PFS of 14.4 months, which was considered no better than historical controls.[246] A trial of cisplatin plus cetuximab in advanced cervical cancer was stopped after only 19 out of a planned 44 patients were accrued because of excessive toxicity, including five deaths (28%).[247] The response rate was 6 of 19 (32%), which was no better than historical controls. In metastatic renal cell cancer, Motzer et al observed a discouraging response rate of 0 of 55 with single-agent cetuximab despite a 17% rate of grade 3- to 4 skin toxicity.[248]

Mechanisms of Antitumor Activity

Sustained blocking of EGFR is believed to be critical for the antitumor effects of cetuximab. Based on randomized trials exploring single doses of 50, 100, 250, 400, or 500 mg/m^2, a dose of 250 mg/m^2 was predicted to nearly saturate EGFRs.[249,250] Skin biopsies in 39 patients, before and after IV infusions of cetuximab, confirmed a dose-dependent relationship with suppression of EGFR expression.[250] In these trials, there was no association between dose and cutaneous rash, but the appearance of rash seemed predictive for clinical benefit. So far, there has been no evidence that chemotherapy alters the pharmacokinetics of cetuximab. Pharmacokinetic trials of cetuximab with irinotecan revealed no change in cetuximab clearance or metabolism when combined with irinotecan compared to infusions of cetuximab alone.[251,252]

Because all preclinical testing of cetuximab and its murine precursors were conducted in animals bearing tumors that strongly expressed EGFR, most early trials restricted patient eligibility to those whose tumors had documentable expression of EGFR by IHC. However, in clinical practice it is now generally accepted that IHC testing for EGFR expression is not necessary for determining appropriateness of cetuximab-based therapy—because of inherent limitations in the assays and potential for sampling error and because responses have been described in patients whose tumors were EGFR-negative by IHC. In eight colorectal cancer patients who were refractory to irinotecan and whose tumors were negative for EGFR by IHC, four responded to cetuximab plus irinotecan therapy.[253] Gene copy number may be a better correlate for the relevance of EGFR because internalization of EGFR after binding of MoAb or ligand may cause misleading results. A small trial of 31 patients suggested that EGFR gene copy number might predict benefit.[254] One group retrospectively analyzed EGFR copy number by FISH in paraffin-embedded tumor blocks from 85 chemorefractory colorectal cancer patients who had been treated with cetuximab.[196] Based on the group's scoring system, the 43 patients who were EGFR positive by FISH had a higher response rate ($p = 0.0001$) and disease PFS ($p = 0.02$) than the 42 patients who were EGFR negative by FISH. However, in a much larger prospective trial using tissue from a variety of different tumors, cell surface expression of EGFR, EGFR kinase domain mutations, and EGFR gene amplification did not predict clinical benefit.[199,255] A pilot study involving tumors from 39 colorectal cancer patients suggested that cyclin D1 A870G and EGF A61G polymorphisms may predict efficacy of single-agent cetuximab.[256]

There is increasing evidence that patients with mutations in the K-ras gene do not benefit from cetuximab therapy. In the trial of supportive care plus cetuximab vs supportive care alone in patients with chemorefractory colorectal cancer,[199] tumor samples were obtained from 394 of 572 patients and analyzed for mutation status of the K-ras gene.[257] At least one mutation in exon 2 of the K-ras gene mutations was detected in 42% of samples. The effectiveness of cetuximab was significantly associated with K-ras mutation status and its interaction with OS ($p = 0.01$) and PFS ($p <0.001$), but in the group of patients receiving best supportive care alone, the mutation status of the K-ras gene was not significantly associated with OS ($p = 0.97$). In patients with wild-type K-ras tumors (no mutations), treatment with cetuximab as compared with supportive care alone significantly improved OS (median = 9.5 vs 4.8 months ($p <0.001$) and PFS (median = 3.7 vs 1.9 months ($p <0.001$). In contrast, among patients with mutated K-ras tumors, there was no significant difference in either survival measurement between cetuximab and supportive care.

Bokemeyer et al came to similar conclusions based on their randomized trial of FOLFOX plus cetuximab vs FOLFOX alone.[211] In patients with unmutated (wild-type) K-ras, the addition of cetuximab to FOLFOX was associated with a higher response rate (61% vs 37%; $p = 0.011$) and a lower risk of disease progression ($p = 0.016$) compared with FOLFOX alone.

Lièvre et al made similar observations in 89 metastatic colorectal cancer patients treated with cetuximab alone after treatment failure with irinotecan-based chemotherapy.[258] In this study, a K-ras mutation was detected in 27% of patients and was associated with lack of benefit from cetuximab. The response rates for cetuximab were 40% among 65 nonmutated patients and 0% among the 24 patients whose tumors were mutated ($p <0.001$). Median PFS for the two groups were 31.4 and 10.1 weeks, respectively ($p = 0.0001$), and median OS was 14.3 and 10.1 months ($p = 0.026$), respectively. A multivariate analysis for all 89 patients revealed that K-ras status was an independent prognostic factor associated with both OS and PFS, whereas skin toxicity was an independent predictor of OS only.

Other investigators have provided additional insight about why not all patients with unmuated K-ras respond to anti-EGFR therapy. Di Nicolantonio et al have suggested that B-raf mutations are also important predictors for whether colorectal cancer patients will benefit from anti-EGFR therapy with cetuximab or panitumumab.[259] The B-raf V600E mutation was found in samples from 11 of 79 patients who did not have K-ras mutations. None of the patients who responded to anti-EGFR MoAb therapy had B-raf mutations, and none of the patients with B-raf mutations responded to treatment ($p = 0.029$). The B-raf-mutated patients had shorter PFS ($p = 0.011$) and OS ($p <0.0001$) than patients with wild-type B-raf. They also found that in-vitro treatment with the tyrosine kinase inhibitor sorafenib, which inhibits B-raf and other tyrosine kinase pathways, converted V600E-mutated cells to sensitivity to cetuximab or panitumumab, providing a rationale for combination therapy. Bibeau et al have provided evidence that Fc polymorphisms may also be important for cetuximab activity in patients with wild-type K-ras.[260] They found that patients with FcγRIIa-131H/H and/or FcγIIIa-158V/V genotypes had longer PFS than FcγRIIa-H131R and FcγRIIIa-V158F polymorphisms.

Toxicity

The toxicities associated with single-agent cetuximab are summarized in Table 12-3. The most common side effect associated with cetuximab and other anti-EGFR therapies is a characteristic acneiform rash, which is most prominent on the face, chest, and upper back and usually appears within a week of starting treatment.[261] In many trials, the prevalence of this side effect was over 80%. Serial punch biopsies in patients revealed two main reaction patterns: a superficial dermal inflammatory cell infiltrate and a superficial folliculitis. The rash can be severe and should be treated to decrease the risk of secondary infection and cellulitis. Grade 3-to-4 dermatitis was reported in 5% to 15% of patients in most trials. Prophylactic topical lubricants are sufficient in many patients, but other patients require treatment with tetracycline antibiotics or clindamycin. A recent, small, double-blinded, placebo-controlled, randomized trial in 61 patients failed to

Table 12-3. Specific Acute Toxicities in Trials of Cetuximab Monotherapy for Colorectal Cancer

Toxicity	Percent of Patients (n = 420)	Toxicity	Percent of Patients (n = 420)
Rash	90	Vomiting	25
Asthenia/malaise	48	Chills/rigors	21
Nausea	29	Diaphoresis	21
Fever	27	Dyspnea	17
Abdominal pain	26	Pruritus	11
Headache	26	Cough	11
Diarrhea	25	Edema	10

support the prophylactic use of tetracycline to prevent the rash.[262] Other common side effects include asthenia and diarrhea. Cetuximab does not appear to increase the toxicity of any of the chemotherapy agents with which it has been combined.

Black-box warnings for cetuximab include infusion reactions and cardiac arrest. The somewhat high rate of severe infusion-related reactions, many of which have been characterized as anaphylactic reactions, is of concern. At this time, it is not clear whether this is the result of cross-reactivity with antigens on circulating cells in some patients, effects of Fc interactions with effector cells, or a true allergic reaction to murine amino acids and/or glycosylation because of the murine plasmacytoma cell line used to produce the product. There was a 2% risk of sudden death in 208 patients with squamous cell cancer of the head and neck who received cetuximab with radiation therapy.[228]

Summary

Cetuximab is widely used in combination with chemotherapy for patients who have relapsed after primary treatment for colorectal cancer. However, based on the comparative strengths and differences of clinical trials, bevacizumab with combination chemotherapy is usually preferred as the initial treatment. Cetuximab is increasingly being used with radiation therapy in patients who are considered poor candidates to receive combined modality treatment with chemotherapy and radiation therapy, which is currently standard for treatment of locoregionally advanced squamous cell cancers of the head and neck. It will be interesting to see randomized comparisons of chemotherapy plus radiation vs cetuximab plus radiation, but there are also trials comparing cetuximab plus chemoradiotherapy to chemoradiotherapy alone. There may be a role for cetuximab with chemotherapy in NSCLC, but, again, bevacizumab with chemotherapy is currently the standard initial therapy.

Panitumumab (Vectibix)

Panitumumab and EGFR

The EGFR MoAb panitumumab [Vectibix (Amgen, Thousand Oaks, CA)] was approved in 2006 based on randomized trials in which the agent was superior to placebo in patients with relapsed, refractory, metastatic colorectal cancer. Formerly known as ABX-EGF, panitumumab was the first fully human MoAb to receive regulatory approval and the first approved for cancer therapy.[263,264] It is a human IgG2. Like the chimeric MoAb cetuximab, the human MoAb panitumumab binds to the extracellular domain of EGFR, causing internalization of the receptor and antibody and "down-regulation" of the receptor with disruption of potential downstream signal transduction that enhances proliferation and resistance to apopotosis in normal and malignant cells. Panitumumab was produced with the hope that its clinical efficacy might be even greater than cetuximab because it is a totally human construct, which may offer advantages in terms of pharmacokinetics, decreased allergenic potential, and possibly enhanced ADCC. The antitumor activity of panitumumab was confirmed in vitro and in vivo against many cancers, including lung, kidney, and colorectal cancer. In these models, it was well tolerated and clinically active both as monotherapy and in combination chemotherapy agents. Panitumumab was originally made in transgenic mice but is manufactured in CHO cells.

Clinical Trials with Panitumumab

A few clinical trials have been published for panitumumab monotherapy and for panitumumab in combination therapy. A pivotal trial for regulatory approval compared panitumumab at 6 mg/kg intravenously every 2 weeks to best supportive care in patients with metastatic colorectal cancer whose disease had progressed during or after standard therapy with fluoropyrimidine-, oxaliplatin-, and irinotecan-containing chemotherapy regimens.[265-268] All patients had EGFR-expressing tumors. Panitumumab produced a 10% objective response rate and and a longer PFS compared to supportive care alone. There was no difference in survival, but approximately 75% of patients in the supportive-care-alone arm crossed over to receive panitumumab after disease progression. Quality of life was also better in the patients who received panitumumab.[269] In 176 patients who progressed on the supportive care arm and subsequently received panitumumab, 12% had an objective response and two patients had complete responses.[268] Hecht et al treated 148 patients whose metastatic colorectal cancer had progressed on chemotherapy that included a fluoropyrimidine and irinotecan or oxaliplatin, or both.[270] Panitumumab was given intravenously at a dose of 2.5 mg/kg weekly for 8 of each 9 weeks until disease progression or excessive toxicity. Skin toxicity occurred in 95%, and 5% were grade 3 or 4. Four patients discontinued therapy because of toxicity, and one patient had an infusion reaction but was able to resume treatment. EGFR of at least 1+ by IHC was an eligibility requirement. There was no difference in response for 105 patients who were judged as having high EGFR by IHC compared to 43 patients who were characterized as having a low EGFR.

Muro et al administered panitumumab to 52 Japanese patients with metastatic colorectal cancer who developed progressive disease during or after fluoropyrimidine, irinotecan, and oxaliplatin chemotherapy.[271] The most common treatment-related adverse events involved the integument, including acne (81%), dry skin (62%), rash (46%), paronychia (33%), and pruritus (33%). Another 33% had hypomagnesemia.

Weiner et al evaluated the safety, pharmacokinetics, and activity of panitumumab in a Phase I trial involving 96 patients. Sequential cohorts were to receive four IV infusions of 1.0 mg/kg weekly, 2.5 mg/kg weekly, 6.0 mg/kg every 2 weeks, and 9.0 mg/kg every 3 weeks.[272] Tumor types were 41% colorectal, 22% prostate, 16% renal, 15% non-small-cell lung, 3% pancreatic, 3% esophageal/gastroesophageal, and 1% anal cancer. There were no infusion reactions, and a maximum tolerated dose was not reached. Five of the 39 colorectal cancer patients had a partial response.

Stephenson et al evaluated safety, pharmacokinetics, and efficacy of panitumumab at two dose schedules and infusion rates: 1) 6 mg/kg every 2 weeks over 60 minutes or a 60-minute infusion for the first dose followed by 30-minute infusions if the first infusion was well tolerated or 2) 9 mg/kg every 3 weeks over 60 minutes.[273] Patients had advanced solid malignancies, not just colorectal cancer, and had failed standard therapies. Treatment-related adverse events were noted in 90% of the 84 patients. There were no differences in toxicity by infusion rates or dose, and peak serum concentrations were similar. Objective responses were seen in 4 patients (5%), one each with colon, rectal, esophageal, and bladder cancer.

Hecht et al conducted a randomized Phase III trial of chemotherapy, bevacizumab, and panitumumab compared with chemotherapy and bevacizumab alone for metastatic colorectal camcer.[274] Panitumumab was discontinued as part of treatment after a planned interim analysis of 812 oxaliplatin-treated patients showed worse efficacy in the panitumumab arm. In the final analysis, median PFS and OS were worse in the treatment arms that included panitumumab. Furthermore, grade 3 or 4 adverse events were more prevalent in the panitumumab arm. Thus, the addition of either of the two anti-EGFR MoAbs, cetuximab or panitumumab, was associated with increased toxicity without evidence of improved efficacy when added to the combination of chemotherapy and bevacizumab in patients with metastatic colorectal cancer.[216,274]

Berlin et al tested the combination of 5-FU, panitumumab, and two different schedules of irinotecan as initial therapy in patients with metastatic colorectal cancer.[275] This was a two-part, multicenter, Phase II study of panitumumab, 2.5 mg/kg weekly, with bolus 5-FU [irinotecan, 5-fluorouracil, leucovorin (IFL)] in the first part of the trial, and infusional 5-FU (FOLFIRI) in the second part. Grade 3-to-4 diarrhea occurred in 11 patients (58%) in part 1 and 6 patients (25%) in part 2. All patients had dermatologic toxicity, but none was grade 4. The authors concluded that panitumumab + FOLFIRI was better tolerated than panitumumab + IFL.

In a recently completed and yet unpublished study, panitumumab + FOLFOX proved superior to FOLFOX alone in patients with unmutated K-ras colon cancer in terms of PFS (2009 results; J. Y. Douillard, unpublished observations).

Toxicities

The toxicities and adverse events associated with panitumumab are summarized in Table 12-4. Panitumumab was developed in the belief that it would be less toxic and more active than cetuximab or other less-than-completely-human antibodies. Even though it is a human MoAb that reacts with EGFR, the toxicity profile is very similar to the anti-EGFR chimeric MoAb in terms of rash and GI symptoms—further evidence that the target rather than the MoAb construct is the more important determinant of toxicity. However, panitumumab was associated with a lower frequency of infusion-related symptoms such as headache, fever, dyspnea, diaphoresis, chills, and rigors. It is unclear

Table 12-4. Specific Acute Toxicities in Trials of Panitumumab Monotherapy in Colorectal Cancer

Toxicity	Percent of Patients (n = 229)	Toxicity	Percent of Patients (n = 229)
Rash	90	Edema	12
Pruritus	57	Chills/rigors	<5
Abdominal pain	25	Diaphoresis	<5
Nausea	23	Dyspnea	<5
Diarrhea	21	Fever	<5
Vomiting	19	Headache	<5
Cough	14	Hypotension	<5

whether the lower frequency of infusion reactions relates to less Fc binding to Fc receptors on circulating cells or endothelial cells or to decreased antigenicity for panitumumab produced in CHO cells as opposed to cetuximab produced in mouse plasmacytoma cells. Like cetuximab, black-box warnings include dermatologic toxicities and infusion reactions.

Panitumumab has been well tolerated whether administered alone or in combination with chemotherapy. However, there was a 1% rate of anaphylaxis in trials submitted for registration of the agent. During eight clinical trials, a very sensitive assay detected anti-panitumumab responses in 25 of 604 subjects (4.1%), and eight developed neutralizing antibodies.[276] At least one patient was reported to have a severe infusion reaction during treatment with cetuximab and was then successfully treated with panitumumab,[277] but because most infusion reactions are seen only with a first infusion, it is not clear that decreased toxicity will be an important benefit.

Similar to other agents targeting the EGFR pathway, skin rash has been the primary toxicity recognized in association with panitumumab therapy and has occurred in 100% of patients receiving doses of 2.5 mg/kg or higher. Hypomagnesemia and diarrhea were also most commonly reported. No severe or life-threatening reactions were noted in the large randomized trial in patients with colorectal cancer.[267,268] Other common adverse events noted were paronychia, fatigue, abdominal pain, and nausea. The most serious adverse events were severe dermatologic toxicity complicated by infectious sequelae and septic death, infusion reactions, pulmonary fibrosis, hypomagnesemia, and GI problems including abdominal pain, nausea, vomiting, diarrhea, and constipation.

Summary

Panitumumab is the first fully human antibody to receive regulatory approval and represents an alternative to cetuximab as an anti-EGFR MoAb. It remains to be seen whether the totally human construct offers any meaningful advantages over the chimeric construct.

Bevacizumab (Avastin)

Bevacizumab and Vascular Endothelial Growth Factor

The anti-VEGF MoAb bevacizumab [Avastin (Genentech, South San Francisco, CA)] was approved in May 2004 based on randomized trials in which the agent was combined with 5-FU-based chemotherapy for the treatment of metastatic colorectal cancer. Subsequently, the agent was granted marketing indications for the following: in combination with FOLFOX for the second-line treatment of metastatic colorectal carcinoma, in combination with paclitaxel and carboplatin chemotherapy in the treatment of metastatic adenocarcinoma of the lung, in combination with taxane chemotherapy for the first-line treatment of metastatic breast cancer, and in the treatment of glioblastoma. Bevacizumab is a recombinant humanized IgG1 MoAb that is manufactured in CHO cells.[278] Unlike other commercially available antibodies that target antigens, bevacizumab binds to the VEGF ligand rather than the VEGF receptor. As discussed earlier in this chapter, VEGF is produced by many tumor cells and is the central mediator of tumor angiogenesis. Various lines of evidence suggest that VEGF would be a useful target for anticancer therapy.[65-69] The binding of bevacizumab to VEGF inhibited its binding to the VEGF receptor in vitro and had anti-angiogenic and antitumor activity in various animal model assay systems.[65,66]

Clinical Trials with Bevacizumab

Exploratory Trials with Bevacizumab

Because VEGF is important in normal angiogenesis, there was concern that the binding of bevacizumab to VEGF might be associated with bleeding. However, in Phase I trials, no grade 3 or 4 bleeding toxicities were observed in 25 patients who received IV doses up to 10 mg/kg.[279] There were no tumor responses, but many patients had stable disease and no significant additive toxicities when bevacizumab was subsequently given in combination with various chemotherapy agents.[280]

Colorectal Cancer

Several Phase II trials with accrual of 50 to 100 patients with metastatic colorectal cancer confirmed the safety of, and suggested the potential efficacy of, bevacizumab in combination with various 5-FU-based combinations. Response rates were as low as 5% in patients treated with 5-FU and leucovorin who had disease that was refractory to irinotecan and oxaliplatin,[281] but as high as 50% to 70% in patients who had not previously received chemotherapy and were then treated with 5-FU/irinotecan or 5-FU/oxaliplatin combinations with bevacizumab.[282,283] The Eastern Cooperative Oncology Group (ECOG) conducted a trial with IFL and bevacizumab in 87 patients with untreated, advanced colorectal cancer.[282] The response rate among 81 evaluable patients was 49%, but the dose of both irinotecan and 5-FU had to be reduced by 20% to 25% because of vomiting, diarrhea, and neutropenia. Bleeding occurred in 37 patients (46%), and nine patients (11%) had grade 3 or 4 thromboembolic events.

FOLFOX and bevacizumab were used to treat 53 patients with previously untreated metastatic colorectal cancer.[283] The response rate was 68%. Hemorrhage was not a problem in this trial, and only one patient had a severe thromboembolic event.

Several randomized clinical trials of bevacizumab in colorectal cancer have been conducted. A three-arm randomized Phase II trial in metastatic colorectal cancer suggested that bevacizumab enhanced 5-FU-based chemotherapy.[284] In this trial, 144 previously untreated patients were randomized to 5-FU and leucovorin (FL) plus low-dose bevacizumab (5 mg/kg every 2 weeks), to FL plus high-dose bevacizumab (10 mg/kg every 2 weeks), or to FL alone (500 mg/m^2 each 5-FU and leucovorin). FL was given weekly for the first 6 weeks of each 8-week cycle. Better results were seen with the addition of bevacizumab, and there appeared to be an advantage for the lower dose. In a randomized trial of initial therapy for patients with metastatic colorectal cancer who were not considered optimal candidates for first-line irinotecan treatment, 209 patients received FL plus becacizumab (FL-BV) at 5 mg/kg or FL plus placebo.[285] The addition of bevacizumab resulted in a better PFS (hazard ratio, or HR = 0.50; p <0.001), higher response rate (p = 0.055), and a trend toward better survival (HR = 0.79; p = 0.16). Hypertension was more frequent with bevacizumab.

In the pivotal trial for regulatory approval, 923 patients with metastatic colorectal cancer were randomized to receive IFL and bevacizumab (IFL-BV), IFL and placebo (control), or FL-BV at a dose of 5 mg/kg every 2 weeks.[286,287] In the first phase, 313 patients were randomly assigned to these three arms; then, following a planned initial analysis of 110 patients, the FL-BV arm was discontinued, not because of inferior results but because IFL had become the standard control arm based on other trials in metastatic colorectal cancer. IFL-BV was superior to IFL-placebo for the 813 patients randomized to treatment with one of these arms, in terms of response rate (p = 0.004), PFS (HR = 0.54; p <0.001), and OS (HR = 0.66; p <0.001).[286] The IFL-BV arm was associated with more grade 3 or 4 hypertension (11% vs 2%). The FL-BV arm also was superior to the IFL-placebo arm.[287]

A meta-analysis was performed using the raw data from three randomized trials that included FL-BV as initial treatment for patients with metastatic colorectal cancer.[288] For the combined data, FL-BV (n = 249) was superior to FL (n = 241) in terms of response rate (34% vs 24%; p = 0.019), PFS (9 vs 6 months; HR = 0.63; p <0.001), and OS (18 vs 15 months; HR = 0.74; p = 0.008). In contrast to these excellent results in previously untreated patients, in an expanded access trial of 350 patients with metastatic colorectal cancer who had relapsed after or progressed during both irinotecan- and oxaliplatin-based therapy, the response rate was only 4% in the first 100 patients enrolled by investigator analysis and only 1% based on blinded central review.[281] A subsequent analysis focused on patients aged 65 years or older who had participated in various randomized trials of bevacizumab and 5-FU-based regimens in chemo-naive patients, and it confirmed safety and therapeutic benefit for this specific subset of patients.[289]

ECOG conducted a three-arm trial in which 829 patients whose cancer had recurred after IFL therapy were randomized to recieve 1) FOLFOX with bevacizumab, 2) FOLFOX alone, or 3) bevacizumab alone.[290] Bevacizumab was given at 10 mg/kg every 2 weeks. Bevacizumab exhibited limited acitivity as a single agent, and FOLFOX plus bevacizumab was superior to FOLFOX alone for all key endpoints, including OS (HR = 0.75; p = 0.001), PFS (HR = 0.61; p <0.0001), and response rate (p <0.0001). There were higher rates of hypertension and bleeding in the FOLFOX plus bevacizumab arm.

In a large randomized trial using a 2 × 2 design, capecitabine plus oxaliplatin (CAPOX) or FOLFOX with bevacizumab was superior to these chemotherapy regimens alone in terms of PFS and possibly OS, but not response rate.[291] Two smaller randomized trials have confirmed the safety and efficacy of capecitabine and bevacizumab in combinations with oxaliplatin or irinotecan. The CAPOX combination appeared to provide efficacy similar to FOLFOX.[292] In a randomized Phase II trial, the combination of CAPOX plus bevacizumab appeared to be more efficacious than CAPOX alone.[293]

Another trial explored the safety and efficacy of bevacizumab in combination with CAPOX as a cytoreductive therapy before resection of colorectal liver metastases as a potentially curative approach.[294] Patients received CAPOX and bevacizumab biweekly for six cycles but did not include bevacizumab in the sixth cycle to allow 5 weeks between the last administration of bevacizumab and surgery. Of 56 patients, 41 (73%) had an objective response to the neoadjuvant therapy, and 52 (93%) underwent resection of liver metastases. There was no increased intraoperative bleeding or wound-healing complications and no postoperative mortality. Three patients (6%) required perioperative blood transfusions, and additional surgery was performed in only one patient. Postoperative liver function and regeneration were normal in all but one patient. The mean postoperative hospitalization duration was 9 days, and 11 patients were considered to have had postoperative morbidity.

There are many unanswered questions regarding the duration of bevacizumab therapy. Some trials examine continuing bevacizumab as a single agent after chemotherapy has been discontinued and the benefit of combining it with another chemotherapy if a patient has experienced progressive disease during or shortly after treatment with a different chemotherapy plus bevacizumab. One study retrospectively analyzed the association between survival and various pre- and posttreatment factors, including the use of bevacizumab beyond first progression in 1445 previously untreated patients with metastatic colorectal cancer who had experienced disease progression during bevacizumab trials.[295] Patients were classified into three groups: treatment with bevacizumab after treatment (n = 642), postprogression treatment without bevacizumab (n = 531), and no postprogression treatment (n = 253). Median OS rates were 32, 20, and 13 months, respectively. Hypertension that required medication was the only bevacizumab-related safety event that occurred more frequently in the bevacizumab arm (25% vs 19%).

Non-Small-Cell Lung Cancer

The second marketing indication for bevacizumab was with chemotherapy in nonsquamous histology, NSCLC. In a three-arm randomized Phase II trial in NSCLC, 99 previously untreated patients were randomized to treatment every 3 weeks with paclitaxel, 200 mg/m^2, and carboplatin (PC; AUC = 6), alone or in combination with bevacizumab at 7.5 or 15 mg/kg.[296] The response rate and PFS were higher for the 15-mg/kg bevacizumab arm compared to chemotherapy alone, with a trend toward better survival. Bleeding was the most significant complication in patients who received bevacizumab. This included not only minor mucocutaneous hemorrhage but, more importantly, major hemoptysis, which was associated with centrally located squamous cell cancers accompanied by tumor necrosis and cavitation.

In a large two-arm pivotal randomized trial, 878 patients with previously untreated nonsquamous NSCLC were randomized to PC plus bevacizumab (15 mg/kg) or PC alone on a 3-week schedule.[297] The bevacizumab arm was associated with a higher response rate (p <0.001), better OS (HR = 0.79; p = 0.003), and PFS (HR = 0.66; p <0.001). Even though patients with squamous cell histology were not enrolled in this trial, there were still 5 hemorrhagic deaths in the bevacizumab arm (1.2%) and significant bleeding was more frequent in the bevacizumab arm (4.4% vs 0.7%; p <0.001). Recently a more detailed review of patients who experienced pulmonary hemorrhages (six from the randomized Phase II trial and 15 from the Phase III trial) was reported.[298] The authors concluded that baseline tumor cavitation might be a risk factor for pulmonary hemorrhage, but no other baseline clinical variables were predictive.

In a large European trial, 1043 patients with previously untreated nonsquamous NSCLC were randomized to gemcitabine plus cisplatin with bevacizumab at 10 mg/kg or 5 mg/kg or placebo.[299] Results favored the bevacizumab arms, although the benefit was not as impressive as in the US trial with PC.

Erlotinib is a tyrosine kinase inhibitor that blocks signal transduction related to the EGFR. In a Phase I/II trial, 40 patients with metastatic nonsquamous NSCLC who had relapsed after previous chemotherapy were treated with bevacizumab, 15 mg/kg intravenously every 2 weeks, and erlotinib, 150 mg orally daily.[300] Eight patients had a partial response. Bevacizumab has also been combined with newer agents such as oxaliplatin and pemetrexed.[301] The most common grade 3 toxicity was hypertension, and there were no episodes of cerebral hemorrhage in nine patients who had known brain metastases. The combination of GEMOX plus bevacizumab was active and had acceptable toxicity in previously untreated nonsquamous NSCLC patients.[302] The most common grade 3 or 4 adverse events attributed to bevacizumab were hypertension (11%) and thromboembolic events (7%), but no pulmonary hemorrhages were reported.

Breast Cancer

The third marketing indication for bevacizumab was with chemotherapy in breast cancer. Miller et al randomized 462 heavily treated patients to oral capecitabine, 2500 mg/m^2 twice daily on days 1 through 14 every 3 weeks, with or without IV bevacizumab, 15 mg/kg on day 1.[303] There was more grade 3 or 4 hypertension requiring treatment (18% vs 0.5%) in patients receiving bevacizumab. The response rate was twice as high for the combination therapy as for capecitabine alone, but this did not result in superior survival, which is not surprising because most of these patients had failed at least three chemotherapy regimens before entering the trial.

In a randomized trial, bevacizumab plus paclitaxel was compared to paclitaxel alone as initial therapy for 722 patients with metastatic breast cancer.[304] There was an improvement in response rate and PFS but not in OS, and there was an increased risk of complications in the bevacizumab arm. The addition of bevacizumab was associated with a prolonged PFS (median = 12 vs 6 months; HR for progression = 0.60; p <0.001) and increased the objective response rate (37% vs 21%; p <0.001). OS, however, was similar in the two groups (median = 27 vs 25 months; HR = 0.88; p = 0.16). Grade 3 or 4 hypertension (15% vs 0%; p <0.001), proteinuria (4% vs 0; p <0.001), headache (2% vs 0; p = 0.008), cerebrovascular ischemia (2% vs 0; p = 0.02), and infection (9% vs 3%; p <0.001) were more frequent in patients receiving paclitaxel plus bevacizumab. A DNA analysis of 363 patients from this trial was used to screen the genotype for selected polymorphisms in VEGF.[305] The VEGF-2578 AA genotype was associated with a better median OS in the patients who received bevacizumab when compared with the alternate genotypes combined (p = 0.023). The VEGF-1154

A allele was also associated with a better survival (p = 0.001). VEGF-634 CC and VEGF-1498 TT genotypes were associated with significantly less grade 3 or 4 hypertension.

Bevacizumab, 10 mg/kg on days 1 and 15 of a 28-day cycle, in combination with docetaxel, 35 mg/m^2 on days 1, 8, and 15, was associated with a 52% response rate in patients with metastatic breast cancer who had not been heavily treated with prior chemotherapy.[306] Only one of 38 previously treated patients responded to the combination of erlotinib plus bevacizumab.[307]

Renal Cell Cancer

Bevacizumab is active as a single agent in renal cell carcinoma, a malignancy in which hypervascularity is common. Most cases of sporadic clear-cell carcinoma of the kidney are associated with loss of heterozygosity in the von Hippel-Lindau (VHL) gene on chromosome 3 and inactivation of the VHL allele. This is associated with a loss of suppressor gene function and induction of genes that are regulated by hypoxia, one of which is the gene associated with production of VEGF. For this reason, renal cell carcinoma was considered an excellent target for bevacizumab trials. In a randomized, double-blind, Phase II trial, bevacizumab at 3 and 10 mg/kg every 2 weeks was compared to placebo in patients with metastatic renal cell cancer.[308] This trial was stopped early after randomization of 116 patients because of significant prolongation of PFS in the 10-mg/kg bevacizumab arm compared with placebo (p <0.001). At the time the study was discontinued, the 5-mg/kg bevacizumab arm also had a slightly longer PFS compared to placebo (p = 0.053). There was no difference in survival, but this analysis was of uncertain significance because crossover to bevacizumab was permitted in the placebo group. Hypertension and asymptomatic proteinuria were the main side effects noted.

Large randomized Phase III trials comparing interferon alpha (IFN) plus bevacizumab with IFN alone in patients with metastatic renal cell cancer have shown an advantage for the addition of the VEGF antibody. IFN was given at a dose of 9 mIU subcutaneously every other day thrice weekly and bevacizumab, 10 mg/kg intravenously every 2 weeks in a large European trial.[90] Hypertension and proteniuria were much more common in the bevacizumab arm. A similar trial conducted in the United States yielded confirmatory results.[309] Toxicity was greater for bevacizumab plus IFN, including significantly more grade 3 hypertension (9% vs 0), anorexia (17% vs 8%), fatigue (35% vs 28%), and proteinuria (13% vs 0%). A subset analysis of the European trial found that 131 patients in the combination arm who had a dose reduction in IFN to 6 or 3 mIU because of toxicity had a comparable PFS.[310]

In a Phase II trial, patients with metastatic clear-cell renal carcinoma were treated with bevacizumab, 10 mg/kg intravenously every 2 weeks, and erlotinib, 150 mg orally daily.[311] The objective response rate was 20%. The most common adverse events were mild-to-moderate rash and diarrhea, which were attributed to erlotinib, and proteinuria, which was attributed to bevacizumab. In dose-finding Phase I-II trials, thalidomide, which also has anti-antigenesis properties, was combined with bevacizumab in patients with metastatic renal cell cancer whose disease had progressed after receiving placebo in another trial.[312] Sequential cohorts of 10 to 12 patients were treated with bevacizumab, 3 mg/kg alone or bevacizumab plus the maximum tolerated dose of thalidomide per dose escalation. The combination was well tolerated, with more than 50% of patients able to escalate their thalidomide dose to at least 500 mg/day. Toxicities were similar for both treatments, and there were no objective responses. PFS was similar between groups: 3.0 months for bevacizumab plus thalidomide and 2.4 months for bevacizumab alone.

In 2009, the FDA approved bevacizumab plus IFN for use in metastatic renal cancer based on a substantial improvement in PFS.

Malignant Gliomas

Bevacizumab received an indication from the FDA for the treatment of glioblastoma multiforme (GBM) in 2009. Early trials of bevacizumab, conducted in colon, lung, breast, and kidney cancer, all excluded patients with brain metastases because of concerns that there might be an increased risk of intracerebral hemorrhage. GBMs are highly vascular, and one issue for these trials is to determine to what extent decreased vascularity is accounting for the decrease in what is interpreted as tumor by magnetic resonance imaging (MRI), because this modality does not readily distinguish tumor from edema, radiation necrosis, or other vascular-related changes.

Because of some enthusiasm for the activity of irinotecan against GBM, several early trials focused on the combination of irinotecan and bevacizumab. In a Phase II trial, adult patients with recurrent anaplastic astrocytoma or GBM (grade III or IV glioma) received bevacizumab at 10 mg/kg and irinotecan intravenously every 2 weeks of a 6-week cycle.[313] The same group subsequently compared to two different schedules of irinotecan with bevacizumab and noted similar results for cohorts of 14 and 24 patients.[314] In both of these trials the dose of irinotecan was determined on the basis of whether patients were taking antiepileptic drugs inducing hepatic enzymes that accelerate metabolism of irinotecan. Patients taking enzyme-inducing antiepileptic drugs received irinotecan at 340 mg/m^2 while other patients received irinotecan at 125 mg/m^2. Based on definitions of response used for such trials, the authors reported an overall response rate of 63% for all patients. There were no instances of central nervous system hemorrhage, but four patients (12%) experienced thromboembolic complications. In another trial, 52 heavily pretreated patients with recurrent high-grade gliomas were treated every 2 weeks with bevacizumab at 10 mg/kg and irinotecan at 340 mg/m^2, for those receiving enzyme-inducing antiepileptic drugs, and 125 mg/m^2 for those not receiving such antiepileptics.[315] Although they reported a lower response rate than observed in many other trials, the PFS and OS were similar. Treatment was discontinued for four patients because of toxicities that included cerebral hemorrhage, cardiac arrhythmia, intestinal perforation, and diarrhea. In a small trial of 13 patients with recurrent glioma, nine (77%) had a radiographic response, but their duration of response and survival was similar to other studies.[316] In this trial, bevacizumab was discontinued in two patients because of intracranial hemorrhage.

Concurrent temozolomide and radiation therapy has become standard treatment for GBM, and bevacizumab has been added to this treatment.[317] Based on encouraging results in the first 10 patients, the trial by Lai et al[317] was planned to continue for accrual of 70 patients.

Other investigators began to examine the effects of bevacizumab as a single agent for the treatment of GBM. Kreisl et al treated 48 patients with bevacizumab, with a response rate of 71%.[318] There were no instances of cerebral hemorrhage, but six patients (12.5%) were removed from study for drug-associated toxicity, including five with thromboembolic events and one with bowel perforation. In accordance with the study design, at relapse, 19 patients were treated with the combination of irinotecan plus bevacizumab, and none had a response. This strongly suggested that the apparent antitumor effects observed in other trials of bevacizumab plus irinotecan may have all been based on the anti-VEGF effects of the MoAb. In May 2009, bevacizumab was granted accelerated approval by the FDA for the treatment of GBM that progresses following standard therapy, based on durable objective responses observed in two single-arm trials of monotherapy. The observed response rate was 26%, with a median duration of response of 4.2 months for the 85 patients in Study AVF3708, and 20% with a median duration of response of 3.9 months for 29 patients in Study NCI 06-C-0064E.[319]

Noncolorectal Gastrointestinal Malignancies

Nonrandomized trials have been conducted involving bevacizumab in various tumor types. The most significant studies have been conducted in patients with pancreatic cancer. In a single-arm trial, patients with previously untreated metastatic pancreatic cancer received gemcitabine, 1000 mg/m² intravenously over 30 minutes on days 1, 8, and 15 every 28 days, and bevacizumab, 10 mg/kg intravenously after gemcitabine on days 1 and 15.[320] Grade 3 and 4 toxicities included hypertension in 19% of the patients, thrombosis in 13%, visceral perforation in 8%, and bleeding in 2%. Results were encouraging enough to take forward into a Phase III trial by the Cancer and Leukemia Group B, in which patients were randomized to receive either gemcitabine plus bevacizumab or gemcitabine plus placebo.[321] There was no advantage for the addition of bevacizumab in terms of reponse rate, PFS, or OS.

In another Phase III trial, patients with metastatic pancreatic adenocarcinoma were treated with the combination of gemcitabine and erlotinib, two products that are approved for the treatment of pancreatic cancer, or with gemcitabine alone.[322] A total of 706 patients were randomized weekly to receive gemcitabine (1000 mg/m²) and daily erlotinib (100 mg) with either bevacizumab (5 mg/kg) intravenously or placebo every 2 weeks. PFS had a statistically significant improvement, but OS was the primary objective endpoint. There was a 1-month difference in median OS for the bevacizumab group, but this was not statistically significant. The 297 patients who received bevacizumab had a higher response rate than the 292 in the placebo arm, and this difference was of borderline significance.

In a single-arm trial of combined modality therapy, 48 patients with inoperable pancreatic adenocarcinoma received bevacizumab 2 weeks before radiotherapy, then every 2 weeks during radiotherapy, and finally after radiotherapy until disease progression.[323] Each cohort included 12 patients at doses of 2.5, 5.0, 7.5, and 10 mg/kg. Capecitabine was administered on days 14 through 52. Four had ulceration and bleeding in the radiation field, possibly related to bevacizumab. Three patients had tumor-associated, bleeding duodenal ulcers, and one had a duodenal perforation.

A few trials have also been reported for GI malignancies other than colorectal or pancreatic malignancies. In one trial, 47 patients with metastatic or unresectable adenocarcinoma of the stomach or gastroesophageal junction were treated every 3 weeks with bevacizumab, 15 mg/kg on day 1; irinotecan, 65 mg/m² on day 1; and cisplatin, 30 mg/m² on days 1 and 8.[324] A response rate of 65% was reported for the 34 patients who had measurable disease. Possible bevacizumab-related toxicity included grade 3 hypertension (28%), grade 3-to-4 thromboembolic events (25%), gastric perforation (6%), myocardial infarction (2%), and significant upper GI bleeding (2%). The primary tumor was unresected in 40 patients, but only one patient had significant upper GI bleeding. Bevacizumab was given to patients with measurable unresectable or metastatic hepatocellular cancer.[325] For cycle 1 (14 days), bevacizumab, 10 mg/kg, was administered alone intravenously on day 1. For cycle 2 and beyond (28 days/cycle), bevacizumab, 10 mg/kg, was administered on days 1 and 15, and gemcitabine, 1000 mg/m², was administered at 10 mg/m²/minute, followed by oxaliplatin, 85 mg/m² on days 2 and 16. The most common treatment-related grade 3-to-4 toxicities included leukopenia/neutropenia, transient elevation of aminotransferases, hypertension, and fatigue. In another trial, 48 patients with hepatocellular cancer had a 25% response rate for the combination of bevacizumab and oral erlotinib.[326] As a single agent, bevacizumab in hepatocellular cancer was associated with a response rate of 13%.[327] Grade 3-to-4 adverse events included hypertension (15%) and thrombosis (6%), including 4% with arterial thrombosis. Significant hemorrhage occurred in 11% of patients, including one fatal variceal bleed.

Gynecologic Malignancies

Single-agent bevacizumab is active in the treatment of ovarian cancer. Response rates of 15% to 20% have been reported in patients who had experienced progressive disease after two or more courses of chemotherapy[328,329] The most frequent serious adverse events that were potentially related to bevacizumab were hypertension (10%) and thromboembolic events (3%) in one ovarian trial,[328] and proteinuria

(16%), GI perforation (11%), hypertension (9%), arterial thromboembolic events (7%), bleeding (2%), and wound-healing complications (2%) in the other.[329] There were also were three treatment-related deaths (7%) in this trial, and the rate of bowel perforation was unusually high.[329] It was noted that bowel perforations occurred in 24% of patients who had received three prior chemotherapy regimens, compared to none in patients who had received less than three prior chemotherapies. The study was stopped early, after two patients had fatal GI perforations in a trial of bevacizumab plus erlotinib and it appeared unlikely that the response rate would be higher than reported for bevacizumab alone.[330]

It has been hypothesized that the high rate of small bowel perforation is the result of rapid elimination of bowel-wall tumor implants and/or an additional insult to the bowel that has been damaged in some manner by chemotherapy. Broader experience based on multiple trials suggests that this complication is observed in only about 5% of all ovarian patients treated with bevzcizumab.[331] The risk of this complication appears to be increased in more heavily treated patients. A three-arm trial has been started, comparing paclitaxel plus carboplatin (PC) to PC and bevacizumab followed by placebo and to PC with bevacizumab followed by bevacizumab for 15 months.

In recurrent cancer of the cervix, bevacizumab produced a response rate of 11% in a trial conducted by the Gynecologic Oncology Group.[332] Grade 3 or 4 adverse events potentially attributable to bevacizumab included hypertension (15%) and thromboembolism (11%), and there was one infectious death. There were no bowel perforations reported in this trial.

Melanoma and Sarcomas

Seventeen patients with metastatic soft-tissue sarcoma were treated with doxorubicin at 75 mg/m^2 intravenously, followed by bevacizumab, 15 mg/kg intravenously every 3 weeks.[333] Dexrazoxane was given as a cardioprotectant once the total doxorubicin dose exceeded 300 mg/m^2. Six patients developed cardiac toxicity of grade 2 or greater despite close monitoring and standard use of dexrazoxane.

Biweekly bevacizumab at 10 mg/kg combined with weekly paclitaxel was associated with a response rate of 17% in 12 patients with previously treated metastatic melanoma.[334] Biweekly bevacizumab at 10 mg/kg was combined with paclitaxel and carboplatin in 53 patients with unresectable metastatic melanoma.[335] The objective response rate was 17%; all were partial responses. Grade 3-or-higher toxicities potentially attributable to bevacizumab included hypertension (9%) and the death of one patient from intracranial hemorrhage in undiagnosed brain metastases after 8 cycles of treatment. The frequency of hematologic toxicities was similar to what is seen when this chemotherapy is given alone.

Head and Neck Cancer

Oral erlotinib, as EGFR signal-transduction inhibitor, and IV bevacizumab at a dose of 15 mg/kg every 3 weeks were given to 48 patients with recurrent squamous cell cancer of the head and neck.[336] The objective response rate was 15%, including four complete responders. Median PFS was 4.1 months, and median OS was 7.1 months.

Prostate Cancer

Bevacizumab at a dose of 10 mg/kg and docetaxel at 60 mg/m^2 every 3 weeks were given to 20 patients with hormone-refractory prostate cancer, all of whom had bone metastases.[337] Substantial decreases in prostate-specific antigen (PSA) were noted in 55%. Three of eight patients who had measurable disease had an objective response.

Bevacizumab was combined with APC8015 (sipuleucel-T) in the treatment of 22 patients with hormone-refractory prostate cancer.[338] Sipuleucel-T is a cellular prostate cancer vaccine containing T lymphocytes and dendritic cells loaded with a recombinant prostatic acid phosphatase and GM-CSF fusion protein. Bevacizumab was given at a dose of 10 mg/kg intravenously on weeks 0, 2, and 4 and every 2 weeks thereafter, while sipuleucel-T was given intravenously on weeks 0, 2, and 4. One patient had a >50% decrease in PSA.

Mechanisms of Anti-Tumor Activity

Bevacizumab probably promotes antitumor effects by a number of mechanisms. The original concept for bevacizumab activity was that it would decrease tumor angiogenesis by blocking VEGF, resulting in a decrease in tumor blood supply, which in turn would lead to cancer cell death. However, it appears that bevacizumab treatment is also associated with afferent vascular dilatation and efferent vascular constriction of tumor vessels, which may help concentrate chemotherapy at the tumor site. One study in patients with rectal cancer showed that the bevacizumab decreased tumor perfusion, vascular volume, interstitial fluid pressure, microvascular density, and circulating endothelial cells while increasing the proportion of blood vessels with percytes.[339] The decrease in interstitial fluid pressure might allow easier penetration for the MoAb itself, which might carry some chemotherapy molecules with it. Another study in patients with inflammatory breast cancer demonstrated a decrease in phosphorylated VEGFR2 in tumor cells, a decrease in vascular permeability, and an increase in tumor cell apoptosis, but no significant changes in microvessel density or VEGF-A expression.[340] In the pivotal trial of IFL and bevacizumab as initial treatment for metastatic colon cancer, levels of epithelial and stromal VEGF, stromal thrombospondin-2, and microvessel density failed to predict clinical benefit associated with the addition of bevacizumab as opposed to placebo.[341]

Toxicities and Adverse Events

The severe toxicities associated with bevacizumab in various monotherapy trials are summarized in Table 12-5. The package insert for the product warns of hemorrhage, hypertension, proteinuria, impaired wound healing, GI perforation, and congestive heart failure. The most serious, and sometimes fatal, bevacizumab-associated toxicities are GI perforation, wound-healing complications, hemorrhage, arterial thromboembolic events, hypertensive crisis, nephrotic syndrome, and congestive heart failure.[109] Consideration of impaired wound-healing has led to the following suggestions: waiting at least 4 to 6 weeks after bevacizumab has been discontinued before taking a patient to surgery, and waiting at least 2 to 3 weeks after surgery before instituting bevacizumab therapy. Bowel perforation has been a

Table 12-5. Severe, Life-Threatening, or Lethal Acute Toxicities* during Bevacizumab Monotherapy in Colorectal Cancer

Toxicity	Percent of Patients (n = 234)	Toxicity	Percent of Patients (n = 234)
Abdominal pain	8%	Ileus	4%
Hypertension	8%	Hemorrhage	4%
Vomiting	6%	Diarrhea	2%
Nausea	6%	Headache	2%
Vomiting	6%	Neurosensory	1%
Asthenia/malaise	5%	Neurologic (other)	1%

*Grade 3 to 5.

problem in the setting of GI and ovarian cancers that are prone to produce tumor implants in the bowel wall, and it may be a result of antitumor effect. However, this complication has also occurred in patients who did not have bowel metastases, and bowel injury from prior chemotherapy may be a contributing factor.

Notably, the adverse events have varied somewhat by tumor types, and some may reflect antitumor effects rather than nonspecific vascular effects. For instance, massive hemoptysis has typically been limited to patients with large, centrally located lung cancers, and bowel perforation has been more common in cancers of the colon and, especially, ovaries—entities often associated with metastatic implants on bowel surfaces. Although patients with brain metastases have been excluded from many studies, in part because of concern about intracranial hemorrhage, bleeding has not been a problem in patients with GBM who have received bevacizumab.

Hypertension and proteinuria occur in all settings and may be caused by effects on small renal vessels because VEGF is involved in repair of glomeruli endothelial cells. Hypertension is usually readily controlled with a single anti-hypertensive agent. As noted earlier in this chapter, a DNA analysis of 363 breast cancer patients, who had been treated with bevacizumab and paclitaxel, found that VEGF-634 CC and VEGF-1498 TT genotypes were associated with significantly less grade 3 or 4 hypertension.[305] Proteinuria can progress to full-blown nephrotic syndrome. Patients should be monitored for proteinuria and treatment discontinued if proteinuria exceeds 2 g/24 hours. Increased rates of epistaxis have been noted in many trials, but increased rates of vascular thrombosis have also been noted.

Summary

Despite some safety concerns, bevacizumab has been a tremendous addition to the therapeutic armamentarium because it is potentially useful in virtually every type of solid tumor as a result of the importance of tumor angiogenesis to tumor growth. Bevacizumab seems to enhance chemotherapy in virtually every tumor type in which chemotherapy is active. It already has been granted marketing indications for the treatment of cancers of the colon, lung, breast, and brain, but it has also shown effectivity in ovarian cancer and renal cell carcinoma. Although its single-agent activity appears limited, bevacizumab alone may be useful in the adjuvant setting, or following complete remission after systemic therapy, because of the inhibition of neoangiogenesis required to develop metastatic tumors.

Conclusions

During the past decade, MoAb "magic bullets" have become standard treatment for many types of solid tumors. Three of these products are limited in their scope of malignant targets because of their specificity for surface antigens on malignant cells, but bevacizumab has the potential to be useful in every cancer setting because of the importance of the VEGF ligand for tumor angiogenesis. So far, cetuximab and panitumumab appear potentially useful in the same patient populations, but at this time it is not clear that the human panitumumab has significant advantages over the chimeric cetuximab. All four of these MoAbs enhance the activity of chemotherapy in various settings. Bevacizumab adds to the beneficial effects of IFNα in renal cell cancer. To date, it has not been determined whether combining these MoAbs results in additive or synergistic effects or whether there is value in combining these MoAbs with tyrosine kinase inhibitors such as erlotinib, sunitinib, or sorafenib.

References

1. Oldham RK. Monoclonal antibodies in cancer therapy. J Clin Oncol 1983;1:582-90.
2. Dillman RO. Monoclonal antibodies in the treatment of cancer. Crit Rev Oncol Hematol 1984;1:357-85.
3. Dillman RO. Monoclonal antibodies for treating cancer. Ann Intern Med 1989;111:592-603.

4. Dillman RO. Antibodies as cytotoxic therapy. J Clin Oncol 1994;12:1497-515.
5. Dillman RO. Magic bullets at last! Finally—approval of a monoclonal antibody for the treatment of cancer!!! Cancer Biother Radiopharm 1997;12:223-5.
6. Oldham RK, Dillman RO. Monoclonal antibodies in cancer therapy: 25 years of progress. J Clin Oncol 2008;26:1774-7.
7. Ehrlich P. Uber den jetzigen stand der Karzinomforschung. In: Ehrlich P, Himmelweit F. The collected papers of Paul Ehrlich. Volume II. London: Pergamon Press, 1956:550-7.
8. Schwartz RS. Paul Ehrlich's magic bullets. N Engl J Med 2004;350:1079-80.
9. Currie GA. Eighty years of immunotherapy: A review of immunobiological methods used in the treatment of cancer. Int J Cancer 1972;26:141-53.
10. Wright PW, Hellstrom KE, Hellstrom IE, Bernstein ID. Serotherapy of malignant disease. Med Clin North Am 1976;60:607-22.
11. Rosenberg SA, Terry WD. Passive immunotherapy of cancer in animals and man. Adv Cancer Res 1977;25:323-88.
12. Kohler G, Milstein C. Continuous cultures of fused cells secreting antibody of predetermined specificity. Nature 1975;256:495-597.
13. Larson SM, Brown, JP, Wright PW, et al. Imaging of melanoma with I-131-labeled monoclonal antibodies. J Nucl Med 1982;24:123-9.
14. Oldham RK, Foon KA, Morgan C, et al. Monoclonal antibody therapy of malignant melanoma: In vivo localization in cutaneous metastases after intravenous administration. J Clin Oncol 1984;2:1235-44.
15. Goodman GL, Beaumier P, Hellstrom I, et al. Pilot trial of murine monoclonal antibodies in patients with advanced melanoma. J Clin Oncol 1985;3:340-52.
16. Halpern SE, Dillman RO, Witztum KF, et al. Radioimmunodetection of melanoma utilizing 111-In-96.5 monoclonal antibody: A preliminary report. Radiology 1985;155:493-9.
17. Houghton AN, Mintzer D, Cordon-Cardo C, et al. Mouse monoclonal IgG3 antibody detecting GD3 ganglioside: A phase I trial in patients with malignant melanoma. Proc Natl Acad Sci U S A 1985;82:1242-6.
18. Murray JL, Rosenblum MG, Lamki K, et al. Clinical parameters related to optimal tumor localization of Indium-111-labeled mouse antimelanoma monoclonal antibody ZME018. J Nucl Med 1987;28:25-33.
19. Kirkwood JM, Neumann RD, Zoghbi SS, et al. Scintigraphic detection of metastatic melanoma using Indium-111/DTPA conjugated anti-gp240 antibody [ZME018]. J Clin Oncol 1987;5:1247-55.
20. Cheung NK, Lazarus H, Miraldi FD, et al. Ganglioside GD2 specific monoclonal antibody 3F8: A phase I study in patients with neuroblastoma and malignant melanoma. J Clin Oncol 1987;5:1430-40.
21. Vadhan-Raj S, Cordon-Cardo C, Carswell E, et al. Phase I trial of mouse monoclonal antibody against GD3 ganglioside in patients with melanoma: Induction of inflammatory responses at tumor sites. J Clin Oncol 1988;6:1636-48.
22. Bajorin DF, Chapman PB, Wong GY, et al. Treatment with high dose mouse monoclonal (anti-GD3) antibody R24 in patients with metastatic melanoma. Melanoma Res 1992;2:355-62.
23. Saleh MN, Khazaeli MB, Wheeler RH, et al. Phase I trial of the murine monoclonal anti-G_{D2} antibody 14G2a in metastatic melanoma. Cancer Res 1992;52:4342-7.
24. Kirkwood JM, Mascari RA, Edington HD, et al. Analysis of therapeutic and immunologic effects of R(24) anti-GD3 monoclonal antibody in 37 patients with metastatic melanoma. Cancer 2000;88:2693-702.
25. Sears HF, Atkinson B, Mattis J, et al. Phase I clinical trial of monoclonal antibody in treatment of gastrointestinal tumors. Lancet 1982;1:762-5.
26. Sears HF, Herlyn D, Steplewski Z, et al. Phase II clinical trial of a murine monoclonal antibody cytotoxic for gastrointestinal adenocarcinoma. Cancer Res 1985;45:5910-13.
27. Halpern SE, Dillman RO, Amox D, et al. Detection of occult tumor using indium 111-labeled anticarcinoembryonic antigen antibodies. Arch Surg 1992;127:1094-100.
28. Weiner LM, Harvey E, Padavic-Shaller K, et al. Phase II multicenter evaluation of prolonged murine monoclonal antibody 17-1A therapy in pancreatic carcinoma. J Immunother 1993;13:110-6.
29. Riethmuller G, Holz E, Schlimok G, et al. Monoclonal antibody therapy for resected Dukes' C colorectal cancer: Seven-year outcome of a multicenter randomized trial. J Clin Oncol 1998;16:1788-94.
30. Mulshine JL, Avis I, Treston AM, et al. Clinical use of a monoclonal antibody to bombesin-like

peptide in patients with lung cancer. Ann N Y Acad Sci 1988;547:360-72.
31. Elias DJ, Hirschowitz L, Kline LE, et al. Phase I clinical comparative study of monoclonal antibody KS1/4 and KS1/4-methotrexate immunoconjugate in patients with non-small cell lung carcinoma. Cancer Res 1990;50:4154-9.
32. Kelley MJ, Linnoila RI, Avis IL, et al. Antitumor activity of a monoclonal antibody directed against gastrin-releasing peptide in patients with small cell lung cancer. Chest 1997;112:256-61.
33. Ryan KP, Dillman RO, DeNardo SJ, et al. Breast cancer imaging with In-111 human IgM monoclonal antibodies. Radiology 1988;167:71-5.
34. Goodman GE, Hellstrom I, Brodzinsky L, et al. Phase I trial of murine monoclonal antibody L6 in breast, colon, ovarian, and lung cancer. J Clin Oncol 1990;8:1083-92.
35. Halpern SE, Dillman RO. Radioimmunodetection with monoclonal antibodies against prostatic acid phosphatase. In: Winkler C, ed. Nuclear medicine in clinical oncology. Berlin/Heidelberg: Springer Verlag, 1986:164-70.
36. Leroy M, Teillac P, Rain JD, et al. Radioimmunodetection of lymph node invasion in prostatic cancer. Cancer 1989;64:1-5.
37. Oosterwijk E, Bander NH, Divgi CR, et al. Antibody localization in human renal cell carcinoma: A phase I study of monoclonal antibody G250. J Clin Oncol 1993;11:738-50.
38. Dillman RO, Beauregard JC, Sobol RE, et al. Lack of radioimmunodetection and complications associated with monoclonal antibody cross-reactivity with an antigen on circulating cells. Cancer Res 1984;44:2213-17.
39. Dillman RO, Dillman JB, Halpern SE, et al. Toxicities and side effects associated with intravenous infusions of murine monoclonal antibodies. J Biol Response Mod 1986;5:73-84.
40. Dillman RO, Beauregard JC, Jamieson M, et al. Toxicities associated with monoclonal antibody infusions in cancer patients. Molec Biother 1988;1:81-5.
41. Schroff RW, Foon KA, Wilburn SB, et al. Human antimurine immunoglobulin responses in patients receiving monoclonal antibody therapy. Cancer Res 1985;45:879-85.
42. Shawler DL, Bartholomew RM, Smith LM, et al. Human immune response to multiple injections of murine monoclonal IgG. J Immunol 1985;135:1530-35.
43. Dillman RO. The human antimouse and anti-globulin responses to monoclonal antibodies. Antibody Immunoconjugates and Radiopharmaceuticals 1990;3:1-15.
44. Dillman RO, Shawler DL, McCallister TJ, et al. Human anti-mouse antibody response in cancer patients following single low-dose injections of radiolabeled murine monoclonal antibodies. Cancer Biother 1994;9:17-28.
45. Khazaeli MB, Conry RM, LoBuglio AF. Human immune response to monoclonal antibodies. J Immunother 1994;15:42-52.
46. DePinho RA, Feldman LB, Scharff MD. Tailor-made monoclonal antibodies. Ann Intern Med 1986;104:225-33.
47. Albrecht H, DeNardo SJ. Recombinant antibodies: From the laboratory to the clinic. Cancer Biother Radiopharm 2006;21:285-303.
48. Scallon BJ, Snyder LA, Anderson GM, et al. A review of antibody therapeutics and antibody-related technologies for oncology. J Immunother 2006;29:351-64.
49. Brown BA, Davis GL, Saltzgaber-Muller J, et al. Tumor specific genetically engineered murine/human chimeric monoclonal antibody. Cancer Res 1987;47:3577-83.
50. Morrison SL, Oi T. Genetically engineered antibody molecules. Adv Immunol 1989;44:65-92.
51. Birch JR, Racher JR. Antibody production. Advanced Drug Delivery Reviews 2006;58:671-85.
52. Bodey B, Bodey B Jr, Siegel SE, Kaiser HE. Genetically engineered monoclonal antibodies for direct anti-neoplastic treatment and cancer cell specific delivery of chemotherapeutic agents. Curr Pharm Des 2000;6:261-76.
53. Eisenberg BI. The polymerase chain reaction. N Engl J Med 1990;322:178-83.
54. Green LL. Antibody engineering via genetic engineering of the mouse: XenoMouse strains are a vehicle for the facile generation of therapeutic human monoclonal antibodies. J Immunol Methods 1999;231:11-23.
55. Langer LF, Clay TM, Morse MA. Update on anti-CTLA-4 antibodies in clinical trials. Expert Opin Biol Ther 2007;7:1245-56.
56. Roskoski R Jr. The ErbB/HER receptor protein-tyrosine kinases and cancer. Biochem Biophys Res Commun 2004;319:1-11.
57. Rowinsky EK, Schwartz GH, Gollob JA, et al. Safety, pharmacokinetics, and activity of ABX-EGF, a fully human anti-epidermal growth factor receptor monoclonal antibody in

patients with metastatic renal cell cancer. J Clin Oncol 2004;22:3003-15.
58. Masui H, Kawamoto T, Sato JD, et al. Growth inhibition of human tumor cells in athymic mice by anti-epidermal growth factor receptor monoclonal antibodies. Cancer Res 1984;44:1002-7.
59. Mendelsohn J. Blockade of receptors for growth factors: An anticancer therapy. Clin Cancer Res 2000;6:747-53.
60. Schecter AL, Stern DF, Vaidanathan L, et al. The neu oncogene: An erb-B-related gene encoding a 185,000-Mr tumor antigen. Nature 1984;312:513-16.
61. Slamon DJ, Clark GM, Wong SG, et al. Human breast cancer: Correlation of relapse and survival with amplification of the HER2-2/neu oncogene. Science 1987;235:177-82.
62. Folkman J. Tumor angiogenesis. Adv Cancer Res 1985;43:175-203.
63. Ferrara N. Molecular and biological properties of vascular endothelial growth factor. J Mol Med 1999;77:527-43.
64. Schlaeppi JM, Wood JM. Targeting vascular endothelial growth factor (VEGF) for antitumor therapy, by anti-VEGF neutralizing monoclonal antibodies or by VEGF receptor tyrosine-kinase inhibitors. Cancer Metastasis Rev 1999;18:473-81.
65. Asano M, Yukita A, Matsumoto T, et al. An anti-human VEGF monoclonal antibody, MV833, that exhibits potent antitumor activity in vivo. Hybridoma 1998;17:185-90.
66. Brekken RA, Overholser JP, Stastny VA, et al. Selective inhibition of vascular endothelial growth factor (VEGF) receptor 2 (KDR/Flk-1) activity by a monoclonal anti-VEGF antibody blocks tumor growth in mice. Cancer Res 2000;60:5117-24.
67. Gerber HP, Kowalski J, Sherman D, et al. Complete inhibition of rhabdomyosarcoma xenograft growth and neovascularization requires blockade of both tumor and host vascular endothelial growth factor. Cancer Res 2000;60:6253-8.
68. Lee CG, Heijn M, di Tomaso E, et al. Anti-vascular endothelial growth factor treatment augments tumor radiation response under normoxic or hypoxic conditions. Cancer Res 2000;60:5565-70.
69. Soh EY, Eigelberger MS, Kim KJ, et al. Neutralizing vascular endothelial growth factor activity inhibits thyroid cancer growth in vivo. Surgery 2000;128:1059-65.
70. Shakib F, ed. Basic and clinical aspects of IgG subclasses. New York: Carger, 1986.
71. Jain RK. Physiological barriers to delivery of monoclonal antibodies and other macromolecules in tumors. Cancer Res 1990;50:814s-19s.
72. Boucher Y, Leunig M, Jain RK. Tumor angiogenesis and interstitial hypertension. Cancer Res 1996;56:4264-6.
73. Davidson MB, Thakkar S, Hix JK, et al. Pathophysiology, clinical consequences, and treatment of tumor lysis syndrome. Am J Med 2004;116:546-54.
74. Tiu RV, Mountantonakis SE, Dunbar AJ, et al. Tumor lysis syndrome. Semin Thromb Haemost 2007;33:397-407.
75. Gessner JE, Heiken H, Tamm A, et al. The IgG Fc receptor family. Ann Haematol 1998;76:231-48.
76. Van Sorge NM, Van der Pol WL, van de Winkel JG. FcgammaR polymorphisms: Implications for function, disease susceptibility and immunotherapy. Tissue Antigens 2003;61:189-202.
77. Nimmerjahn F, Ravetch JV. Antibodies, Fc receptors and cancer. Curr Opin Immunol 2007;19:239-45.
78. Stevenson FK, Wrightham M, Glennie MJ, et al. Antibodies to shared idiotypes as agents for analysis and therapy for human B cell tumors. Blood 1986;68:430-6.
79. Siberil S, Dutertre CA, Fridman WH, et al. FcgammaR: The key to optimize therapeutic antibodies? Crit Rev Oncol Hematol 2007;62:26-33.
80. Weiner LM, Steplewski Z, Koprowski H, et al. Divergent dose-related effects of gamma-interferon therapy on in vitro antibody-dependent cellular and nonspecific cytotoxicity by human peripheral blood monocytes. Cancer Res 1988;48:1042-6.
81. Weiner LM, Moldofsky PJ, Gatenby RA, et al. Antibody delivery and effector cell activation in a phase II trial of recombinant gamma-interferon and the murine monoclonal antibody CO17-1A in advanced colorectal carcinoma. Cancer Res 1988;48:2568-73.
82. Saleh MN, LoBuglio AF, Wheeler RH, et al. A phase II trial of murine monoclonal antibody 17-1A and interferon-gamma: Clinical and immunological data. Cancer Immunol 1990;32:185-90.
83. Tempero MA, Sivinski C, Steplewski Z, et al. Phase II trial of interferon gamma and mono-

clonal antibody 17-1A in pancreatic cancer: Biologic and clinical effects. J Clin Oncol 1990; 8:2019-26.
84. Ziegler LD, Palazzolo P, Cunningham J, et al. Phase I trial of murine monoclonal antibody L6 in combination with subcutaneous interleukin-2 in patients with advanced carcinoma of the breast, colorectum, and lung. J Clin Oncol 1992;10:1470-8.
85. Sosman JA, Weiss GR, Margolin KA, et al. Phase IB clinical trial of anti-CD3 followed by high dose bolus interleukin-2 in patients with metastatic melanoma and advanced renal cell carcinoma; clinical and immunologic effects. J Clin Oncol 1993;11:1496-505.
86. Soiffer RJ, Chapman PB, Murray C, et al. Administration of R24 monoclonal antibody and low-dose interleukin-2 for malignant melanoma. Clin Cancer Res 1997;3:17-24.
87. Repka T, Chiorean EG, Gay J, et al. Trastuzumab and interleukin-2 in HER2-positive metastatic breast cancer: A pilot study. Clin Cancer Res 2003;9:2440-6.
88. Choi BS, Sondel PM, Hank JA, et al. Phase I trial of combined treatment with ch14.18 and R24 Mab and interleukin-2 for patients with melanoma or sarcoma. Cancer Immunol Immunother 2006;55:761-74.
89. Caulfield MJ, Barna B, Murthy S, et al. Phase Ia/Ib trial of an anti-GD3 monoclonal antibody (R24) in combination with interferon alpha (rHuIFNa-2a) in patients with malignant melanoma. J Biol Response Mod 1990;9:319-28.
90. Escudier B, Pluzanska A, Koralewski P, et al. Bevacizumab plus interferon alfa-2a for treatment of metastatic renal cell carcinoma: A randomised, double-blind phase III trial. Lancet 2007;370:2103-11.
91. Ragnhammar P, Pagerberg J, Frodin JE, et al. Effect of monoclonal antibody 17-1A and GM-CSF in patients with advanced colorectal carcinoma: Long-lasting complete remissions can be induced. Int J Cancer 1993;53:751-8.
92. Hjelm Skog A, Ragnhammar P, Fagerberg J, et al. Clinical effects of monoclonal antibody 17-1A combined with granulocyte/macrophage-colony-stimulating factor and interleukin-2 for treatment of patients with advanced colorectal carcinoma. Cancer Immunol Immunother 1999;48:463-70.
93. Fiedler W, Krüger W, Laack E, et al. A clinical trial of edrecolomab, interleukin-2 and GM-CSF in patients with advanced colorectal cancer. Oncol Rep 2001;8:225-31.
94. James ND, Atherton PJ, Jones J, et al. A phase II study of the bispecific antibody MDX-H210 (anti-HER2 x CD64) with GM-CSF in HER2+ advanced prostate cancer. Br J Cancer 2001; 85:152-6.
95. Dillman RO, Shawler DL, Sobol RE, et al. Murine monoclonal antibody therapy in two patients with chronic lymphocytic leukemia. Blood 1982;59:1036-45.
96. Byrd JC, Waselenko JK, Maneatis TA, et al. Rituximab therapy in hematologic malignancy patients with circulating blood tumor cells: Association with increased infusion-related side effects and rapid tumor clearance. J Clin Oncol 1999;17:791-5.
97. Lim LC, Koh LP, Tan P. Fatal cytokine release syndrome with chimeric anti-CD20 monoclonal antibody rituximab in a 71-year old patient with chronic lymphocytic leukemia. J Clin Oncol 1999;17:1962-3.
98. Dillman RO. Infusion reactions associated with the therapeutic use of monoclonal antibodies in the treatment of malignancy. Cancer Metastasis Rev 1999;18:465-71.
99. Winkler U, Jensen M, Manzke O, et al. Cytokine-release syndrome in patients with B-cell chronic lymphocytic leukemia and high lymphocyte counts after treatment with an anti-CD20 monoclonal antibody (rituximab, IDEC-C2B8). Blood 1999;94:2217-24.
100. Dillman RO, Hendrix CS. Unique aspects of supportive care using monoclonal antibodies in cancer treatment. Support Cancer Ther 2003; 1:38-48.
101. Jacot W, Bessis D, Jorda E, et al. Acneiform eruption induced by epidermal growth factor receptor inhibitors in patients with solid tumours. Br J Dermatol 2004;151:238-41.
102. Perez-Soler R, Delord JP, Halpern A, et al. HER1/EGFR inhibitor-associated rash: Future directions for managment and investigation outcomes for the HER1/EGFR inhibitor rash management forum. Oncologist 2005;10:345-56.
103. Seagaert S, van Cutsem E. Clinical signs, pathophysiology, and management of skin toxicity during therapy with epidermal growth factor receptor inhibitors. Ann Oncol 2005;16:1425-33.
104. Keefe DL. Trastuzumab-associated cardiotoxicity. Cancer 2002;95:1592-600.

105. Seidman A, Hudis C, Pierri MK, et al. Cardiac dysfunction in the trastuzumab clinical trials experience. J Clin Oncol 2002;20:1215-21.
106. Smith KL, Dang C, Seidman AD. Cardiac dysfunction associated with trastuzumab. Expert Opin Drug Saf 2006;5:619-29.
107. Ostendorf T, Kunter U, Eitner F, et al. VEGF(165) mediates glomerular endothelial repair. J Clin Invest 1999;104:913-23.
108. Sugimoto H, Hamano Y, Charytan D, et al. Neutralization of circulating vascular endothelial growth factor (VEGF) by anti-VEGF antibodies and soluble VEGF receptor 1 (sFlt-1) induces proteinuria. J Biol Chem 2003;278:12605-8.
109. Eskens FA, Verweij J. The clinical toxicity profile of vascular endothelial growth factor (VEGF) and vascular endothelial growth factor receptor (VEGFR) targeting angiogenesis inhibitors; a review. Eur J Cancer 2006;42:3127-39.
110. Dillman RO. Perceptions of Herceptin: A monoclonal antibody for the treatment of breast cancer. Cancer Biother Radiopharm 1999;14:5-10.
111. Carter P, Presta L, Gorman C, et al. Humanization of an anti-p185Her2 antibody for human cancer. Proc Natl Acad Sci U S A 1992;89:4285-9.
112. Sliwkowski MX, Lofgren JA, Lewis GC, et al. Nonclinical studies addressing the mechanism of action of trastuzumab (Herceptin). Semin Oncol 1999;26(Suppl 12):60-70.
113. Masui H, Kamrath H, Apell G, et al. Cytotoxicity against human tumor cells mediated by the conjugate of anti-epidermal growth factor receptor monoclonal antibody to recombinant ricin A chain. Cancer Res 1989;49:3482-8.
114. Arnould L, Gelly M, Penault-Llorca F, et al. Trastuzumab-based treatment of HER2-positive breast cancer: An antibody-dependent cellular cytotoxicity mechanism? Br J Cancer 2006;94:259-67.
115. Leyland-Jones B, Gelmon K, Ayoub JP, et al. Pharmacokinetics, safety, and efficacy of trastuzumab administered every three weeks in combination with paclitaxel. J Clin Oncol 2003;21:3965-71.
116. Baselga J, Carbonell X, Castaneda-Soto NJ, et al. Phase II study of efficacy, safety, and pharmacokinetics of trastuzumab monotherapy administered on a 3-weekly schedule. J Clin Oncol 2005;23:2162-71.
117. Pauletti G, Dandekar S, Rong HM, et al. Assessment of methods for tissue-based detection of the HER-2/neu alteration in human breast cancer: A direct comparison of fluorescence in situ hybridization and immunohistochemistry. J Clin Oncol 2000;18:3651-64.
118. Tubbs RR, Pettay JD, Roche PC, et al. Discrepancies in clinical laboratory testing of eligibility for trastuzumab therapy: Apparent immunohistochemical false-positives do not get the message. J Clin Oncol 2001;19:2714-21.
119. Dowsett M, Bartlett J, Ellis IO, et al. Correlation between immunohistochemistry (HercepTest) and fluorescence in situ hybridization (FISH) for HER-2 in 426 breast carcinomas from 37 centres. J Pathol 2003;199:418-23.
120. Perez EA, Suman VJ, Davidson NE, et al. HER2 testing by local, central, and reference laboratories in specimens from the North Central Cancer Treatment Group N9831 intergroup adjuvant trial. J Clin Oncol 2006;24:3032-8.
121. Paik S, Bryant J, Tan-Chiu E, et al. Real-world performance of HER2 testing—National Surgical Adjuvant Breast and Bowel Project experience. J Natl Cancer Inst 2002;94:852-4.
122. Hudis CA. Trastuzumab—mechanisms of action and use in clinical practice. N Engl J Med 2007;357:39-51.
123. Baselga J, Tripathy D, Mendelsohn, et al. Phase II study of weekly intravenous recombinant hmanized anti-p185^{HER2} monoclonal antibody in patients with HER2/neu-overexpressing metastatic breast cancer. J Clin Oncol 1996;14:737-44.
124. Cobleigh MA, Vogel CL, Tripathy D, et al. Multinational study of the efficacy and safety of humanized anti-HER2 monoclonal antibody in women who have HER2-overexperessing metastatic breast cancer that has progressed after chemotehrapy for metastatic disease. J Clin Oncol 1999;17:2639-48.
125. Vogel CL, Cobleigh MA, Tripathy D, et al. Efficacy and safety of trastuzumab as a single agent in first-line treatment of HER2-overexpressing metastatic breast cancer. J Clin Oncol 2002;20:719-26.
126. Burris H 3rd, Yardley D, Jones S, et al. Phase II trial of trastuzumab followed by weekly paclitaxel/carboplatin as first-line treatment for patients with metastatic breast cancer. J Clin Oncol 2004;22:1621-9.
127. Baselga J, Norton L, Albanell J, et al. Recombinant humanized anti-HER2 antibody (Hercep-

tin) enhances the antitumor activity of paclitaxel and doxorubicin against HER/neu overexpressing human breast cancer xenografts. Cancer Res 1998;58:2825-31.
128. Pegram MD, Konecny GE, O'Callaghan C, et al. Rational combinations of trastuzumab with chemotherapeutic drugs used in the treatment of breast cancer. J Natl Cancer Inst 2004;96:739-49.
129. Esteva FJ, Valero V, Booser D, et al. Phase II study of weekly docetaxel and trastuzumab for patients with HER-2-overexpressing metastatic breast cancer. J Clin Oncol 2002;20:1800-8.
130. Montemurro F, Choa G, Faggiuolo R, et al. Safety and activity of docetaxel and trastuzumab in HER2 overexpressing metastatic breast cancer: A pilot phase II study. Am J Clin Oncol 2003;26:95-7.
131. Tedesco KL, Thor AD, Johnson DH, et al. Docetaxel combined with trastuzumab is an active regimen in HER-2 3+ overexpressing and fluorescent in situ hybridization-positive metastatic breast cancer: A multi-institutional phase II trial. J Clin Oncol 2004;22:1071-7.
132. Sato N, Sano M, Tabei T, et al. Combination docetaxel and trastuzumab treatment for patients with HER-2-overexpressing metastatic breast cancer: A multicenter, phase-II study. Breast Cancer 2006;13:166-71.
133. Fountzilas G, Tsavdaridis D, Kalogera-Fountzila A, et al. Weekly paclitaxel as first-line chemotherapy and trastuzumab in patients with advanced breast cancer. A Hellenic Cooperative Oncology Group phase II study. Ann Oncol 2001;12:1545-51.
134. Seidman AD, Fornier MN, Esteva FJ, et al. Weekly trastuzumab and paclitaxel therapy for metastatic breast cancer with analysis of efficacy by HER2 immunophenotype and gene amplification. J Clin Oncol 2001;19:2587-95.
135. Gori S, Colozza M, Mosconi AM, et al. Phase II study of weekly paclitaxel and trastuzumab in anthracycline- and taxane-pretreated patients with HER2-overexpressing metastatic breast cancer. Br J Cancer 2004;90:36-40.
136. Robert N, Leyland-Jones B, Asmar L, et al. Randomized phase III study of trastuzumab, paclitaxel, and carboplatin compared with trastuzumab and paclitaxel in women with HER-2-overexpressing metastatic breast cancer. J Clin Oncol 2006;24:2786-92.
137. Jahanzeb M, Mortimer JE, Yunus F, et al. Phase II trial of weekly vinorelbine and trastuzumab as first-line therapy in patients with HER2(+) metastatic breast cancer. Oncologist 2002;7:410-7.
138. Burstein HJ, Kuter I, Campos SM, et al. Clinical activity of trastuzumab and vinorelbine in women with HER2-overexpressing metastatic breast cancer. J Clin Oncol 2001;19:2722-30.
139. Burstein HJ, Harris LN, Marcom PK, et al. Trastuzumab and vinorelbine as first-line therapy for HER2-overexpressing metastatic breast cancer: Multicenter phase II trial with clinical outcomes, analysis of serum tumor markers as predictive factors, and cardiac surveillance algorithm. J Clin Oncol 2003;21:2889-95.
140. De Maio E, Pacilio C, Gravina A, et al. Vinorelbine plus 3-weekly trastuzumab in metastatic breast cancer: A single-centre phase 2 trial. BMC Cancer 2007;7:50.
141. Bartsch R, Wenzel C, Altorjai G, et al. Results from an observational trial with oral vinorelbine and trastuzumab in advanced breast cancer. Breast Cancer Res Treat 2007;102:375-81.
142. Chan A, Martin M, Untch M, et al. Vinorelbine plus trastuzumab combination as first-line therapy for HER 2-positive metastatic breast cancer patients: an international phase II trial. Br J Cancer 2006;95:788-93.
143. Bayo-Calero JL, Mayordomo JI, Sánchez-Rovira P, et al. A phase II study of weekly vinorelbine and trastuzumab in patients with HER2-positive metastatic breast cancer. Clin Breast Cancer 2008;8:264-8.
144. Papaldo P, Fabi A, Ferretti G, et al. A phase II study on metastatic breast cancer patients treated with weekly vinorelbine with or without trastuzumab according to HER2 expression: Changing the natural history of HER2-positive disease. Ann Oncol 2006;17:630-6.
145. Chia S, Clemons M, Martin LA, et al. Pegylated liposomal doxorubicin and trastuzumab in HER-2 overexpressing metastatic breast cancer: A multicenter phase II trial. J Clin Oncol 2006;24:2773-8.
146. Christodoulou C, Kostopoulos I, Kalofonos HP, et al. Trastuzumab combined with pegylated liposomal doxorubicin in patients with metastatic breast cancer. Phase II Study of the Hellenic Cooperative Oncology Group (HeCOG) with biomarker evaluation. Oncology 2009;76:275-85.
147. Pegram MD, Lipton A, Hayes DF, et al. Phase II study of receptor-enhanced chemosensitivity using recombinant humanized anti-p185HER2/

neu monoclonal antibody plus cisplatin in patients with HER2/neu-overexpressing metastatic breast cancer refractory to chemotherapy treatment. J Clin Oncol 1998; 16:2659-71.
148. O'Shaughnessy JA, Vukelja S, Marsland T, et al. Phase II study of trastuzumab plus gemcitabine in chemotherapy-pretreated patients with metastatic breast cancer. Clin Breast Cancer 2004;5:142-7.
149. Yamamoto D, Iwase S, Kitamura K, et al. A phase II study of trastuzumab and capecitabine for patients with HER2-overexpressing metastatic breast cancer: Japan Breast Cancer Research Network (JBCRN) 00 Trial. Cancer Chemother Pharmacol 2008;61:509-14.
150. Nishimura R, Okumura Y, Arima N. Trastuzumab monotherapy versus combination therapy for treating recurrent breast cancer: Time to progression and survival. Breast Cancer 2008;15:57-64.
151. Perez EA, Suman VJ, Rowland KM, et al. Two concurrent phase II trials of paclitaxel/carboplatin/trastuzumab (weekly or every-3-week schedule) as first-line therapy in women with HER2-overexpressing metastatic breast cancer: NCCTG study 983252. Clin Breast Cancer 2005;6:425-32.
152. Pegram MD, Pienkowski T, Northfelt DW, et al. Results of two open-label, multicenter phase II studies of docetaxel, platinum salts, and trastuzumab in HER2-positive advanced breast cancer. J Natl Cancer Inst 2004;96:759-69.
153. Infante JR, Yardley DA, Burris HA 3rd, et al. Phase II trial of weekly docetaxel, vinorelbine, and trastuzumab in the first-line treatment of patients with HER2-positive metastatic breast cancer. Clin Breast Cancer 2009;9:23-8.
154. Miller KD, Sisk J, Ansari R, et al. Gemcitabine, paclitaxel, and trastuzumab in metastatic breast cancer. Oncology 2001;15(Suppl 3):38-40.
155. Yardley DA, Burris HA 3rd, Simons L, et al. A phase II trial of gemcitabine/carboplatin with or without trastuzumab in the first-line treatment of patients with metastatic breast cancer. Clin Breast Cancer 2008;8:425-31.
156. Loesch D, Asmar L, McIntyre K, et al. Phase II trial of gemcitabine/carboplatin (plus trastuzumab in HER2-positive disease) in patients with metastatic breast cancer. Clin Breast Cancer 2008;8:178-86.
157. Fountzilas G, Christodoulou C, Tsavardaridis D, et al. Paclitaxel and gemcitabine, as first-line chemotherapy, combined with trastuzumab in patients with advanced breast cancer: A phase II study conducted by the Hellenic Cooperative Oncology Group (HeCOG). Cancer Invest 2004; 22:655-62.
158. Morabito A, Longo R, Gattuso D, et al. Trastuzumab in combination with gemcitabine and vinorelbine as second-line therapy for HER-2/neu overexpressing metastatic breast cancer. Oncol Rep 2006;16:393-8.
159. Stemmler HJ, Kahlert S, Brudler O, et al. High efficacy of gemcitabine and cisplatin plus trastuzumab in patients with HER2-overexpressing metastatic breast cancer: A phase II study. Clin Oncol 2005;17:630-5.
160. Cortes J, Di Cosimo S, Climent MA, et al. Nonpegylated liposomal doxorubicin (TLC-D99), paclitaxel, and trastuzumab in HER-2-overexpressing breast cancer: A multicenter phase I/II study. Clin Cancer Res 2009;15:307-14.
161. Nisticò C, Bria E, Vaccaro V, et al. Trastuzumab plus weekly epirubicin and paclitaxel for locally advanced and metastatic breast cancer: Preliminary results of a feasibility-phase II study aimed at cardiotoxicity. Anticancer Drugs 2009;20:109-14.
162. Venturini M, Bighin C, Monfardini S, et al. Multicenter phase II study of trastuzumab in combination with epirubicin and docetaxel as first-line treatment for HER2-overexpressing metastatic breast cancer. Breast Cancer Res Treat 2006;95:45-53.
163. Dang C, Fornier M, Sugarman S, et al. The safety of dose-dense doxorubicin and cyclophosphamide followed by paclitaxel with trastuzumab in HER-2/neu overexpressed/amplified breast cancer. J Clin Oncol 2008;26: 1216-22.
164. Slamon DJ, Leyland-Jones B, Shak S, et al. Use of chemotherapy plus a monoclonal antibody against HER2 for metastatic breast cancer that overexpresses HER2. N Engl J Med 2001; 344:783-92.
165. Marty M, Cognetti F, Maraninchi D, et al. Randomized phase II trial of the efficacy and safety of trastuzumab combined with docetaxel in patients with human epidermal growth factor receptor 2-positive metastatic breast cancer administered as first-line treatment: The M77001 study group. J Clin Oncol 2005;23: 4265-74.
166. Piccart-Gebhart MJ, Procter M, Leyland-Jones B, et al. Trastuzumab after adjuvant chemotherapy in HER2-positive breast cancer. N Engl J Med 2005;353:1659-72.

167. Romond EH, Perez EA, Bryant J, et al. Trastuzumab plus adjuvant chemotherapy for operable HER2-positive breast cancer. N Engl J Med 2005;353:1673-84.
168. Joensuu H, Kellokumpu-Lehtinen PL, Bono P, et al. Adjuvant docetaxel or vinorelbine with or without trastuzumab for breast cancer. N Engl J Med 2006;354:809-20.
169. Smith I, Procter M, Gelber RD, et al. 2-year follow-up of trastuzumab after adjuvant chemotherapy in HER2-positive breast cancer: A randomised controlled trial. Lancet 2007;369:29-36.
170. Perez EA, Suman VJ, Davidson NE, et al. Cardiac safety analysis of doxorubicin and cyclophosphamide followed by paclitaxel with or without trastuzumab in the North Central Cancer Treatment Group N9831 adjuvant breast cancer trial. J Clin Oncol 2008;26:1231-8.
171. Burstein HJ, Harris LN, Gelman R, et al. Preoperative therapy with trastuzumab and paclitaxel followed by sequential adjuvant doxorubicin/cyclophosphamide for HER2 overexpressing stage II or III breast cancer: A pilot study. J Clin Oncol 2003;21:46-53.
172. Buzdar AU, Ibrahim NK, Francis D, et al. Significantly higher pathologic complete remission rate after neoadjuvant therapy with trastuzumab, paclitaxel, and epirubicin chemotherapy: Results of a randomized trial in human epidermal growth factor receptor 2-positive operable breast cancer. J Clin Oncol 2005;23:3676-85.
173. Buzdar AU, Valero V, Ibrahim NK, et al. Neoadjuvant therapy with paclitaxel followed by 5-fluorouracil, epirubicin, and cyclophosphamide chemotherapy and concurrent trastuzumab in human epidermal growth factor receptor 2-positive operable breast cancer: An update of the initial randomized study population and data of additional patients treated with the same regimen. Clin Cancer Res 2007;13:228-33.
174. Mohsin SK, Weiss HL, Gutierrez MC, et al. Neoadjuvant trastuzumab induces apoptosis in primary breast cancers. J Clin Oncol 2005;23:2460-8.
175. Hurley J, Doliny P, Reis I, et al. Docetaxel, cisplatin, and trastuzumab as primary systemic therapy for human epidermal growth factor receptor 2-positive locally advanced breast cancer. J Clin Oncol 2006;24:1831-8.
176. Coudert BP, Largillier R, Arnould L, et al. Multicenter phase II trial of neoadjuvant therapy with trastuzumab, docetaxel, and carboplatin for human epidermal growth factor receptor-2-overexpressing stage II or III breast cancer: Results of the GETN(A)-1 trial. J Clin Oncol 2007;25:2678-84.
177. Marcom PK, Isaacs C, Harris L, et al. The combination of letrozole and trastuzumab as first or second-line biological therapy produces durable responses in a subset of HER2 positive and ER positive advanced breast cancers. Breast Cancer Res Treat 2007;102:43-9.
178. Bookman MA, Darcy KM, Clarke-Pearson D, et al. Evaluation of monoclonal humanized anti-HER2 antibody, trastuzumab, in patients with recurrent or refractory ovarian or primary peritoneal carcinoma with overexpression of HER2: A phase II trial of the Gynecologic Oncology Group. J Clin Oncol 2003;21:283-90.
179. Clamon G, Herndon J, Kern J, et al. Lack of trastuzumab activity in nonsmall cell lung carcinoma with overexpression of erb-B2: 39810: A phase II trial of Cancer and Leukemia Group B. Cancer 2005;103:1670-5.
180. Lara PN Jr, Laptalo L, Longmate J, et al. Trastuzumab plus docetaxel in HER2/neu-positive non-small-cell lung cancer: A California Cancer Consortium screening and phase II trial. Clin Lung Cancer 2004;5:231-6.
181. Ziada A, Barqawi A, Glode LM, et al. The use of trastuzumab in the treatment of hormone refractory prostate cancer; phase II trial. Prostate 2004;60:332-7.
182. Gatzemeier U, Groth G, Butts C, et al. Randomized phase II trial of gemcitabine-cisplatin with or without trastuzumab in HER2-positive non-small-cell lung cancer. Ann Oncol 2004;15:19-27.
183. Safran H, Iannitti D, Ramanathan R, et al. Herceptin and gemcitabine for metastatic pancreatic cancers that overexpress HER-2/neu. Cancer Invest 2004;22:706-12.
184. Zinner RG, Glisson BS, Fossella FV, et al. Trastuzumab in combination with cisplatin and gemcitabine in patients with Her2-overexpressing, untreated, advanced non-small cell lung cancer: Report of a phase II trial and findings regarding optimal identification of patients with Her2-overexpressing disease. Lung Cancer 2004;44:99-110.
185. Krug LM, Miller VA, Patel J, et al. Randomized phase II study of weekly docetaxel plus trastuzumab versus weekly paclitaxel plus trastuzumab in patients with previously untreated

advanced nonsmall cell lung carcinoma. Cancer 2005;104:2149-55.
186. Hussain MH, MacVicar GR, Petrylak DP, et al. Trastuzumab, paclitaxel, carboplatin, and gemcitabine in advanced human epidermal growth factor receptor-2/neu-positive urothelial carcinoma: Results of a multicenter phase II National Cancer Institute trial. J Clin Oncol 2007; 25:2218-24.
187. Safran H, Diepetrillo T, Akerman P, et al. Phase I/II study of trastuzumab, paclitaxel, cisplatin and radiation for locally advanced, HER2 overexpressing, esophageal adenocarcinoma. Int J Radiat Oncol Biol Phys 2007;67: 405-9.
188. Fleming GF, Meropol NJ, Rosner GL, et al. A phase I trial of escalating doses of trastuzumab combined with daily subcutaneous interleukin 2: Report of Cancer and Leukemia Group B 9661. Clin Cancer Res 2002;8:3718-27.
189. Tripathy D, Seidman A, Keefe D, et al. Effect of cardiac dysfunction on treatment outcomes in women receiving trastuzumab for HER2-overexpressing metastatic breast cancer. Clin Breast Cancer 2004;5:293-8.
190. Telli ML, Hunt SA, Carlson RW, et al. Trastuzumab-related cardiotoxicity: Calling into question the concept of reversibility. J Clin Oncol 2007;25:3525-33.
191. Dillman RO, Shawler DL, Johnson DE, et al. Preclinical trials with combinations and conjugates of T101 and doxorubicin. Cancer Res 1986;46:4886-91.
192. Tan-Chiu E, Yothers G, Romond E, et al. Assessment of cardiac dysfunction in a randomized trial comparing doxorubicin and cyclophosphamide followed by paclitaxel, with or without trastuzumab as adjuvant therapy in node-positive, human epidermal growth factor receptor 2-overexpressing breast cancer: NSABP B-31. J Clin Oncol 2005;23:7811-19.
193. Kelly H, Kimmick G, Dees EC, et al. Response and cardiac toxicity of trastuzumab given in conjunction with weekly paclitaxel after doxorubicin/cyclophosphamide. Clin Breast Cancer 2006;7:237-43.
194. Lee KF, Simon H, Chen H, et al. Requirement for neuregulin receptor erbB2 in neural and cardiac development. Nature 1995;378:394-8.
195. Prewett M, Rolthman M, Walsal H, et al. Mouse-human chimeric anti-epidermal growth factor receptor antibody C225 inhibits the growth of human renal cell carcinoma xenografts in nude mice. Clin Cancer Res 1998;4:2957-66.
196. Cappuzzo F, Finocchiaro G, Rossi E, et al. EGFR FISH assay predicts for response to cetuximab in chemotherapy refractory colorectal cancer patients. Ann Oncol 2008;19:717-23.
197. Italiano A, Follana P, Caroli FX, et al. Cetuximab shows activity in colorectal cancer patients with tumors for which FISH analysis does not detect an increase in EGFR gene copy number. Ann Surg Oncol 2008;15:649-54.
198. Lenz HJ, Van Cutsem E, Khambata-Ford S, et al. Multicenter phase II and translational study of cetuximab in metastatic colorectal carcinoma refractory to irinotecan, oxaliplatin, and fluoropyrimidines. J Clin Oncol 2006;24: 4914-21.
199. Jonker DJ, O'Callaghan CJ, Karapetis et al. Cetuximab for the treatment of colorectal cancer. N Engl J Med 2007;357:2040-8.
200. Cunningham D, Humblet Y, Siena S, et al. Cetuximab monotherapy and cetuximab plus irinotecan in irinotecan-refractory metastatic colorectal cancer. N Engl J Med 2004;351: 337-45.
201. Saltz LB, Meropol NJ, Loehrer PJ Sr, et al. Phase II trial of cetuximab in patients with refractory colorectal cancer that expresses the epidermal growth factor receptor. J Clin Oncol 2004;22:1201-8.
202. Pessino A, Artale S, Sciallero S, et al. First-line single-agent cetuximab in patients with advanced colorectal cancer. Ann Oncol 2008; 19:711-6.
203. Sobrero AF, Maurel J, Fehrenbacher L, et al. EPIC: Phase III trial of cetuximab plus irinotecan after fluoropyrimidine and oxaliplatin failure in patients with metastatic colorectal cancer. J Clin Oncol 2008;26:2311-19.
204. Wilke H, Glynne-Jones R, Thaler J, et al. Cetuximab plus irinotecan in heavily pretreated metastatic colorectal cancer progressing on irinotecan: MABEL Study. J Clin Oncol 2008; 26:5335-43.
205. Gamucci T, Nelli F, Cianci G, et al. A phase II study of cetuximab/irinotecan in patients with heavily pretreated metastatic colorectal cancer: Predictive value of early specific toxicities. Clin Colorectal Cancer 2008;7:273-9.
206. Gebbia V, Del Prete S, Borsellino N, et al. Efficacy and safety of cetuximab/irinotecan in chemotherapy-refractory metastatic colorectal

adenocarcinomas: A clinical practice setting, multicenter experience. Clin Colorectal Cancer 2006;5:422-8.
207. Vincenzi B, Santini D, Rabitti C, et al. Cetuximab and irinotecan as third-line therapy in advanced colorectal cancer patients: A single centre phase II trial. Br J Cancer 2006;94: 792-7.
208. Martín-Martorell P, Roselló S, Rodríguez-Braun E, et al. Biweekly cetuximab and irinotecan in advanced colorectal cancer patients progressing after at least one previous line of chemotherapy: Results of a phase II single institution trial. Br J Cancer 2008;99:455-8.
209. Tahara M, Shirao K, Boku N, et al. Multicenter Phase II study of cetuximab plus irinotecan in metastatic colorectal carcinoma refractory to irinotecan, oxaliplatin and fluoropyrimidines. Jpn J Clin Oncol 2008;38:762-9.
210. Van Cutsem E, Köhne CH, Hitre E, et al. Cetuximab and chemotherapy as initial treatment for metastatic colorectal cancer. N Engl J Med 2009;360:1408-17.
211. Bokemeyer C, Bondarenko I, Makhson A, et al. Fluorouracil, leucovorin, and oxaliplatin with and without cetuximab in the first-line treatment of metastatic colorectal cancer. J Clin Oncol 2009;27:663-71.
212. Tabernero J, Van Cutsem E, Diaz-Rubio E, et al. Phase II trial of cetuximab in combination with fluorouracil, leucovorin, and oxaliplatin in the first-line treatment of metastatic colorectal cancer. J Clin Oncol 2007;25:5225-32.
213. Arnold D, Höhler T, Dittrich C, et al. Cetuximab in combination with weekly 5-fluorouracil/folinic acid and oxaliplatin (FUFOX) in untreated patients with advanced colorectal cancer: A phase Ib/II study of the AIO GI Group. Ann Oncol 2008;19:1442-9.
214. Cartwright T, Kuefler P, Cohn A, et al. Results of a phase II trial of cetuximab plus capecitabine/irinotecan as first-line therapy for patients with advanced and/or metastatic colorectal cancer. Clin Colorectal Cancer 2008;7:390-7.
215. Borner M, Koeberle D, Von Moos R, et al. Adding cetuximab to capecitabine plus oxaliplatin (XELOX) in first-line treatment of metastatic colorectal cancer: A randomized phase II trial of the Swiss Group for Clinical Cancer Research SAKK. Ann Oncol 2008;19:1288-92.
216. Tol J, Koopman M, Cats A, et al. Chemotherapy, bevacizumab, and cetuximab in metastatic colorectal cancer. N Engl J Med 2009;360: 563-72.
217. Machiels JP, Sempoux C, Scalliet P, et al. Phase I/II study of preoperative cetuximab, capecitabine, and external beam radiotherapy in patients with rectal cancer. Ann Oncol 2007; 18:738-44.
218. Hofheinz RD, Horisberger K, Woernle C, et al. Phase I trial of cetuximab in combination with capecitabine, weekly irinotecan, and radiotherapy as neoadjuvant therapy for rectal cancer. Int J Radiat Oncol Biol Phys 2006;66:1384-90.
219. Bertolini F, Chiara S, Bengala C, et al. Neoadjuvant treatment with single-agent cetuximab followed by 5-FU, cetuximab, and pelvic radiotherapy: A phase II study in locally advanced rectal cancer. Int J Radiat Oncol Biol Phys 2009;73:466-72.
220. Rödel C, Arnold D, Hipp M, et al. Phase I-II trial of cetuximab, capecitabine, oxaliplatin, and radiotherapy as preoperative treatment in rectal cancer. Int J Radiat Oncol Biol Phys 2008;70:1081-6.
221. Vermorken JB, Trigo J, Hitt R, et al. Open-label, uncontrolled, multicenter phase II study to evaluate the efficacy and toxicity of cetuximab as a single agent in patients with recurrent and/or metastatic squamous cell carcinoma of the head and neck who failed to respond to platinum-based therapy. J Clin Oncol 2007;25: 2171-7.
222. Herbst RS, Arquette M, Shin DM, et al. Phase II multicenter study of the epidermal growth factor receptor antibody cetuximab and cisplatin for recurrent and refractory squamous cell carcinoma of the head and neck. J Clin Oncol 2005;23:5578-87.
223. Baselga J, Trigo JM, Bourhis J, et al. Phase II multicenter study of the antiepidermal growth factor receptor monoclonal antibody cetuximab in combination with platinum-based chemotherapy in patients with platinum-refractory metastatic and/or recurrent squamous cell carcinoma of the head and neck. J Clin Oncol 2005;23:5568-77.
224. Pfister DG, Su YB, Kraus DH, et al. Concurrent cetuximab, cisplatin, and concomitant boost radiotherapy for locoregionally advanced, squamous cell head and neck cancer: A pilot phase II study of a new combined-modality paradigm. J Clin Oncol 2006;24:1072-8.
225. Bourhis J, Rivera F, Mesia R, et al. Phase I/II study of cetuximab in combination with cispl-

atin or carboplatin and fluorouracil in patients with recurrent or metastatic squamous cell carcinoma of the head and neck. J Clin Oncol 2006;24:2866-72.
226. Chan AT, Hsu MM, Goh BC, et al. Multicenter, phase II study of cetuximab in combination with carboplatin in patients with recurrent or metastatic nasopharyngeal carcinoma. J Clin Oncol 2005;23:3568-76.
227. Robert F, Ezekiel MP, Spencer SA, et al. Phase I study of anti-epidermal growth factor receptor antibody cetuximab in combination with radiation therapy in patients with advanced head and neck cancer. J Clin Oncol 2001;19: 3234-43.
228. Bonner JA, Harari PM, Giralt J, et al. Radiotherapy plus cetuximab for squamous-cell carcinoma of the head and neck. N Engl J Med 2006;354:567-78.
229. Burtness B, Goldwasser MA, Flood W, et al. Phase III randomized trial of cisplatin plus placebo compared with cisplatin plus cetuximab in metastatic/recurrent head and neck cancer: An Eastern Cooperative Oncology Group study. J Clin Oncol 2005;23:8646-54.
230. Vermorken JB, Mesia R, Rivera F, et al. Platinum-based chemotherapy plus cetuximab in head and neck cancer. N Engl J Med 2008; 359:1116-27.
231. Hanna N, Lilenbaum R, Ansari R, et al. Phase II trial of cetuximab in patients with previously treated non-small-cell lung cancer. J Clin Oncol 2006;24:5253-8.
232. Borghaei H, Langer CJ, Millenson M, et al. Phase II study of paclitaxel, carboplatin, and cetuximab as first line treatment, for patients with advanced non-small cell lung cancer (NSCLC): Results of OPN-017. J Thorac Oncol 2008;3:1286-92.
233. Thienelt CD, Bunn PA Jr, Hanna N, et al. Multicenter phase I/II study of cetuximab with paclitaxel and carboplatin in untreated patients with stage IV non-small-cell lung cancer. J Clin Oncol 2005;23:8786-93.
234. Belani CP, Schreeder MT, Steis RG, et al. Cetuximab in combination with carboplatin and docetaxel for patients with metastatic or advanced-stage non small cell lung cancer: A multicenter phase 2 study. Cancer 2008;113: 2512-17.
235. Robert F, Blumenschein G, Herbst RS, et al. Phase I/IIa study of cetuximab with gemcitabine plus carboplatin in patients with chemotherapy-naive advanced non-small-cell lung cancer. J Clin Oncol 2005;23:9089-96.
236. Pirker R, Pereira JR, Szczesna A, et al. Cetuximab plus chemotherapy in patients with advanced non-small-cell lung cancer (FLEX): An open-label randomised phase III trial. Lancet 2009;373:1525-31.
237. Rosell R, Robinet G, Szczesna A, et al. Randomized phase II study of cetuximab plus cisplatin/vinorelbine compared with cisplatin/vinorelbine alone as first-line therapy in EGFR-expressing advanced non-small-cell lung cancer. Ann Oncol 2008;19:362-9.
238. Han SW, Oh DY, Im SA, et al. Phase II study and biomarker analysis of cetuximab combined with modified FOLFOX6 in advanced gastric cancer. Br J Cancer 2009;100:298-304.
239. Pinto C, Di Fabio F, Siena S, et al. Phase II study of cetuximab in combination with FOLFIRI in patients with untreated advanced gastric or gastroesophageal junction adenocarcinoma (FOLCETUX study). Ann Oncol 2007; 18:510-7.
240. Asnacios A, Fartoux L, Romano O, et al. Gemcitabine plus oxaliplatin (GEMOX) combined with cetuximab in patients with progressive advanced stage hepatocellular carcinoma: Results of a multicenter phase 2 study. Cancer 2008;112:2733-9.
241. Xiong HQ, Rosenberg A, LoBuglio A, et al. Cetuximab, a monoclonal antibody targeting the epidermal growth factor receptor, in combination with gemcitabine for advanced pancreatic cancer: A multicenter phase II Trial. J Clin Oncol 2004;22:2610-6.
242. Kullmann F, Hollerbach S, Dollinger MM, et al. Cetuximab plus gemcitabine/oxaliplatin (GEMOXCET) in first-line metastatic pancreatic cancer: A multicentre phase II study. Br J Cancer 2009;100:1032-6.
243. Philip PA, Benedetti J, Fenoglio-Preiser C, et al. Phase III study of gemcitabine plus cetuximab versus gemcitabine in patients with locally advanced or metastatic pancreatic adenocarcinoma (abstract). Proc Am Soc Clin Oncol 2007;25:199s.
244. Cascinu S, Berardi R, Labianca R, et al. Cetuximab plus gemcitabine and cisplatin compared with gemcitabine and cisplatin alone in patients with advanced pancreatic cancer: A randomised, multicentre, phase II trial. Lancet Oncol 2008;9:39-44.

245. Secord AA, Blessing JA, Armstrong DK, et al. Phase II trial of cetuximab and carboplatin in relapsed platinum-sensitive ovarian cancer and evaluation of epidermal growth factor receptor expression: A Gynecologic Oncology Group study. Gynecol Oncol 2008;108:493-9.
246. Konner J, Schilder RJ, DeRosa FA, et al. A phase II study of cetuximab, paclitaxel, carboplatin for the initial treatment of advanced-stage ovarian, primary peritoneal, or fallopian tube cancer. Gynecol Oncol 2008;110:140-5.
247. Kurtz JE, Hardy-Bessard AC, Deslandres M, et al. Cetuximab, topotecan and cisplatin for the treatment of advanced cervical cancer: A phase II GINECO trial. Gynecol Oncol 2009; 113:16-20.
248. Motzer RJ, Amato R, Todd M, et al. Phase II trial of antiepidermal growth factor receptor antibody C225 in patients with advanced renal cell carcinoma. Invest New Drugs 2003;21: 99-101.
249. Tan AR, Moore DF, Hidalgo M, et al. Pharmacokinetics of cetuximab after administration of escalating single dosing and weekly fixed dosing in patients with solid tumors. Clin Cancer Res 2006;12:6517-22.
250. Fracasso PM, Burris H 3rd, Arquette MA, et al. A phase 1 escalating single-dose and weekly fixed-dose study of cetuximab: Pharmacokinetic and pharmacodynamic rationale for dosing. Clin Cancer Res 2007;13:986-93.
251. Delbaldo C, Pierga JY, Dieras V, et al. Pharmacokinetic profile of cetuximab (Erbitux) alone and in combination with irinotecan in patients with advanced EGFR-positive adenocarcinoma. Eur J Cancer 2005;41:1739-45.
252. Ettlinger DE, Mitterhauser M, Wadsak W, et al. In vivo disposition of irinotecan (CPT-11) and its metabolites in combination with the monoclonal antibody cetuximab. Anticancer Res 2006;26:1337-41.
253. Hebbar M, Wacrenier A, Desauw C, et al. Lack of usefulness of epidermal growth factor receptor expression determination for cetuximab therapy in patients with colorectal cancer. Anticancer Drugs 2006;17:855-7.
254. Moroni M, Veronese S, Benvenuti S, et al. Gene copy number for epidermal growth factor receptor (EGFR) and clinical response to anti-EGFR treatment in colorectal cancer: A cohort study. Lancet Oncol 2005;6:279-86.
255. Lenz G, Dreyling M, Hoster E, et al. Immunochemotherapy with rituximab and cyclophosphamide, doxorubicin, vincristine, and prednisone significantly improves response and time to treatment failure, but not long-term outcome in patients with previously untreated mantle cell lymphoma: Results of a prospective randomized trial of the German Low Grade Lymphoma Study Group (GLSG). J Clin Oncol 2005;23:1984-92.
256. Zhang W, Gordon M, Press OA, et al. Cyclin D1 and epidermal growth factor polymorphisms associated with survival in patients with advanced colorectal cancer treated with cetuximab. Pharmacogenet Genomics 2006;16: 475-83.
257. Karapetis CS, Khambata-Ford S, Jonker DJ, et al. K-ras mutations and benefit from cetuximab in advanced colorectal cancer. N Engl J Med 2008;359:1757-65.
258. Lièvre A, Bachet JB, Boige V, et al. KRAS mutations as an independent prognostic factor in patients with advanced colorectal cancer treated with cetuximab. J Clin Oncol 2008; 26:374-9.
259. Di Nicolantonio F, Martini M, Molinari F, et al. Wild-type BRAF is required for response to panitumumab or cetuximab in metastatic colorectal cancer. J Clin Oncol 2008;26:5705-12.
260. Bibeau F, Lopez-Crapez E, Di Fiore F, et al. Impact of Fc{gamma}RIIa-Fc{gamma}RIIIa polymorphisms and KRAS mutations on the clinical outcome of patients with metastatic colorectal cancer treated with cetuximab plus irinotecan. J Clin Oncol 2009;27:1122-9.
261. Busam KJ, Capodieci P, Motzer R, et al. Cutaneous side-effects in cancer patients treated with the antiepidermal growth factor receptor antibody C225. Br J Dermatol 2001;144: 1169-76.
262. Jatoi A, Rowland K, Sloan JA, et al. Tetracycline to prevent epidermal growth factor receptor inhibitor-induced skin rashes: Results of a placebo-controlled trial from the North Central Cancer Treatment Group (N03CB). Cancer 2008;113:847-53.
263. Chua YJ, Cunningham D. Panitumumab. Drugs Today 2006;42:711-19.
264. Cohenuram M, Saif MW. Panitumumab the first fully human monoclonal antibody: From the bench to the clinic. Anticancer Drugs 2007;18:7-15.
265. Gibson TB, Ranganathan A, Grothey A. Randomized phase III trial results of panitumumab, a fully human anti-epidermal growth factor receptor monoclonal antibody, in meta-

static colorectal cancer. Clin Colorectal Cancer 2006;6:29-31.
266. Giusti RM, Shastri KA, Cohen MH, et al. FDA drug approval summary: Panitumumab (Vectibix). Oncologist 2007;12:577-83.
267. Van Cutsem E, Peeters M, Siena S, et al. Open-label phase III trial of panitumumab plus best supportive care compared with best supportive care alone in patients with chemotherapy-refractory metastatic colorectal cancer. J Clin Oncol 2007;25:1658-64.
268. Van Cutsem E, Siena S, Humblet Y, et al. An open-label, single-arm study assessing safety and efficacy of panitumumab in patients with metastatic colorectal cancer refractory to standard chemotherapy. Ann Oncol 2008;19:92-8.
269. Siena S, Peeters M, Van Cutsem E, et al. Association of progression-free survival with patient-reported outcomes and survival: Results from a randomised phase 3 trial of panitumumab. Br J Cancer 2007;97:1469-74.
270. Hecht JR, Patnaik A, Berlin J, et al. Panitumumab monotherapy in patients with previously treated metastatic colorectal cancer. Cancer 2007;110:980-8.
271. Muro K, Yoshino T, Doi T, et al. A phase 2 clinical trial of panitumumab monotherapy in Japanese patients with metastatic colorectal cancer. Jpn J Clin Oncol 2009;39:321-6.
272. Weiner LM, Belldegrun AS, Crawford J, et al. Dose and schedule study of panitumumab monotherapy in patients with advanced solid malignancies. Clin Cancer Res 2008;14:502-8.
273. Stephenson JJ, Gregory C, Burris H, et al. An open-label clinical trial evaluating safety and pharmacokinetics of two dosing schedules of panitumumab in patients with solid tumors. Clin Colorectal Cancer 2009;8:29-37.
274. Hecht JR, Mitchell E, Chidiac T, et al. A randomized phase IIIB trial of chemotherapy, bevacizumab, and panitumumab compared with chemotherapy and bevacizumab alone for metastatic colorectal cancer. J Clin Oncol 2009;27:672-80.
275. Berlin J, Posey J, Tchekmedyian S, et al. Panitumumab with irinotecan/leucovorin/5-fluorouracil for first-line treatment of metastatic colorectal cancer. Clin Colorectal Cancer 2007;6:427-32.
276. Lofgren JA, Dhandapani S, Pennucci JJ, et al. Comparing ELISA and surface plasmon resonance for assessing clinical immunogenicity of panitumumab. J Immunol 2007;178:7467-72.
277. Huen J, Holen K. Treatment with panitumumab after a severe infusion reaction to cetuximab in a patient with metastatic colorectal cancer: A case report. Clin Colorectal Cancer 2007;6:529-31.
278. Presta LG, Chen H, O'Connor SJ, et al. Humanization of an anti-vascular endotherlial growth factor monoclonal antibody for the therapy of solid tumors and other disorders. Cancer Res 1997;57:4593-9.
279. Gordon MS, Margolin K, Talpaz M, et al. Phase I safety and pharmacokinetic study of recombinant human anti-vascular endothelial growth factor in patients with advanced cancer. J Clin Oncol 2001;19:843-50.
280. Margolin K, Gordon MS, Holmgren E, et al. Phase Ib trial of intravenous recombinant humanized monoclonal antibody to vascular endothelial growth factor in combination with chemotherapy in patients with advanced cancer: Pharmacologic and long-term safety data. J Clin Oncol 2001;19:851-6.
281. Chen HX, Mooney M, Boron M, et al. Phase II multicenter trial of bevacizumab plus fluorouracil and leucovorin in patients with advanced refractory colorectal cancer: An NCI Treatment Referral Center Trial TRC-0301. J Clin Oncol 2006;24:3354-60.
282. Giantonio BJ, Levy DE, O'dwyer PJ, et al. A phase II study of high-dose bevacizumab in combination with irinotecan, 5-fluorouracil, leucovorin, as initial therapy for advanced colorectal cancer: Results from the Eastern Cooperative Oncology Group study E2200. Ann Oncol 2006;17:1399-403.
283. Emmanouilides C, Sfakiotaki G, Androulakis N, et al. Front-line bevacizumab in combination with oxaliplatin, leucovorin and 5-fluorouracil (FOLFOX) in patients with metastatic colorectal cancer: A multicenter phase II study. BMC Cancer 2007;7:91.
284. Kabbinavar F, Hurwitz HI, Fehrenbacher L, et al. Phase II, randomized trial comparing bevacizumab plus fluorouracil (FU)/leucovorin (LV) with FU/LV alone in patients with metastatic colorectal cancer. J Clin Oncol 2003;21:60-5.
285. Kabbinavar FF, Schulz J, McCleod M, et al. Addition of bevacizumab to bolus fluorouracil and leucovorin in first-line metastatic colorectal cancer: Results of a randomized phase II trial. J Clin Oncol 2005;23:3697-705.

286. Hurwitz H, Fehrenbacher L, Novotny W, et al. Bevacizumab plus irinotecan, fluorouracil, and leucovorin for metastatic colorectal cancer. N Engl J Med 2004;350:2335-42.
287. Hurwitz HI, Fehrenbacher L, Hainsworth JD, et al. Bevacizumab in combination with fluorouracil and leucovorin: An active regimen for first-line metastatic colorectal cancer. J Clin Oncol 2005;23:3502-8.
288. Kabbinavar FF, Hambleton J, Mass RD, et al. Combined analysis of efficacy: The addition of bevacizumab to fluorouracil/leucovorin improves survival for patients with metastatic colorectal cancer. J Clin Oncol 2005;23:3706-12.
289. Kabbinavar FF, Hurwitz HI, Yi J, et al. Addition of bevacizumab to fluorouracil-based first-line treatment of metastatic colorectal cancer: Pooled analysis of cohorts of older patients from two randomized clinical trials. J Clin Oncol 2009;27:199-205.
290. Giantonio BJ, Catalano PJ, Meropol NJ, et al. Bevacizumab in combination with oxaliplatin, fluorouracil, and leucovorin (FOLFOX4) for previously treated metastatic colorectal cancer: Results from the Eastern Cooperative Oncology Group Study E3200. J Clin Oncol 2007; 25:1539-44.
291. Saltz LB, Clarke S, Díaz-Rubio E, et al. Bevacizumab in combination with oxaliplatin-based chemotherapy as first-line therapy in metastatic colorectal cancer: A randomized phase III study. J Clin Oncol 2008;26:2013-9.
292. Hochster HS, Hart LL, Ramanathan RK, et al. Safety and efficacy of oxaliplatin and fluoropyrimidine regimens with or without bevacizumab as first-line treatment of metastatic colorectal cancer: Results of the TREE Study. J Clin Oncol 2008;26:3523-9.
293. Moehler M, Sprinzl MF, Abdelfattah M, et al. Capecitabine and irinotecan with and without bevacizumab for advanced colorectal cancer patients. World J Gastroenterol 2009;15:449-56.
294. Gruenberger B, Tamandl D, Schueller J, et al. Bevacizumab, capecitabine, and oxaliplatin as neoadjuvant therapy for patients with potentially curable metastatic colorectal cancer. J Clin Oncol 2008;26:1830-5.
295. Grothey A, Sugrue MM, Purdie DM, et al. Bevacizumab beyond first progression is associated with prolonged overall survival in metastatic colorectal cancer: Results from a large observational cohort study (BRiTE). J Clin Oncol 2008;26:5326-34.
296. Johnson DH, Fehrenbacher L, Novotny WF, et al. Randomized phase II trial comparing bevacizumab plus carboplatin and paclitaxel with carboplatin and paclitaxel alone in previously untreated locally advanced or metastatic non-small-cell lung cancer. J Clin Oncol 2004;22: 2184-91.
297. Sandler A, Gray R, Perry MC, et al. Paclitaxel-carboplatin alone or with bevacizumab for non-small-cell lung cancer. N Engl J Med 2006;355:2542-50.
298. Sandler AB, Schiller JH, Gray R, et al. Retrospective evaluation of the clinical and radiographic risk factors associated with severe pulmonary hemorrhage in first-line advanced, unresectable non-small-cell lung cancer treated with carboplatin and paclitaxel plus bevacizumab. J Clin Oncol 2009;27:1405-12.
299. Reck M, von Pawel J, Zatloukal P, et al. Phase III trial of cisplatin plus gemcitabine with either placebo or bevacizumab as first-line therapy for nonsquamous non-small-cell lung cancer: AVAil. J Clin Oncol 2009;27:1227-34.
300. Herbst RS, Johnson DH, Mininberg E, et al. Phase I/II trial evaluating the anti-vascular endothelial growth factor monoclonal antibody bevacizumab in combination with the HER-1/epidermal growth factor receptor tyrosine kinase inhibitor erlotinib for patients with recurrent non-small-cell lung cancer. J Clin Oncol 2005;23:2544-55.
301. Heist RS, Fidias P, Huberman M, et al. A phase II study of oxaliplatin, pemetrexed, and bevacizumab in previously treated advanced non-small cell lung cancer. J Thorac Oncol 2008;3: 1153-8.
302. Lilenbaum R, Raez L, Tseng J, et al. Efficacy and safety of oxaliplatin and gemcitabine with bevacizumab in advanced non-small cell lung cancer. J Thorac Oncol 2008;3:511-5.
303. Miller KD, Chap LI, Holmes FA, et al. Randomized phase III trial of capecitabine compared with bevacizumab plus capecitabine in patients with previously treated metastatic breast cancer. J Clin Oncol 2005;23:792-9.
304. Miller K, Wang M, Gralow J, et al. Paclitaxel plus bavacizumab versus paclitaxel alone for metastatic breast cancer. N Engl J Med 2007; 357:2666-76.
305. Schneider BP, Wang M, Radovich M, et al. Association of vascular endothelial growth factor and vascular endothelial growth factor receptor-2 genetic polymorphisms with outcome in a trial of paclitaxel compared with

327. Siegel AB, Cohen EI, Ocean A, et al. Phase II trial evaluating the clinical and biologic effects of bevacizumab in unresectable hepatocellular carcinoma. J Clin Oncol 2008;26:2992-8.
328. Burger RA, Sill MW, Monk BJ, et al. Phase II trial of bevacizumab in persistent or recurrent epithelial ovarian cancer or primary peritoneal cancer: A Gynecologic Oncology Group study. J Clin Oncol 2007;25:5165-71.
329. Cannistra SA, Matulonis UA, Penson RT, et al. Phase II study of bevacizumab in patients with platinum-resistant ovarian cancer or peritoneal serous cancer. J Clin Oncol 2007;25: 5180-6.
330. Nimeiri HS, Oza AM, Morgan RJ, et al. Efficacy and safety of bevacizumab plus erlotinib for patients with recurrent ovarian, primary peritoneal, and fallopian tube cancer: A trial of the Chicago, PMH, and California Phase II Consortia. Gynecol Oncol 2008;110:49-55.
331. Han ES, Monk BJ. What is the risk of bowel perforation associated with bevacizumab therapy in ovarian cancer? Gynecol Oncol 2007; 105:3-6.
332. Monk BJ, Sill MW, Burger RA, et al. Phase II trial of bevacizumab in the treatment of persistent or recurrent squamous cell carcinoma of the cervix: A Gynecologic Oncology Group study. J Clin Oncol 2009;27:1069-74.
333. D'Adamo DR, Anderson SE, Albritton K, et al. Phase II study of doxorubicin and bevacizumab for patients with metastatic soft-tissue sarcomas. J Clin Oncol 2005;23:7135-42.
334. González-Cao M, Viteri S, Díaz-Lagares A, et al. Preliminary results of the combination of bevacizumab and weekly paclitaxel in advanced melanoma. Oncology 2008;74:12-16.
335. Perez DG, Suman VJ, Fitch TR, et al. Phase 2 trial of carboplatin, weekly paclitaxel, and biweekly bevacizumab in patients with unresectable stage IV melanoma: A North Central Cancer Treatment Group study, N047A. Cancer 2009;115:119-27.
336. Cohen EE, Davis DW, Karrison TG, et al. Erlotinib and bevacizumab in patients with recurrent or metastatic squamous-cell carcinoma of the head and neck: A phase I/II study. Lancet Oncol 2009;10:247-57.
337. Di Lorenzo G, Figg WD, Fossa SD, et al. Combination of bevacizumab and docetaxel in docetaxel-pretreated hormone-refractory prostate cancer: A phase 2 study. Eur Urol 2008;54: 1089-94.
338. Rini BI, Weinberg V, Fong L, et al. Combination immunotherapy with prostatic acid phosphatase pulsed antigen-presenting cells (Provenge) plus bevacizumab in patients with serologic progression of prostate cancer after definitive local therapy. Cancer 2006;107:67-74.
339. Willett CG, Boucher Y, di Tomaso E, et al. Direct evidence that the VEGF-specific antibody bevacizumab has antivascular effects in human rectal cancer. Nat Med 2004;10:145-7.
340. Wedam SB, Low JA, Yang SX, et al. Antiangiogenic and antitumor effects of bevacizumab in patients with inflammatory and locally advanced breast cancer. J Clin Oncol 2006;24:769-77.
341. Jubb AM, Hurwitz HI, Bai W, et al. Impact of vascular endothelial growth factor-A expression, thrombospondin-2 expression, and microvessel density on the treatment effect of bevacizumab in metastatic colorectal cancer. J Clin Oncol 2006;24:217-27.

Index

Page numbers in italics refer to tables or figures

A

Abortion
    anti-D in, 178
    IVIG in, 47, 48, 53, *114,* 128
ABX-EGF. *See* Panitumumab
Acneiform rash, 233-235, 238
Acute myeloid leukemia, 200-201
ADAMTS13, 194-195
Adhesion molecules, 50, 56, 81-82
Adverse effects
    of anti-D, 182-183
    of IVIG, 14, 18, 74, 79, 93-95
    of monoclonal antibodies, 222-223
        alemtuzumab, 197-198
        bevacizumab, 250-251
        cetuximab, 238-239
        eculizumab, 199
        gemtuzumab ozogamicin, 201, 204
        ibritumomab tiuxetan, 205-206
        panitumumab, 240-242
        rituximab, 195-196
        tositumomab, 207
        trastuzumab, 226, 230-231
Affinity chromatography, 25-26
Agammaglobulinemia, 3, 14
Albumin, 14
Alemtuzumab, 196-198
Allergic reactions, 222-223, 239
Allergies, use of IVIG in, 47
Alloimmunization to D antigen, 141-142
    after transfusion of D+ blood components, 180-181
    antenatal prophylaxis, 178-180
    postnatal prophylaxis, 177-178
Alzheimer disease, 35, 55, 92, *114,* 128-129
Amniocentesis, 180
Amyotrophic lateral sclerosis, 87
Anal cancer, 240
Anaphylactic/anaphylactoid reactions
    to IVIG, 74, 94
    to monoclonal antibodies, 222-223, 239
ANCA-associated systemic necrotizing vasculitides, *10, 114,* 116-117
Anemia, autoimmune hemolytic, 51
Anti-B1. *See* Tositumomab
Anti-D immunoglobulin
    animal model studies of, 142-143, 161
    clinical indications for, *176*
        after transfusion of D+ blood products, 180-181
        antenatal prophylaxis, 178-180
        immune thrombocytopenia, 9-10, 35, 69, 159-168, 181-183
        postnatal immune prophylaxis, 177-178
    dosage of, 142, 177-179
    historical overview of, 140-141, 175
    human studies of, 142
    infectious risk of, 176
    intramuscular vs intravenous administration, 177
    mechanisms of
        antigen clearance, 146-147
        B-cell inhibition, 147-150
        cytokines in, 161, 163-164, *165*
        epitope masking, 148-149
        idiotypic antibodies in, 165-166
        overview of, 145-146
        reticuloendothelial system blockade, 161, *162*
        signaling mechanism alterations, 166
        T cells in, 147, 149-150
    monoclonal, 141, 143-144, 167
    pharmacology of, 176-177
    production of, 160, 176
    recombinant, 141, 143-144, 167-168
    and weak D/partial D phenotype, 178
Antibodies. *See also* Monoclonal antibodies
    GM1, 83
    human anti-chimeric, 196, 220
    human anti-human, 220
    human mouse, 187, 207, 220

idiotypic, 47-48, 80-81, 165-166
in IVIG, 55
MAG, 87-88
recombinant polyclonal, 167-168
to sphingoglycolipids, 87-88
in virus inactivation of IVIG, 32
Antibody-enhanced nanofiltration, 31
Antibody-mediated immune suppression, 144-145
  defined, 139-140, 144
  mechanisms of, 145-150
    antigen clearance, 146-147
    B-cell inhibition, 148-150
    epitope masking, 149
    T cells in, 147, 149-150
Antigen clearance mechanism, 145-147
Antineutrophil cytoplasmic autoantibody vasculitis, 10, *114*, 116-117
Antiphospholipid antibody syndrome, 47, *114*, 117
Apoptosis, 48-49
Argentine hemorrhagic fever, 108
Arthritis, rheumatoid
  IVIG in, 35, 50, 52, 53, *114*, 116
  rituximab in, 190, 195
Aseptic meningitis, 94
Asthma, 55, *114*, 127-128
Atherosclerosis, 51
Atopic dermatitis, *114*, 119-120
Autoimmune blistering disorders, *114*, 117-119
Autoimmune congenital heart block, 116
Autoimmune diabetes mellitus, *114*, 126-127
Autoimmune disorders, 10, 47, 190. *See also* specific disorders
Autoimmune Graves ophthalmopathy, *114*, 126
Autoimmune hemolytic anemia, 51, 73, 194
Autoimmune liver disease, *114*, 127
Autoimmune neutropenia, 51, 72-73
Autoimmune uveitis, *114*, 126

B

B-cell acute lymphoblastic leukemia, 193
B-cell chronic lymphocytic leukemia, 192, 196-197
B-cell depletion, 189-190, 207
B-cell inhibition, 145, 147-150
B-raf mutations, 238
Bacterial sepsis, 51, 55, 102, 104-105
Beta-amyloid protein, 55
$Beta_2$-microglobulin, 51, 52
Bevacizumab, *224*, 242-251
  antitumor mechanisms of, 250
  clinical trials in
    breast cancer, 245-246
    colorectal cancer, 241, 243-244
    exploratory, 242-243

gynecologic malignancies, 248-249
head and neck cancers, 249
malignant gliomas, 246-247
melanoma, 249
non-small-cell lung cancer, 244-245
noncolorectal gastrointestinal malignancies, 247-248, 250-251
prostate cancer, 249-250
renal cell cancer, 246
sarcomas, 249
  toxicities and adverse events with, 250-251
  and vascular endothelial growth factor, 242, 250
Birdshot retinochoroidopathy, 126
Bladder cancer, 241
Bleeding toxicity, 242, 244-245
Blistering disorders, autoimmune, 117-119
Bovine spongiform encephalopathy, 29, 33
Bowel perforation, 249-251
Brain damage, ischemic, 51
Breast cancer clinical trials
  adjuvant treatments, 228-229
  bevacizumab in, 242, 245-246
  chemotherapy with or without trastuzumab, 228
  neoadjuvant treatments, 229
  trastuzumab alone, 225-226
  trastuzumab and hormonal therapy, 229-230
  trastuzumab plus combination chemotherapy, 227-228
Bronchospasm, 223
Bullous pemphigoid, 118
Burn patients, 102, *103*

C

C-type lectin domain family 10, member A, 86
Campylobacter jejuni infection, 83
Cardiac disorders
  IVIG in, 124-125
  and trastuzumab, 227-231
Cardiac transplantation, *114*, 122
Cardiomyopathy, dilated, *114*, 125
"Cascade" technology, 27
Cerebellar degeneration, 127
Cervical cancer, 237, 249
Cetuximab, *224*, 232-239
  antitumor mechanisms of, 237-238
  clinical trials in, 235-237
  and epidermal growth factor receptor, 232-233
  toxicity to, 234-236, 238-239
Chemotherapy
  and alemtuzumab, 197
  and bevacizumab, 242-250
  and cetuximab, 232-237

and gemtuzumab ozogamicin, 201, *202-203*
and ibritumomab tiuxetan, 205
and panitumumab, 240-241
and rituximab, 190-193
and trastuzumab, 226-228
Children
 chronic inflammatory demyelinating polyneuropathy in, 86-87
 Guillain-Barré syndrome in, 84
 immune thrombocytopenia in, 68-72
 juvenile dermatomyositis in, 116
 Kawasaki disease in, 93, 124-125
 neonatal alloimmune neutropenia in, 73
 neonatal hemachromatosis in, 125-126
 preventing infection in, 102
 rheumatoid arthritis in, 116
 sepsis in, 102, 104-105
 systemic lupus erythematosus in, 116
Chills, 74, 93
Chimeric antibodies, 187-188, 218
Chorionic villus sampling, 180
Chromatographic methods, 15, 22-27
 affinity chromatography, 25-26
 base matrices in, 23-24
 ion exchange media in, 24-25
 membrane chromatography, 27
 multimodal chromatography, 26-27
Chronic fatigue syndrome, *114,* 128
Chronic inflammatory demyelinating polyneuropathy, 84-87
 and diabetes, 85
 IVIG in, 79, 84-87
  in children, 86-87
  cost of therapy, 86
  FDA approval of, 79, 85
  maintenance therapy, 85
  mechanism of, 50, 51, 81
  predictors of response to, 86
  starting therapy, 86
 plasmapheresis in treatment of, 84, 86
 steroids in treatment of, 84-86
 variants of, 85
Chronic lymphocytic leukemia, 192, 196-197
Churg-Strauss syndrome, 49
Cicatricial pemphigoid, 118-119
CIDP. *See* Chronic inflammatory demyelinating polyneuropathy
Clinical trials
 with alemtuzumab, 197
 with anti-D, 69, 140, 142, 168, 181
 with bevacizumab, 242-250
 with cetuximab, 233-237
 with eculizumab, 199
 with gemtuzumab ozogamicin, 201, *202-203*

with ibritumomab tiuxetan, 205
with IVIG, 11, 20
 in cardiac disorders, 124-125
 in dermatologic disorders, 117-120
 in infection and inflammatory response syndromes, 102, *103-104,* 104-108
 in manufacturing process, 35
 in miscellaneous disorders, 125-129
 in neuromuscular disorders, 82-93
 in rheumatic diseases, 115-117
 in solid organ transplantation, 120-123
with panitumumab, 240-241
with rituximab, 190-195
with tositumomab, 206-206
with trastuzumab, 225-230
Clostridium difficile-associated disease, 106
Cohn ethanol fractionation, 22, *23*
 history of, 1, 13-14
 virus removal and inactivation in, 16, 32
Cold agglutinin syndrome, 194
Colorectal cancer
 bevacizumab in, 241-244
 cetuximab in, 233-235
 panitumumab in, 240-241
Combined variable immune deficiency, 72, 73
Complement
 activation of, by IgG aggregates, 1-2, 14
 inhibition of, by IVIG, 50-51, 81
 interaction with antibodies, 221
Congestive heart failure, 227, 230-231
Cordocentesis, 180
Corticosteroids
 in CIDP, 84-86
 in dermatomyositis, 91
 in Guillain-Barré syndrome, 83
 in ITP, 6-7, *8*
Creutzfeldt-Jakob disease, 15, 33, 34, 176
Critically ill patients, 102, *103-104*
CSF-1, 52
Cystic fibrosis, *114,* 128
Cytokines
 in anti-D mechanism, 145-146, 161, 163-164, *165*
 and dendritic cells, 52, 53
 in IVIG mechanism, 49-50, 52-53, 81-82, 163
Cytomegalovirus, 198
Cytomegalovirus immune globulin, 122, 123

D

D antigen
 alloimmunization to, 141-142
  after transfusion of D+ blood components, 180-181

    with antenatal prophylaxis, 178-180
    with postnatal immune prophylaxis, 177-178
  fetal, 180
  weak and/or partial, 178
Demyelinating polyneuropathies, 87-88
Dendritic cells
  and cytokines, 53
  interactions with natural killer cells, 53
  in mechanism of IVIG, 46-48, 52-54
  and T-regulatory cells, 54
Dengue fever, 107
Dermatitis, atopic, *114,* 119-120
Dermatologic disorders, *114,* 117-120. *See also* specific disorders
Dermatologic reactions
  to cetuximab, 233-235, 238-239
  to IVIG, 94
  to panitumumab, 241, 242
Dermatomyositis, 115-116
    IVIG in treatment of, *10,* 79, 90-91, *115*
    IVIG mechanism in, 50, 51, 81, 82
    juvenile, 116
    steroids in treatment of, 91
Deutsch fractionation scheme, *24*
Diabetes
  and CIDP, 85
  IVIG in, 46, 53, *114,* 126
Diffuse intravascular coagulation, 182
Diffuse large B-cell lymphoma, 192, 193
Diphtheria, 107
Donors, plasma
  "qualified," 30
  selection of, 16, 28-29
  testing, 16, 29-30
Dosage
  of anti-D immunoglobulin, 142, 177-179
  of IVIG
    in Guillain-Barré syndrome, 83
    in ITP, 6, 69-70
    in Kawasaki disease, 93
    in neurologic disorders, 93
    studies for, 10-11
  of monoclonal antibodies, 222, 223, 225

E

Eculizumab, 198-199
Eczema, 119-120
EGFR. *See* Epidermal growth factor receptors
Electrolytes, precipitation by, 21
Embolism, pulmonary, 93
Encephalitis, limbic, 127
Encephalomyelitis, experimental autoimmune, 50, 54-56

Endocytosis, 166
Epidermal growth factor receptors, 219
  and cetuximab, 232-233
  and panitumumab, 239-240
Epilepsy, 46
Epitope-masking mechanism, 145, 148-149
Erythrocyte sedimentation rate, 94
Esophageal cancer, 240, 241
Ethanol fractionation, 1, 13-14, 22, *23*
Euglobulin precipitation, 21
Evans syndrome, 73, 182

F

F(ab')$_2$ fragments, 1, *2,* 45, 47, 52
Fallopian tube cancer, 237
Fatty acids, precipitation with, 15, 21-22
Fc fragments, 1, *2,* 48, 52
Fc receptor, neonatal, 51-52
Fcã receptor, 161, *162,* 189-190
  in anti-D mechanism, 143
  in IVIG mechanism, 44-46, 54, 81, 83
Fcã receptor IIB, inhibitory receptor
  in anti-D mechanism, 143, 147-148
  in chronic inflammatory demyelinating polyneuropathy, 86
  in IVIG mechanism, 46-47, 54, 81, 83
Fetal alloimmune thrombocytopenia, 70-71
Fetomaternal hemorrhage, 141, 177-178
Fever, 74, 93
Flaviviral infection, 107-108
Follicular lymphoma, 190-192, 207
Fractionation and purification methods, 20-27
  challenges of, 20-21
  chromatographic, 15, 22-27
  history of, 1, 13-14
  precipitation
    with ethanol, 1, 13-14, 22, *23-26,* 31-32
    with fatty acids, 15, 21-22
    with inorganic salts, 21
    by polyethylene glycol, 15, 21
    by removal of electrolytes, 21
  in virus removal, 31-32

G

Gastric cancer, 236, 248
Gastroesophageal cancer, 240
Gastrointestinal malignancies, noncolorectal
  bevacizumab in, 247-248, 250-251
  cetuximab in, 236
  panitumumab in, 240-241
Gastrointestinal side effects
  of cetuximab, 234, 239
  of panitumumab, 241, 242

Gemtuzumab ozogamicin, 199-204
    mechanism of, 200
    pharmacokinetics of, 200
    safety of, 201, 204
    structure of, 199, *200*
    therapeutic efficiency for, 201, *202-203*
Gliomas, malignant, 242, 246-247
GM1 antibodies, 83
"Gradiflow" technology, 27
Graft-vs-host disease, 49
Graves ophthalmopathy, *114,* 126
Guillain-Barré syndrome, IVIG in, 79, 82-84
    in children, 84
    dosing, 83
    early relapses after, 83
    markers of response to, 83-84
    mechanism of
        blockade of Fc receptors in, 45-46, 81
        complement in, 51, 81
        cytokine modulation in, 49-50, 82
        dendritic cells in, 54
        idiotypic antibodies in, 47, 80-81
        immunomodulation, 48
    second infusion of, 83
Gynecologic malignancies
    bevacizumab in, 248-249, 251
    cetuximab in, 237

H

HACA. *See* Human anti-chimeric antibodies
HAHA. *See* Human anti-human antibodies
HAMA. *See* Human mouse antibodies
Head and neck cancers, squamous cell, 235-236, 249
Headache, 74, 93, 94
Heart block, autoimmune congenital, 116
Heart failure, chronic, 50
Heart transplantation, *114,* 122
Heat treatments, in IVIG manufacturing, 31
Hemachromatosis, neonatal, 125-126
Hematologic disorders, *10,* 67-73. *See also* specific disorders
Hematopoietic stem cell transplantation, 73, 197
Hemoglobinuria, paroxysmal nocturnal, 198-199
Hemolysis, extravascular, 182-183
Hemolytic anemia, autoimmune, 51, 73, 194
Hemolytic disease of the fetus and newborn
    anti-D immunoglobulin in, 139-150
        antenatal prophylaxis, 178-180
        postnatal immune prophylaxis, 177-178
    IVIG in, 73
Hemophilia, 47
Hepatitis, autoimmune, 127

Hepatitis A, 107
Hepatitis B, 107, 195
Hepatitis C, 15
Hepatocellular cancer, 248
HER2. *See* Human epidermal growth factor receptor-2
HLA sensitization, 120, 121
Hormonal therapy, 229-230
Human anti-chimeric antibodies, 196, 220
Human anti-human antibodies, 220
Human antibodies, 187-188, 218
Human epidermal growth factor receptor-2, 219
    and breast cancer, 224-230
    in other tumors, 230
    testing for, 225
Human immunodeficiency virus, 27, 29, 72
Human mouse antibodies, 187, 207, 220
Humanized antibodies, 187-188, 218
Hyaluronidase, 35
Hypereosinophilic syndrome, 49
Hypersensitivity reactions, 222-223
Hypertension, 243-246, 248, 251
Hypogammaglobulinemia, 3, 14, 49, 73, 74
Hypomagnesemia, 233, 242
Hyponatremia, 94-95

I

^{131}I-tositumomab, 206-207
Ibritumomab tiuxetan, 204-206
ICAM-1, 50, 56, 81
ICAM-3, 144
Idiotypic antibodies
    in anti-D mechanism, 165-166
    in IVIG mechanism, 47-48, 80-81
IgG
    after IVIG and corticosteroid therapy, 6-7, *8, 9,* 48
    after IVIG in Guillain-Barré syndrome, 84
    binding with Fc γRs, 143,144
    structure and function of, 1, *2*
IgM, 6-7, *8, 9,* 48
IgM paraproteinemic polyneuropathy, 47, 87-88
IL-1, 83
IL-1Ra, 49, 50, 53, 55, 163-164, *165*
IL-2, 52, 230
IL-4, 52
IL-6, 50-52
IL-7, 52
IL-8, 50
IL-10, 52-55, *191*
IL-12, 51, 52, 54
IL-15, 52
IL-21, 52

Immune complexes, 45, 46, 54, 223
Immune deficiencies, 55
Immune effector cells, 221
Immune response, to D antigen, 141-142
Immune serum globulin, 1-2
Immune thrombocytopenia, 67-70
   acute, 68, 160, 181
   in adults, 68-70, 181
   anti-D in, 69, 159-168
     adverse effects of, 182-183
     efficacy of, 181-182
     mechanism of, 9-10, 161, 163-166
     monoclonal/recombinant, 167-168
   in children, 68, 69, 181
   chronic, 68, 70, 160, 194
   IVIG in
     clinical trials for, 11
     compared to anti-D, 181-182
     dosage of, 6, 69-70
     evolution of use of, 3, 6, 43, 69-70
     mechanisms of, 44-56, 67-68
     platelet counts after, 3, 6, 7
     serum IgG and IgM after, 6-7, *8*, 9
   pathophysiology of, 3, 68, 181
   primary, 68, 160, 181, 194
   rituximab in, 190, 194
   secondary, 68
   severe, 160
Immunoconjugates, 188
Immunomodulation, 48-49
Inclusion body myositis, 79, 91, *114,* 116
Infections, 101-108
   after stem cell transplants, 73
   and alemtuzumab, 198
   and cetuximab, 233
   Clostridium difficile-associated disease, 106
   meningococcal, 199
   methicillin-resistant *S. aureus,* 106
   necrotizing pneumonia, 106
   preventing in critically ill and surgical patients, 102, *103-104*
   preventing in neonates, 102
   and rituximab, 195
   sepsis and septic shock, 102, 104-105
   toxic shock syndromes, 105-106
   viral, 106-108
Infectious safety
   of anti-D, 176
   of IVIG, 2, 15-16, 27-34
Inflammatory myopathies, 45-46, 90-91, 115-116
Inflammatory response syndromes. *See* Infections
Infusion reactions
   to alemtuzumab, 197-198
   to cetuximab, 233-235, 239
   to gemtuzumab ozogamicin, 201, 204
   to monoclonal antibodies, 222
   to panitumumab, 240-242
   to rituximab, 195
   to trastuzumab, 230
Inorganic salts, precipitation with, 21
Interferon, 50, 52, 246
Interleukins
   in anti-D mechanism, 163-164, *165*
   in IVIG mechanism, 49-50, 52, 53
International Quality Plasma Program, 29
Intramuscular administration products, 1, 14, 19-20
Intravenous immunoglobulin
   clinical trials of, 11
   clinical uses of
     cardiac disorders, 124-125
     dermatologic disorders, 117-120
     hematologic disorders, 67-75
     immune thrombocytopenia, 3, 6-10
     infections, 101-108
     miscellaneous disorders, 125-129
     neurologic disorders, 79-95
     off-label, 10, 34, 43, 113, 115
     rheumatologic diseases, 115-117
     solid organ transplantation, 120-124
   commercial products, *4-5*, 16-17
   developmental history of, 1-2
   dosage of, 6, 10-11
   formulation of, 18
   future directions for, 11
   immunomodulatory effects of, 3, 6-10
   kinetic studies of, 82
   manufacturing, *4-5*, 13-36
   market supply of, 18-19
   mechanisms of action, 44-56
     activating Fcγ receptor in, 44-46
     complement in, 50-51
     cytokine modulation in, 49-50
     dendritic cells in, 52-54
     idiotypic antibodies in, 47-48
     immunomodulation and apoptosis in, 48-49
     inhibitory receptor FcγRIIB in, 46-47
     neonatal Fc receptor in, 51-52
   molecular target of, 54
   preventing virus transmission in, 2, 15-16, 27-34
   process efficiency, 18-19
   regulatory requirements for, 19-20
   safety of, 27-34
   tolerability of, 2-3, 17-18, 20
   toxicity to, 1, 74
   unresolved issues with, 10-11
Inventory hold, 30
Ion exchange chromatography, 15, 24-25

ITP. *See* Immune thrombocytopenia
IVIG. *See* Intravenous immunoglobulin

J-K

Juvenile dermatomyositis, 116
Juvenile rheumatoid arthritis, 116
Juvenile systemic lupus erythematosus, 116
K-ras mutations, 237-238
Kawasaki disease, 124-125
    dosage of IVIG in, 93
    IVIG guidelines for use, *114*
    mechanism of IVIG in, 46, 47, 49, 50
Kidney cancer. *See* Renal cell cancer
Kidney transplantation, *114,* 121-123
Kinetic studies of infused IVIG, 82
Kistler and Nitschmann fractionation scheme, *26*
Kleihauer-Betke test, 177-178

L

Lambert-Eaton myasthenic syndrome, 79, 90
Leukemia
    acute lymphoblastic, 193
    acute myeloid, 200-201
    chronic lymphocytic, 192, 196-197
Ligands, affinity, 25-27
Limbic encephalitis, 127
Liquid products, 16-20
Liver disease, autoimmune, *114,* 127
Liver toxicity, 204
Liver transplantation, *114,* 123
Low-pH treatments, 30-31
Lung cancer, non-small-cell
    bevacizumab in, 242, 244-245
    cetuximab in, 236
    panitumumab in, 240
    trastuzumab in, 230
Lung transplantation, *114,* 123
Lymphoma, non-Hodgkin. *See also* specific lymphomas
    alemtuzumab in, 197
    ibritumomab tiuxetan in, 205
    rituximab in, 190-193
    tositumomab in, 206, 207
Lymphoplasmacytic lymphoma, 193
Lyophilized products, 16-18

M

MAG antibodies, 87-88
Mantle cell lymphoma, 190, 192
Manufacturing of IVIG
    clinical trials in, 20
    commercial products, *4-5,* 16-17
    development strategy in, 17-20
    future outlook for, 34-36
    history of, 13-17
    market supply in, 18-19
    preclinical investigations in, 20
    prevention of virus transmission in, 15-16, 27-34
    process efficiency in, 18-19, 34-35
    processes for, 20-27
    requirements for, 17-20
Market supply of IVIG, 18-19
Matrix metalloproteinases, 48-49
Mechanisms of anti-D
    antigen clearance, 146-147
    B-cell inhibition, 147-148
    cytokines in, 161-164, *165*
    epitope masking, 148-149
    idiotypic antibodies in, 165-166
    overview of, 145-146
    reticuloendothelial system blockade, 161, *162*
    signaling mechanism alterations, 166
    T cells in, 147
Mechanisms of IVIG
    activating Fcγ receptor, 44-46, 81
    apoptosis, 48-49
    complement inhibition, 50-51, 81
    cytokine modulation, 49-50, 81-82
    dendritic cells in, 52-54
    enhanced steroid sensitivity, 55
    idiotypic antibodies, 47-48, 80-81
    immunomodulation, 48-49
    inhibition of cell migration, 55-56
    inhibitory receptor FcγRIIB, 46-47, 81
    molecular target of IVIG, 54
    neonatal Fc receptor in, 51-52
    remyelination, 55, 82
    repopulation of normal antibody spectrum, 55
Melanoma, 218, 249
Membrane chromatography, 27
Membranolytic attack complex, 81, 90
Meningitis, aseptic, 94
Meningococcal infections, 199
4-MEP chromatography resin, 27
Methicillin-resistant *S. aureus,* 106
Migraine headache, 94
Monoclonal antibodies
    affinity and avidity of, 220
    anti-D, 141, 143-144, 167
    antitumor mechanism of, 218-219
    binding to cellular targets by, 220
    development of, 187-188
    dosing and schedules of, 222
    and epidermal growth factor, 219
    future directions of, 207
    generations of, 187-188

for hematologic disorders
  alemtuzumab, 196-198
  eculizumab, 198-199
  gemtuzumab ozogamicin, 199-204
  ibritumomab tiuxetan, 204-206
  ocrelizumab, 207
  ofatumumab, 207
  rituximab, 188-196
  tositumomab, 206-207
  veltuzumab, 207
historical background of, 217-218
immunoglobulin class and subclass of, 220
infusion rates of, 221-222
interaction with complement, 221
interaction with immune cells, 221
nomenclature for, 218
relative specificity of, 220
for solid tumors
  bevacizumab, *224*, 242-251
  cetuximab, *224*, 232-239
  panitumumab, *224*, 239-242
  trastuzumab, 224-232
toxicity and side effects of, 222-223
tumor penetration by, 220-221
unconjugated (naked), 188
and vascular endothelial growth factor, 219
Mucous membrane pemphigoid, 118-119
Multifocal motor neuropathy, 35, 79, 87
Multimodal chromatography, 26-27
Multiple sclerosis, 50, 55-56, 92
Murine antibodies, 187-188, 218
Myasthenia gravis, 48, 51, 79, 81, 88-90
Myocardial infarction, 93
Myocarditis, 50, 107, *114*, 125
Myopathies, inflammatory, 45-46, 90-91, 115-116

N

Nanofiltration, 31
Natural killer cells, 48, 53
Neck cancers, squamous cell, 235-236, 249
Necrotizing pneumonia, 106
Neonatal Fc receptor, 51-52
Neonates
  alloimmune neutropenia in, 73
  alloimmune thrombocytopenia in, 70-71
  congenital heart block (neonatal lupus) in, 116
  hemachromatosis in, 125-126
  immune thrombocytopenia in, 71-72
  preventing infections in, 102
  sepsis in, 102, 104-105
Nephropathy, IgA, 51
Neuritis, autoimmune, 55
Neuroinflammation, 92

Neurologic disorders, IVIG in, *10*, 79-95
  adverse reactions and risk factors of, 79, 93-95
  in Alzheimer disease, 35, 92
  in chronic inflammatory demyelinating polyneuropathy, 84-87
  in dermatomyositis, 90-91
  dose for, 93
  in Guillain-Barré syndrome, 82-84
  in inclusion body myositis, 91
  kinetic studies of, 82
  in Lambert-Eaton myasthenic syndrome, 90
  mechanisms of action, 45-46, 80-82
  in multifocal motor neuropathy, 35, 87
  in multiple sclerosis, 92
  in myasthenia gravis, 88-90
  in other neuropathies, 88
  in paraproteinemic demyelinating polyneuropathies, 87-88
  in post-polio syndrome, 93
  in stiff-person syndrome, 91-92
  unresolved issues with, 79-80
Neuropathy
  associated with Sjogren syndrome, 88
  chronic inflammatory demyelinating polyneuropathy, 84-87
  diabetic amyotrophy, 88
  Guillain-Barré syndrome, 82-84
  mechanism of IVIG in, 48-50
  multifocal motor, 35, 79, 87
  paraproteinemic demyelinating polyneuropathies, 87-88
  vasculitic peripheral, 88
Neutropenia
  and alemtuzumab, 198
  autoimmune, 51, 72-73
  and gemtuzumab ozogamicin, 204
  and tositumomab, 207
  and trastuzumab, 228
Non-Hodgkin lymphoma. *See also* specific lymphomas
  alemtuzumab in, 197
  ibritumomab tiuxetan in, 205
  rituximab in, 190-193
  tositumomab in, 206, 207
Non-small-cell lung cancer
  bevacizumab in, 242, 244-245
  cetuximab in, 236
  panitumumab in, 240
  trastuzumab in, 230
Nucleic acid amplification, 29

O

Ocrelizumab, 207
Ofatumumab, 207

Oncley fractionation scheme, 25
Ophthalmopathy, Graves, *114,* 126
Opsoclonus myoclonus, 127
Organ transplantation. *See* Transplantation
Ovarian cancer
    bevacizumab in, 248-249, 251
    cetuximab in, 237
    trastuzumab in, 230

P

Pancreatic cancer
    bevacizumab in, 247-248
    cetuximab in, 236-237
    panitumumab in, 240
PANDAS, *114,* 127
Panitumumab, *224,* 239-242
    clinical trials with, 240-241
    and epidermal growth factor receptor, 239-240
    toxicities to, 241-242
Paraneoplastic disorders, 127
Paraproteinemic demyelinating polyneuropathies, 79, 87-88
Paroxsymal nocturnal hemoglobinuria, 198-199
Partial D phenotype, 178
Parvovirus B19, 29, 30, 32, 108
Pediatric and Adult Registry on Chronic ITP, 11
Pemphigoid, 117-118
    bullous, 117
    cicatricial, 118-119
    guidelines for IVIG use in, *114*
Pemphigus, 117-118
    foliaceus, 119
    guidelines for IVIG use in, *114*
    vulgaris, 47, 48, 50, 119
Peripheral neuropathy. *See* Neuropathy
Peritoneal cancer, primary, 237
pH, low, treatment with, 30-31
Phagocytosis, Fc receptor-mediated, 3, 44-45, 161, 163-164, 166
Plasma, recovered, and source, 29-30
Plasma exchange. *See* Plasmapheresis
Plasma Protein Therapeutics Association, 17, 29
Plasmapheresis
    in chronic inflammatory demyelinating polyneuropathy, 84, 86
    donors for, 16, 28-30
    in Guillain-Barré syndrome, 82-83
    in kidney transplantation, 121-123
    in myasthenia gravis, 88-90
    in rheumatoid arthritis, 116
    in solid organ transplantation, 120, 124
    vs IVIG, in neurologic disorders, 80

Platelet concentrates, D+ positive, 180-181
Platelet counts, response to IVIG, 3, 6, 7
Pneumonia, necrotizing, 106
Polyethylene glycol, precipitation by, 15, 21
Polymysitis, *114*
Polyneuropathy, IgM paraproteinemic, 47, 87-88
Post-polio syndrome, 93
Posttransfusion purpura, 72
Potassium channel antibody-associated, nonneoplastic limbic encephalitis, 127
Precipitation methods
    with ethanol, 1, 13-14, 22, *23*
    with fatty acids, 15, 21-22
    with inorganic salts, 21
    by polyethylene glycol, 15, 21
    by removal of electrolytes, 21
Preclinical studies, 20
Prions, 33-34
Process efficiency, 18-19, 34-35
Products, commercial, *4-5,* 16-17
    formulation of, 18
    lyophilized and liquid, 16-18
    market supply of, 18-19
    process efficiency of, 18-19
    regulatory requirements for, 19-20
    tolerability of, 2-3, 17-18, 20
Prostate cancer
    bevacizumab in, 249-250
    panitumumab in, 240
    trastuzumab in, 230
Proteinuria, 245, 246, 248, 251
Pruritus, 223
Psoriasis, 120
Pulmonary embolism, 93
Purification methods. *See* Fractionation and purification methods
Pyoderma gangrenosum, 120

R

RAADP (Routine antenatal anti-D prophylaxis), 178-180
Rash, skin
    and cetuximab, 233-235, 238
    and panitumumab, 241, 242
Reactions, infusion-related
    to alemtuzumab, 197-198
    to cetuximab, 233-235, 239
    to gemtuzumab ozogamicin, 201, 204
    to monoclonal antibodies, 222
    to panitumumab, 240-242
    to rituximab, 195
    to trastuzumab, 230
Reactive oxygen species, 164, *165*

Recombinant products
    anti-D, 141, 143-144, 167-168
    to replace IVIG, 35-36
Rectal cancer, 234-235, 241
Regulations, 19-20, 28
Remyelination, 55, 82
Renal cell cancer
    bevacizumab in, 246
    cetuximab in, 237
    panitumumab in, 240
Renal failure, 74
Renal transplantation, *114,* 121-123
Renal tubular necrosis, 94
Requirements for IVIG, 17-20
    formulation, 18
    market supply, 18-19
    process efficiency, 18-19
    quality regulations, 19-20
    safety regulations, 28
    tolerability, 17-18, 20
Resins, chromatographic, 23-27
Reticuloendothelial system, 161, 166-167
Retinochoroidopathy, birdshot, 126
Rheumatoid arthritis
    IVIG in, *114,* 116
    monoclonal antibodies in, 35
    rituximab in, 190, 195
Rheumatologic diseases, 115-117
    ANCA-associated systemic necrotizing vasculitides, 116-117
    antiphospholipid antibody syndrome, 117
    inflammatory myopathies, 115-116
    rheumatoid arthritis, 116
    sclerosis (scleroderma), 116
    Sjogren syndrome, 117
    systemic lupus erythematosus, 116
Rituximab, 188-196
    in autoimmune hemolytic anemia, 194
    B-cell depletion induced by, 189-190
    in chronic lymphocytic leukemia, 192
    and ibritumomab tiuxetan, 204
    in immune thrombocytopenia, 181-182, 194
    maintenance therapy with, 191-192
    in non-Hodgkin lymphoma
        aggressive, 192-193
        indolent, 190-192
    in other lymphoproliferative disorders, 193
    safety of, 195-196
    structure of, 188-189
    in thrombotic thrombocytopenic purpura, 194-195
Routine antenatal anti-D prophylaxis, 178-180

S

Safety
    of anti-D, 176, 182-183
    of IVIG, 2, 14, 15-16, 18, 27-34
    of monoclonal antibodies
        alemtuzumab, 197-198
        bevacizumab, 250-251
        cetuximab, 238-239
        eculizumab, 198-199
        gemtuzumab ozogamicin, 201, 204
        ibritumomab tiuxetan, 204-206
        panitumumab, 240-242
        rituximab, 195-196
        tositumomab, 207
        trastuzumab, 226
Salting out, 21
Sarcoma, 249
Scleroderma, 116
Sclerosis, systemic, 116
Sepsis
    in adults, 105
    IVIG mechanism in, 51, 55
    in neonates, 102, 104-105
Serum sickness, 196, 223
Serum viscosity, 93-94
SHIP1, 46
Shock, septic, 105
Side effects. *See* Adverse effects
Siglecs, 49
SIGN-R1, 54, 144
Single nucleotide polymorphisms, 86
Sjogren syndrome, 117
Skin reactions
    to cetuximab, 233-235, 238-239
    to IVIG, 94
    to panitumumab, 241, 242
Sodium, 94-95
Solvent/detergent treatment, 30
Sphingoglycolipids, antibodies to, 87-88
Spontaneous abortion, 47, 48, 53, *114,* 128
Squamous cell cancers of head and neck, 235-236, 249
Stability studies, 20
Staphylococcal toxic shock syndrome, 105-106
Staphylococcus aureus, methicillin-resistant, 106
Stem cell transplantation, 73, 197
Steric-hindrance mechanism, 145, 148-149
Steroids. *See* Corticosteroids
Stevens-Johnson syndrome, *114,* 118
Stiff-person syndrome, 79, 91-92, *114,* 126
Stomach cancer, 236, 248
Streptococcal toxic shock syndrome, 105-106
Stroke, 93

Index

Subcutaneous administration products
   history of, 1, 3, 14
   interest in, 18, 35
   requirements for, 19-20
Surgical patients, preventing infection in, 102, *103-104*
Systemic juvenile idiopathic arthritis, 116
Systemic lupus erythematosus, 54, *114*, 116

T

T-cell non-Hodgkin lymphoma, 197
T-cells
   in anti-D mechanism, 147, 149-150
   in IVIG mechanism, 48, 52, 54
TAG-1 (transient axonal glycoprotein 1), 86
TGF-β, 51, 52, 83
Thrombocytopenia. *See also* Immune thrombocytopenia
   and alemtuzumab, 198
   in aplastic anemia, 3
   fetal/neonatal alloimmune, 70-71
   and gemtuzumab ozogamicin, 204
   HIV-associated, 72
   neonatal immune, 51, 71-72
   posttransfusion purpura, 72
   and tositumomab, 207
   in Wiskott-Aldrich syndrome, 3
Thrombosis, 74, 93-94, 248-249
Thrombotic thrombocytopenic purpura, 194-195
TNF-α, 51, 52
Tolerability, 2-3, 17-18, 20
Tositumomab, 206-207
Toxic epidermal necrolysis, 49, *114*, 118
Toxic shock syndromes, 105-106
Toxicity. *See also* Adverse effects
   to bevacizumab, 250-251
   to cetuximab, 233-236, 238-239
   to IVIG, 74
   to monoclonal antibodies, 222-223
   to panitumumab, 240-242
   to trastuzumab, 230-231
Transfusion, of D+ blood components, 180-181
Transient axonal glycoprotein 1, 86
Transmissible spongiform encephalopathy, 33-34
Transplantation
   solid organ, 120-124
      ABO-incompatible, 120-124
      cardiac, *114*, 122
      HLA sensitization in, 120, 121
      kidney, *114*, 121-122
      liver, *114*, 123
      lung, *114*, 123
      recommendations for, 123-124
      rejection of, 120-124
   stem cell, 73, 197
Trastuzumab, 224-232
   clinical trials with
      in breast cancer, 225-230
      with other biologicals, 230
      in other tumor types, 230
   dose and schedule of, 225, 226
   mechanism of, 224-225
   structure of, 224
   toxicity and side effects of, 226, 230-231
Trauma patients, preventing infection in, 102, *103-104*
Tumor growth factor beta, 51, 52, 83
Tumor lysis syndrome, 221
Tumor necrosis factor, 49-52, 81

U-V

Urticaria
   IVIG in, 47, *114*, 120
   and monoclonal antibodies, 223
Uveitis, autoimmune, *114*, 126
Vaccinations, 145, 196
Varicella zoster virus, 107
Vascular endothelial growth factor, 52, 219, 242, 250
Vascular cell adhesion molecule. *See* VCAM-1
Vasculitides, ANCA-associated, *114*, 116-117
VCAM-1, 56
VEGF. *See* Vascular endothelial growth factor
Veltuzumab, 207
Viral infections, 106-108
Viral testing, 16
Virus inactivation and removal, 16, 30-32
Virus transmission prevention, 27-34
   in anti-D immunoglobulin, 176
   donor selection in, 16, 28-29
   of emerging viruses, 32-33, 35
   history of, 14, 15-16
   regulatory guidelines for, 28
   testing donor plasma in, 16, 29-30
   TSE (prion) safety, 33-34
   virus inactivation and removal in, 16, 30-32
Viscosity, serum, 93-94

W-X

Waldenström macroglobulinemia, 193
Weak D phenotype, 178
West Nile virus, 32, 33, 107-108
Wiskott-Aldrich syndrome, 3
X-linked agammaglobulinemia, 3, 14
X-linked hyper-IgM syndrome, 73

paclitaxel plus bevacizumab in advanced breast cancer: ECOG 2100. J Clin Oncol 2008;26:4672-8.
306. Ramaswamy B, Elias AD, Kelbick NT, et al. Phase II trial of bevacizumab in combination with weekly docetaxel in metastatic breast cancer patients. Clin Cancer Res 2006;12:3124-9.
307. Dickler MN, Rugo HS, Eberle CA, et al. A phase II trial of erlotinib in combination with bevacizumab in patients with metastatic breast cancer. Clin Cancer Res 2008;14:7878-83.
308. Yang JC, Haworth L, Sherry RM, et al. A randomized trial of bevacizumab, an anti-vascular endothelial growth factor antibody, for metastatic renal cancer. N Engl J Med 2003;349: 427-34.
309. Rini BI, Halabi S, Rosenberg JE, et al. Bevacizumab plus interferon alfa compared with interferon alfa monotherapy in patients with metastatic renal cell carcinoma: CALGB 90206. J Clin Oncol 2008;26:5422-8.
310. Melichar B, Koralewski P, Ravaud A, et al. First-line bevacizumab combined with reduced dose interferon-alpha2a is active in patients with metastatic renal cell carcinoma. Ann Oncol 2008;19:1470-6.
311. Hainsworth JD, Sosman JA, Spigel DR, et al. Treatment of metastatic renal cell carcinoma with a combination of bevacizumab and erlotinib. J Clin Oncol 2005;23:7889-96.
312. Elaraj DM, White DE, Steinberg SM, et al. A pilot study of antiangiogenic therapy with bevacizumab and thalidomide in patients with metastatic renal cell carcinoma. J Immunother 2004;27:259-64.
313. Vredenburgh JJ, Desjardins A, Herndon JE 2nd, et al. Phase II trial of bevacizumab and irinotecan in recurrent malignant glioma. Clin Cancer Res 2007;13:1253-9.
314. Desjardins A, Reardon DA, Herndon JE 2nd, et al. Bevacizumab plus irinotecan in recurrent WHO grade 3 malignant gliomas. Clin Cancer Res 2008;14:7068-73.
315. Poulsen HS, Grunnet K, Sorensen M, et al. Bevacizumab plus irinotecan in the treatment patients with progressive recurrent malignant brain tumours. Acta Oncol 2009;48:52-8.
316. Ali SA, McHayleh WM, Ahmad A, et al. Bevacizumab and irinotecan therapy in glioblastoma multiforme: A series of 13 cases. J Neurosurg 2008;109:268-72.
317. Lai A, Filka E, McGibbon B, et al. Phase II pilot study of bevacizumab in combination with temozolomide and regional radiation therapy for up-front treatment of patients with newly diagnosed glioblastoma multiforme: Interim analysis of safety and tolerability. Int J Radiat Oncol Biol Phys 2008;71:1372-80.
318. Kreisl TN, Kim L, Moore K, et al. Phase II trial of single-agent bevacizumab followed by bevacizumab plus irinotecan at tumor progression in recurrent glioblastoma. J Clin Oncol 2009; 27:740-5.
319. Food and Drug Administration. Bevacizumab injection. (May 5, 2009) Rockville, MD: Office of Oncology Drug Products, 2009. [Available at http://www.fda.gov/AboutFDA/CentersOffices/CDER/ucm149364.htm (accessed April 24, 2010).]
320. Kindler HL, Friberg G, Singh DA, et al. Phase II trial of bevacizumab plus gemcitabine in patients with advanced pancreatic cancer. J Clin Oncol 2005;23:8033-40.
321. Kindler HL, Niedzwiecki D, Hollis E, et al. A double-blind, placebo-controlled, randomized phase III trial of gemcitabine plus bevacizumab versus gemcitabine plus placebo in patients with advanced pancreatic cancer: A preliminary analysis of Cancer and Leukemia Group B (abstract). Proc Am Soc Clin Oncol 2007;25:1992.
322. Van Cutsem E, Vervenne WL, Bennouna J, et al. Phase III trial of bevacizumab in combination with gemcitabine and erlotinib in patients with metastatic pancreatic cancer. J Clin Oncol 2009;27:2231-7.
323. Crane CH, Ellis LM, Abbruzzese JL, et al. Phase I trial evaluating the safety of bevacizumab with concurrent radiotherapy and capecitabine in locally advanced pancreatic cancer. J Clin Oncol 2006;24:1145-51.
324. Shah MA, Ramanathan RK, Ilson DH, et al. Multicenter phase II study of irinotecan, cisplatin, and bevacizumab in patients with metastatic gastric or gastroesophageal junction adenocarcinoma. J Clin Oncol 2006;24:5201-6.
325. Zhu AX, Blaszkowsky LS, Ryan DP, et al. Phase II study of gemcitabine and oxaliplatin in combination with bevacizumab in patients with advanced hepatocellular carcinoma. J Clin Oncol 2006;24:1898-903.
326. Thomas MB, Morris JS, Chadha R, et al. Phase II trial of the combination of bevacizumab and erlotinib in patients who have advanced hepatocellular carcinoma. J Clin Oncol 2009;27: 843-50.